PROBLEM-BASED
IMMUNOLOGY

PROBLEM-BASED IMMUNOLOGY

Reginald Gorczynski, MD, PhD

Professor
Departments of Surgery and Immunology
University of Toronto and The Toronto Hospital
Toronto, Canada

Jacqueline Stanley, PhD

Course Director and Professor of Immunology
St. George's University School of Medicine
St. George's, Grenada

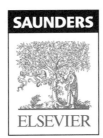

SAUNDERS

ELSEVIER

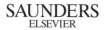

SAUNDERS
ELSEVIER

1600 John F. Kennedy Blvd.
Ste 1800
Philadelphia, PA 19103-2899

Problem-Based Immunology

ISBN-13: 978-1-4160-2416-3
ISBN-10: 1-4160-2416-6

Notice

Immunology is an ever-changing field. Standard safety precautions must be followed, but as new research and clinical experience broaden our knowledge, changes in treatment and drug therapy may become necessary or appropriate. Readers are advised to check the most current product information provided by the manufacturer of each drug to be administered to verify the recommended dose, the method and duration of administration, and contraindications. It is the responsibility of the treating physician, relying on experience and knowledge of the patient, to determine dosages and the best treatment for each individual patient. Neither the Publisher nor the editor assumes any liability for any injury and/or damage to persons or property arising from this publication.

The Publisher

Library of Congress Cataloging-in-Publication Data

Gorczynski, Reginald M.
   Problem-based immunology / Reginald Gorczynski, Jacqueline Stanley.
       p. ;   cm.
   Includes bibliographical references.
   ISBN 1-4160-2416-6
   1. Clinical immunology—Case studies.   I. Stanley, Jacqueline.   II. Title.
   [DNLM: 1. Immune System Diseases—Case Reports.   2. Immunization—Case Reports.   3.
Neoplasms—immunology—Case Reports.   4. Psychoneuroimmunology—methods—Case Reports.
5. Transplantation Immunology—Case Reports.   WD 300 G661p 2006]
   RC582.G67 2006
   616.07'9—dc22   2005056314

Acquisitions Editor: William R. Schmitt
Developmental Editor: Kevin Kochanski
Publishing Services Manager: Tina Rebane
Design Direction: Louis J. Forgione

Printed in China

Last digit is the print number: 9   8   7   6   5   4   3   2   1

To Pat, Christopher, and Laura

To David and Brian

Preface

The pace of advancement of knowledge in the basic science of immunology and the application of that knowledge into the clinical realms continue to amaze even the most enthusiastic of scientists in the field. Some thirty years ago we had just become used to thinking in terms of acquired immune responses developing from an interaction between two separate lymphocyte populations, B cells and T cells. The old adage from Shaw's popular play that we should "pay attention to the phagocytes," presaged by Metchnikoff's earlier characterization of the importance of these cells in host resistance, seemed "old hat." In the intervening years, how much has changed. Acquired immunity is now understood to be an extraordinarily complex beast, many of whose secrets unquestionably still remain untold. And our evolving understanding of the innate immune system, with the documentation of the intricacy and heterogeneity of newly described receptors on and in cells contributing to innate immunity ("toll-like receptors" [TLRs] and "nuclear oligomerization domain" containing proteins [NODs]) has rightly restored Metchnikoff (and Shaw) to a position of preeminence.

The rationale for this volume, as it was for our earlier publication, *Clinical Immunology*, was based on a need to supply medical students and graduate students with an up-to-date understanding of immunology as it is applied to clinical practice. Our experience, both as students and as teachers, convinced us that a "problem-based" approach was an ideal one to generate most interest during the learning process itself, and to ensure that what was learned would prove to have some long-lasting value. This new volume represents a major improvement over our earlier book, in that we have now endeavored even more to curtail the introductory basic concepts included in each section and incorporated/embedded most of our objectives into the clinical cases used to highlight the science. Accordingly, the cases described are richer in material and interest, and while many of them highlight comparatively esoteric clinical scenarios, the basic immunobiology behind those scenarios continues to be all the more intelligible because it is seen in these contexts.

We have in addition added one novel section on psychoneuroimmunbiology into this book. This we are sure is new to any clinical immunology text, and especially to one such as ours, using a case-based approach. Given the growing worldwide interest in alternative medicines and the scientific evidence that documents the impact of many physiological systems on the functioning of the immune system itself, the rationale for this new section is, we feel, self-evident.

As before, we hope the reader enjoys working through the problems as much as we enjoyed collating them. We have endeavored to correct errors in fact and typography—but are happy to receive feedback should others strongly disagree with statements they find herein. We would like to acknowledge the help of both Kevin Kochanski and Tina Rebane at Elsevier for their tireless efforts to ensure the publication would be as timely and professional as possible.

Finally, if the reader completes the journey and remains hungry for more knowledge in any or all of the subjects he/she finds herein, we shall have been successful in our goals.

Reg Gorczynski & Jacqueline Stanley

Contents

ix

SECTION I

Immunodeficiency Disorders

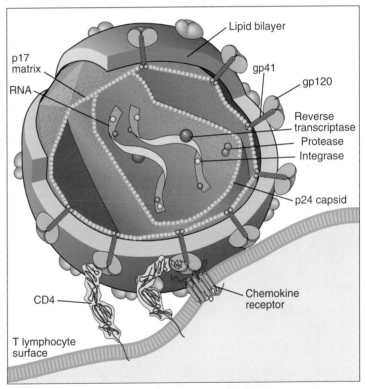

Lipid bilayer

p17 matrix

RNA

gp41

gp120

Reverse transcriptase

Protease

Integrase

p24 capsid

CD4

Chemokine receptor

T lymphocyte surface

   Immunodeficiency disorders can be classified in terms of whether they are inherited (primary) or acquired (secondary), and whether they affect the innate immune system or the adaptive immune system. The complexity of cells and molecules that function in normal host resistance mechanisms of both innate and acquired immunity is covered in brief. Given the significant redundancy in the mechanisms by which normal host resistance to bacterial infection, for instance, is achieved, it should come as no surprise that there is in turn a considerable heterogeneity in the origin (at the cellular and molecular level) of apparently similar clinical presentations. This often makes determination of the etiology of a clinical disorder a puzzle worthy of a Holmes novel.

   The cases presented in this section range from the comparatively common (selective IgA deficiency; AIDS) to the seemingly esoteric (bare lymphocyte syndrome). However, in all cases there are a number of details whose mastery will continue to provide the student with an important background understanding of the nature of the development of a normal working mammalian immune system. It is against that background of understanding, that the later sections of the book will have a greater meaning.

Immunodeficiency disorders (IDs) are classified as "primary" or "secondary" depending on whether they are inherited or acquired. Primary IDs are inherited and include defects in cellular, antibody, or complement arms of the immune system (Fig. I–1). In contrast, secondary IDs are the result of extrinsic causes, including drugs, infection, aging, and other miscellaneous (often unknown) causes.

PRIMARY IMMUNODEFICIENCY DISORDERS

For the most part, patients with a primary immunodeficiency have a genetic defect in T cells, B cells, natural killer (NK) cells, phagocytes, or the complement system (Fig. I–2). Whether patients show increased susceptibility to bacterial, viral, fungal, or parasitic infection depends on the nature of the defect and the role that the cells or system component plays in immunity (Fig. I–3). When these genetic defects affect stem cells that give rise to several cell lineages, as occurs in hematopoiesis, an understanding of the general hematopoietic development pathways provides insight into the magnitude of the problem and the cell phenotypes affected (Fig. I–4).

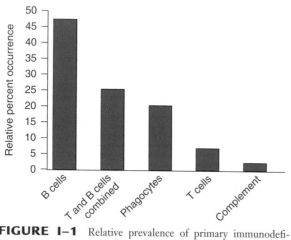

FIGURE I–1 Relative prevalence of primary immunodeficiency disorders. Immunodeficiency disorders include defects in cellular, antibody, and complement arms of the immune system. (Modified with permission from Gorczynski R, Stanley J: Clinical Immunology. Austin, Landes, 1999.)

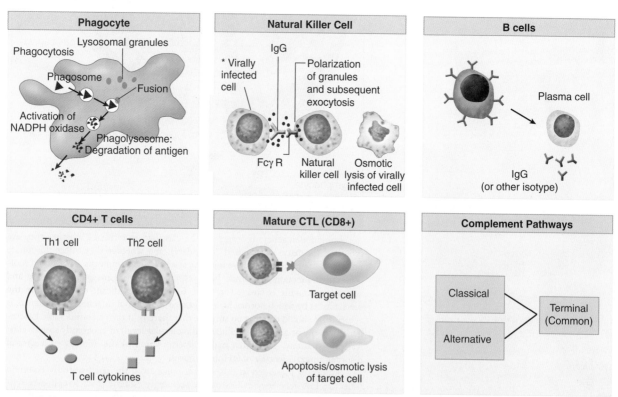

FIGURE I–2 Defects in some components of the immune system lead to immunodeficiency disorders. Defects in phagocytes, NK cells, B cells, T cells, or complement can lead to immunodeficiency disorders. (Modified with permission from Gorczynski R, Stanley J: Clinical Immunology. Austin, Landes, 1999.)

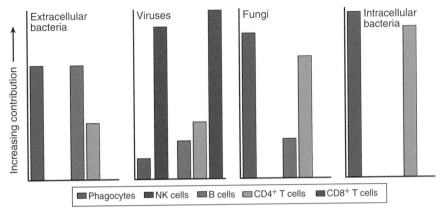

FIGURE I–3   Different components of the immune system are recruited in host defense against various pathogens. Whether an individual has increased bacterial, viral, fungal, or parasitic infections will depend on the particular immune component that is defective. (Modified with permission from Gorczynski R, Stanley J: Clinical Immunology. Austin, Landes, 1999.)

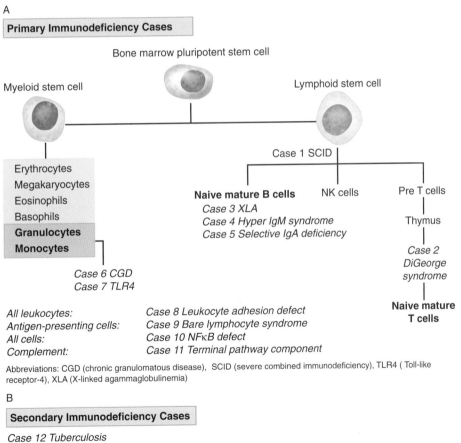

FIGURE I–4   Immunodeficiency disorders arise when cells or cellular components are deficient. Inherited defects in various cells or systems of the immune system are referred to as primary immunodeficiencies (**A**), whereas acquired defects are referred to as secondary immunodeficiencies (**B**). The scope of the primary immunodeficiency disorder will depend on where (or whether) the defect occurs during hematopoiesis. Acquired immunodeficiency diseases have many causes.

Stem Cell Disorders

Defects that arise in pluripotent, lymphoid, and myeloid stem cells can have profound effects because each of these cells gives rise to several cell types. As can be seen in Figure I–4, pluripotent stem cell defects are the most devastating because these cells give rise to both lymphoid and myeloid stem cells. One disease arising from a disorder in pluripotent stem cells is reticular dysgenesis, an autosomal recessive disorder that leads to a deficiency in both myeloid and lymphoid stem cells, and the cells that derive from them. In contrast, lymphoid stem cell defects will affect T cells, B cells, and NK cells but will not affect cells arising from myeloid stem cells (see Case 1). Because T cells, B cells, and NK cells are affected, such a patient may be susceptible to all infectious agents.

T Cell Disorders

T cell disorders occur much less frequently than B cell disorders. The classic T cell ID is DiGeorge syndrome, in which defective thymus maturation leads to a deficiency of mature T cells (see Case 2). In addition to increased susceptibility to viral infections, these patients have an overall decrease in immune function because cytokines derived from CD4+ T cells are required for virtually all aspects of immunity.

Other diseases exist in which there are antigen-specific T cell defects (especially of CD4+ cells). One such example is chronic mucocutaneous candidiasis, in which individuals lack T cells specific for *Candida* antigen. These individuals have increased susceptibility to yeast infections (e.g., *Candida albicans*).

B Cell Disorders

B cell defects represent 45% to 50% of all IDs and generally present at about 6 months of age when passive immunity acquired from maternal immunoglobulin G (IgG) antibodies crossing the placenta wanes.

X-Linked Agammaglobulinemia

The most severe B cell ID is X-linked agammaglobulinemia, a disorder in which B cells fail to mature beyond the pre–B cell stage (see Case 3). The molecular changes responsible for this disorder have been elucidated. The disease is now known to result from a defect in Btk, a protein tyrosine kinase (encoded on the X-chromosome) whose function is crucial for transmitting signals involved in lymphoid differentiation.

Transient Hypogammaglobulinemia of Infancy

A classic B cell disorder arising from a maturational delay is so-called transient hypogammaglobulinemia of infancy. Although this disorder manifests as diminished IgG production, the impairment results from decreased production of T cell–derived cytokines needed for B cell activation. Patients usually recover without treatment. However, in severe cases intravenous immunoglobulin (IVIG) is required for particular infections.

Hyper IgM Syndrome

Hyper IgM syndrome (also referred to as immunoglobulin deficiency with increased IgM) results from a deficiency of molecules required for isotype switching, a process that leads to the secretion of IgG, IgE, or IgA instead of IgM (see Case 4). As is apparent from the alternate name for this disorder, patients in general have a decrease in all antibody isotypes but an increase in IgM.

Selective IgA Deficiency

Selective IgA deficiency is common in whites (approximately 0.1% prevalence) (see Case 5). Individuals show an increased incidence of recurrent sinopulmonary infection, in association with an increased incidence of celiac disease. These individuals generally are treated symptomatically (with antibiotics) rather than with passive IgA. The reason for this is that there are only low levels of IgA in serum. It does not get to target sites, and recipients quickly form antibodies to donor IgA.

NK Cell Disorders

Chédiak-Higashi syndrome is a disorder that affects a number of cell types, including NK cells. It is characterized by the presence of large granules, platelet-dense antibodies, and a defect in the lysosomal trafficking gene regulator (LYST). Consequently, exocytosis of granules (containing perforin) does not occur, a process that is required for NK cell–mediated killing. Individuals with Chédiak-Higashi syndrome generally have decreased pigmentation of the skin and eyes. Additionally, they are susceptible to bleeding disorders as well as recurrent and severe bacterial and viral infections.

Phagocytic Cell Defects

Phagocytic cell defects represent about 20% of all IDs. There are two essential causes of phagocytic cell defects: those due to extrinsic factors (e.g., the absence of activating cytokines) and those resulting from intrinsic defects in intracellular "killing" pathways (e.g., chronic granulomatous disease). In this latter case, decreased NADPH oxidase activity reduces the generation of H_2O_2 and superoxide radicals, both of which are needed to kill ingested intracellular organisms (see Case 6 and Fig. I–5). Individuals suffering from phagocytic disorders generally need antifungal and antibacterial agents as treatment. Long-term treatment might include bone marrow transplantation. Defects in toll-like receptor expression, molecules now known to act as primitive recognition receptors for conserved antigens on pathogens, can also hamper the innate immune response (see Case 7 and Fig. I–5). Chédiak-Higashi syndrome also affects phagocytes in that large cytoplasmic granules accumulate, trafficking is impaired, and so lysosomal granules do not fuse with phagosomes.

Other Leukocyte Defects

Other leukocyte defects are much rarer. Included among these is so-called leukocyte adhesion deficiency (LAD) disease, in which impaired trafficking to sites of infection leads to increased necrotic infections (see Case 8 and Fig. I–5). Bone marrow transplantation is the treatment of choice. Defects that lead to reduced expression of antigen-presenting molecules on antigen-presenting cells (see Case 9 and Fig. I–5) can lead to severe IDs, as can defects in signaling pathways (see Case 10 and Fig. I–6).

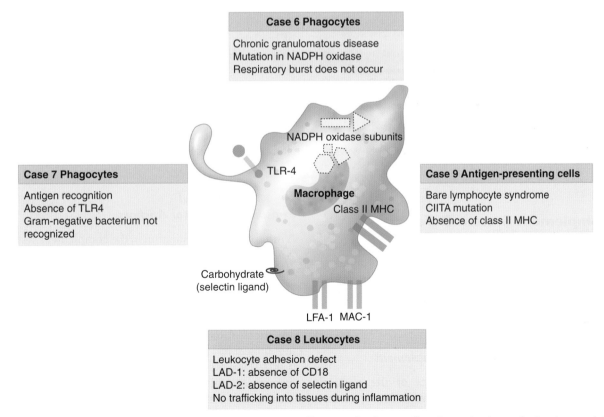

FIGURE I–5 Defects in cell receptors, enzyme components, adhesion molecules, or cell surface molecules can lead to immunodeficiency disorders. Known phagocytic defects include those that result in a decrease in the production of enzymatic activity (NADPH oxidase), recognition (toll-like receptors), transcription (CIITA), or adhesion molecules (leukocyte adhesion molecules). Some of these defects also manifest in other leukocytes.

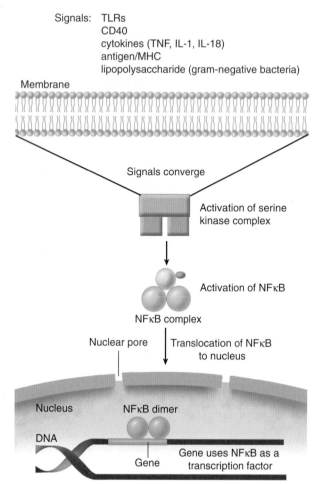

Signals: TLRs
          CD40
          cytokines (TNF, IL-1, IL-18)
          antigen/MHC
          lipopolysaccharide (gram-negative bacteria)

Membrane

Signals converge

Activation of serine kinase complex

Activation of NFκB

NFκB complex

Nuclear pore   Translocation of NFκB to nucleus

Nucleus   NFκB dimer

DNA

Gene   Gene uses NFκB as a transcription factor

FIGURE 1–6 A single mutation can affect various signaling pathways. Defects in signaling pathways can affect transcription of several genes whose products are required for immune responses.

Complement System Defects

Complement system defects constitute 2% to 3% of IDs and are frequently associated with bacterial infection and autoimmunity. Several distinct categories have been described, depending on the complement components that are absent (see Case 11).

Defects in Components of Complement

Defects in the early components of the classical pathway are associated with autoimmune complex diseases (e.g., systemic lupus erythematosus), whereas individuals with defects in the terminal pathway components present with recurrent neisserial infections. A deficiency in the complement protein C3, a central

molecule for both the alternative and classical complement pathways, is associated with chronic nephritis, an immune complex–type disorder resulting from deposition of so-called C3 nephritic factor (an IgG autoantibody that stabilizes an enzymatic complex in the alternative complement pathway). Deficiencies in C3 are the most profound of all complement defects because both complement pathways are affected. As a result, the proteolytic fragments of C3 that function as opsonins are not produced.

Defects in Regulatory Protein, C1 (Esterase) Protein

Defects in complement regulatory proteins may also be inherited. The most common regulatory protein mutations are those that involve C1 (esterase) inhibitor. The molecule regulates activation of the classical pathway by complexing with C1, the protein that attaches to immune complexes to initiate complement activation. Mutations in C1 (esterase) inhibitor result in uncontrolled activation of C1, C2, and C4. C1 (esterase) inhibitor also inhibits kallikrein, an enzyme whose action on kininogen leads to release of bradykinin, a molecule that acts to increase vascular permeability. The combined action of the C2 proteolytic fragment C2b (a kinin) along with bradykinin (produced in the absence of kallikrein inhibition) leads to an often life-threatening edema in C1 (esterase) protein deficiency, which is referred to as hereditary angioedema. Treatment of this disorder involves infusion of C1 esterase inhibitor.

Defects in Glycosyl Phosphatidylinositol Anchors

A different type of mutation in the complement system is associated with alteration in the ability of regulatory molecules to anchor to the cell membrane. Many complement regulatory proteins, including decay accelerating factor (DAF) and CD59, are not integrated into the membrane through transmembrane domains but are attached to the red blood cell surface by anchoring molecules such as glycosyl phosphatidylinositol (GPI). Patients who are unable to synthesize these linkages do not express DAF and CD59 on their cell surface and so are unable to deactivate the proteolytic complement complexes that form on their cell surface, resulting in an increased spontaneous susceptibility of red blood cells to lysis (triggered by low levels of spontaneously produced C3, so-called C3 "tickover"). The prototypical disease resulting from defects in GPI linkages is paroxysmal nocturnal hemoglobinuria (PNH).

SECONDARY IMMUNODEFICIENCY DISORDERS

The etiology of secondary immunodeficiency disorders is manifold (see Cases 12 and 13). Acquired immunodeficiency diseases have many causes, including bacterial (e.g., *Mycobacterium tuberculosis*, see Case 12); viral (e.g., human immunodeficiency virus [HIV], see Case 13); drugs (e.g., post-transplantation immunosuppression; treatment of neoplastic disease); lifestyle (e.g., alcohol, a profound immunosuppressant); and other chronic disorders (e.g., aging, diabetes; Fig. I–7, see Case 24).

Secondary ID disorders are often associated with abnormal production of immune components. Included among these are the so-called monoclonal gammopathies, in which overproduction of clonal immunoglobulin occurs, with a relative deficiency of other antigen-specific immunoglobulins. Waldenström's macroglobulinemia (an IgM gammopathy) is one such disorder, which is also associated with a hyperviscosity syndrome and hypogammaglobulinemia. Multiple myeloma (with increased urinary excretion of free light chains, Bence Jones proteins) is yet

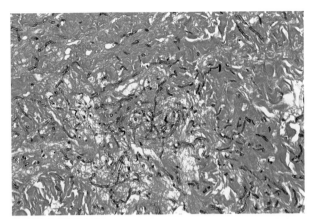

FIGURE I–7 Histologic section from a case of **mucormycosis**, such as can be seen in nasolabial lesions in rare cases of poorly controlled diabetes (with chronic immunosuppression). Ribbon-like, broad, nonseptate hyphae (stained with Gomori methenamine silver) are shown. (From Murray P, Rosenthal K, Kobayashi G, Pfaller M: Medical Microbiology, 4th ed. St. Louis, Mosby, 2002.)

another secondary ID disorder. Finally, in principle, any B cell and/or T cell malignancy in which abnormal random oncogene insertion occurs that subverts subsequent lymphoid development and "freezes" differentiation at a stage that results in diminished "downstream" production of antigen-specific effector cells can be classified as a secondary ID disease.

Mark is a 7-month-old boy who was born at term (40 weeks) weighing 4 kg, physically normal and apparently healthy. Although Mark was well the first couple of months of life, the last 3 months have shattered the illusion that Mark is healthy and normal. In the last few months, Mark has been plagued with fungal (diaper rash, oral candidiasis), viral (upper respiratory tract infections), and bacterial (otitis media) infections, all of which resolved with appropriate pharmacologic intervention. Mark has received routine childhood immunization, which his mother hoped would reduce the number of infections. Not surprising, Mark has not thrived and is well below the 50% percentile for weight. Mark was referred to a pediatrician who noted that Mark had (once again) a diaper rash and candidiasis (Fig. 1-1) and an upper respiratory tract infection. Despite these infections, his tonsils and lymph nodes were barely detectable. The pediatrician ordered a number of tests that included a complete blood cell count with differential, serum immunoglobulin (IgG), and a chest radiograph. The blood cell count indicated a low leukocyte count, profound lymphopenia, and very low serum IgG value.

QUESTIONS FOR GROUP DISCUSSION

1. When taking a family history, why is it important to determine whether both male and female members of the family have been affected?
2. This patient has a history of infection with bacteria, viruses, and fungi. What lymphoid defect is suggested when a patient has a history of bacterial infection? What lymphoid defect is suggested when a patient has a history of viral and fungal infections?
3. With what type of infection history would a patient with a myeloid progenitor cell defect present?
4. What is the rationale for requesting a complete blood cell count with differential? Given the information presented in this case, what would you expect a blood test to reveal?
5. A history of bacterial, viral, and fungal infections suggests that both T cell and B cell function are affected. What laboratory technique is used to determine the relative numbers of B cells and T cells in circulation?
6. What is the significance of small tonsils and barely detectable lymph nodes? This could have been predicted given the very low levels of serum immunoglobulin. Explain.
7. How can the fact that this child has been immunized be used to determine if B cell function is intact?
8. NK cells are also derived from a lymphoid stem cell. What cell surface marker can be used to quantitate circulating NK cells by flow cytometry? What type(s) of infections would a patient have if he or she had a deficiency of NK cells?

9. On the basis of the listed tests, the patient was shown to have a defect in T cells, B cells, and NK cells, suggesting a defect at the level of a lymphoid progenitor cell. Such defects give rise to severe combined immunodeficiency disorder (SCID). There are several mutations or defects that can give rise to SCID. Explain how mutations or defects in each of the following would result in SCID phenotype: (a) adenosine deaminase; (b) CD132-γ common chain present in several cytokine receptors, (c) recombinase activating genes RAG1 and RAG2; and (d) JAK 3.
10. Describe potential therapeutic interventions.

RECOMMENDED APPROACH

Implications/Analysis of Family History

Immunodeficiency disorders present as recurrent and persistent infections. Because these disorders may be inherited or acquired, a family history indicating that other members have been affected similarly would indicate a genetic basis for the infections. A history indicating that only male infants have been affected directs the physician toward a defect in a gene encoded on the X chromosome. Genetic defects in which both male and female family members are also affected generally indicate an autosomal recessive mode of inheritance. In this particular case, Mark's family history indicated that both sexes have been affected and so the cause of these infections is unlikely to be an X-linked disorder.

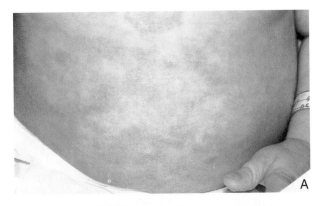

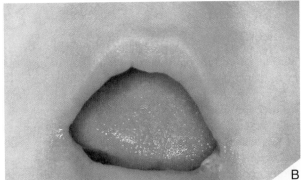

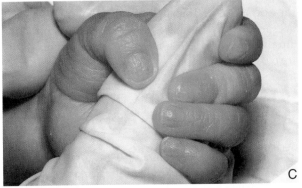

FIGURE 1–1   Severe disseminated candidal infection (**A**) on the trunk, (**B**) in the mouth, and (**C**) on the nails of a child. (From Fireman P, Slavin R: Atlas of Allergies, 2nd ed. St. Louis, Mosby, 1996.)

Implications/Analysis of Clinical History

Mark has presented with viral, fungal, and bacterial infections, suggesting that his problem is not limited solely to a B cell or a T cell defect. Although defects in components of the innate immune system can lead to increased susceptibility to these types of infections, adaptive immune defects that result in increased susceptibility to bacterial infections indicate a B cell defect whereas viral and fungal infections typify a T cell defect. Small tonsils and lymph nodes in the presence of active infection would suggest a B cell defect.

Implications/Analysis of Laboratory Investigation

Although the chest radiograph did indicate that Mark has pneumonia, there is no mention of an anomaly regarding the thymic shadow, suggesting the organ of differentiation for T cells is intact (see Case 2). Laboratory investigations should focus on both T cell and B cell numbers and function.

Additional Laboratory Tests

A total blood cell count and differential indicated a gross deficiency in lymphocyte numbers. Quantification of serum IgG and response to immunization confirmed the B cell deficiency, as did the flow cytometry analysis. Given the B cell defect, it was not surprising that serum IgG was low and tonsils/lymph nodes were barely detectable. The low serum IgG levels, despite immunization, also indicate a B cell defect. Flow cytometry results also indicated that both T cell (CD3+) and NK cell (CD3−, CD56+) numbers were drastically decreased. B cells, T cells, and NK cells are derived from a lymphoid stem cell during hematopoiesis.

DIAGNOSIS

On the basis of the test results, Mark was diagnosed with a form of severe combined immunodeficiency (SCID) in which there is a deficiency of both T cells and B cells. However, a number of primary/genetic defects can lead to SCID (see Etiology).

THERAPY

Bone Marrow Transplant

SCID is often referred to as the "bubble boy" disease, in reference to David Vetter, a young boy who lived for 12 years in a plastic, sterile bubble but succumbed to infection after a bone marrow transplant from his sister who carried a latent Epstein-Barr virus (human herpesvirus 4) infection.

For both SCID and XSCID (and Omenn syndrome) bone marrow transplantation is the treatment of choice if a matched donor can be identified. Because the graft (bone marrow) is a source of lymphohematopoietic cells capable of recognizing the host as foreign, development of graft versus host disease can potentially occur except for grafts between identical twins (see Introduction, Transplantation Immunology, Section V).

Enzyme Therapy (Depending on Etiology)

For SCID secondary to a deficiency in adenosine deaminase (ADA), regular injections of ADA linked to polyethylene glycol (PEG-ADA) are often effective. PEG is linked to the ADA to delay degradation of the ADA.

Pharmacologic Treatment

In some cases there is a very leaky syndrome (incomplete loss of T cells and B cells); and for these cases, lifelong treatment of infections "as they appear" is possible. However, for more severe cases, other forms of therapy must be considered.

Gene Therapy

Because the gene products absent in all of the aforementioned causes of SCID and XSCID have been identified, a gene therapy approach may be the treatment of choice in the future. Gene therapy for ADA-SCID was introduced in 1990 when three physicians working at the National Institutes of Health infused T cells carrying a normal ADA gene into Ashanthi Desilva, a 4-year-old girl for whom PEG-ADA was not optimally effective. Today, she is alive and well but continues to receive injections of PEG-ADA, albeit at much lower doses.

In the early gene therapy clinical trials, a genetically altered retrovirus carrying a normal ADA gene was allowed to infect the patient's T cells *in vitro* and then the T cells were activated to proliferate. When a sufficient number of T cells had been generated, they were infused into the patient at regular intervals for 2 years. Because retroviruses integrate (randomly) into host chromosomes, the normal ADA gene was now an integral part of the DNA in the transfected T cells and was present in all their progeny after T cell activation.

More recently, physicians from the Hospital Necker in Paris have treated children with XSCID by infusing genetically altered stem cells isolated from their bone marrow, instead of using mature T cells to carry the vector. Consequently, all myeloid and lymphoid cells generated during hematopoiesis will carry the normal gene. To date, these patients are doing well and are reported to have developed serum antibodies after pediatric DPT (diphtheria, pertussis, and tetanus toxoid) immunization.

ETIOLOGY: SEVERE COMBINED IMMUNODEFICIENCY

Adenosine Deaminase

One of the earliest defects identified in SCID patients was a deficiency in ADA, an enzyme required for purine metabolism and which is most active in lymphocytes, particularly T lymphocytes. In the absence of this enzyme, toxic metabolites accumulate and inhibit DNA synthesis so proliferation does not occur in response to polyclonal activators.

Deficiency in CD132 (Common γ Chain)

CD132, a signaling molecule in several cytokine receptor complexes, is encoded on the X chromosome and so this immunodeficiency is referred to as XSCID. Receptor complexes, in which CD132 is a component, bind the following interleukins: IL-2, IL-4, IL-7, IL-9, and IL-15 (Fig. 1–2). IL-7 plays an important role in the development of lymphoid progenitors during hematopoiesis; however, knockout mice for IL-7 are grossly deficient in T cells and only moderately deficient in B cells, suggesting that IL-7 is required for T cell maturation in the thymus.

Mutations, ranging from nonsense mutations to deletion of entire exons, in the gene encoding CD132 lead to SCID because multiple cytokine systems are simultaneously affected. One of the diagnostic procedures for identifying these individuals is genomic sequencing of CD132. Because CD132 is encoded on the X chromosome, males are predominantly affected.

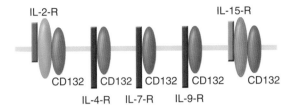

Receptors That Share the Gamma (CD132) Chain

FIGURE 1–2 Defects in CD132 lead to X-linked severe combined immunodeficiency disorder (XSCID). Receptor complexes through which cytokines IL-2, IL-4, IL-7, IL-9, and IL-15 signal all have CD132 as a component of that complex. Defects in this protein, therefore, have a significant impact on immune responses because so many cytokine receptors are affected. (Modified with permission from Gorczynski R, Stanley J: Clinical Immunology. Austin, Landes, 1999.)

Mark's family history indicated that both males and females had presented with this disorder; therefore, it is unlikely that Mark has XSCID. Furthermore, the white blood cell differential indicated a gross deficiency of both B cells and T cells.

Deficiency in JAK 3

CD132 is a transmembrane protein whose cytoplasmic domain interacts with JAK 3 (Janus tyrosine kinase 3) after cytokine binding (Table 1–1). JAK 3 activates, by phosphorylation, the latent transcription factor, STAT 5 (signal transducer and activator of transcription), which then translocates to the nucleus. Stable T cell lines derived from patients with a deficiency in JAK 3 do not proliferate in response to IL-2, a T cell growth factor that signals via a receptor complex that includes CD132. An *in vitro* reconstitution study, in which a retroviral vector encoding JAK 3 was introduced into these cell lines, restored JAK 3 expression and proliferation of T cells in response to IL-2. Not surprisingly, JAK 3–deficient patients have a clinical phenotype virtually identical to that of XSCID, even though JAK 3 is encoded on chromosome 19 and not on the X chromosome.

Defect in Recombinase Activation Gene

Theoretically, in any given individual, it is possible to generate 10^{12} different T cell (or B cell) clones each bearing antigen specific receptors that consist of a unique variable and a constant region. This uniqueness is made possible because the variable regions are made up of sections of DNA referred to as variable (V), diversity (D), and joining (J) segments. Multiple versions of each segment are present in the germline genes (see Case 2). In the construction of a gene encoding any variable region, the gene segments are recombined in a different sequence from that present in germline DNA. This process, termed *somatic recombination*, requires the activation of recombinases, nucleoprotein products of the RAG1 and RAG2 genes (recombination-activating genes).

Mutations in RAG1 and RAG2 have been identified. Although many of the mutations are missense mutations, deletional or splice mutations have also been identified. Patients with a total defect in these recombinase activation genes are unable to construct variable regions for the B cell and T cell antigen receptors, which results in an SCID phenotype. However, some mutations impair but do not totally abolish the recombination activity such that a very restricted repertoire of T cells is generated. Patients with this rare form of SCID, called Omenn syndrome, present with symptoms of graft versus host disease. In the absence of an allograft, this clinical presentation can be explained by the generation of an autoreactive T cell population that was not negatively selected during development in the thymus. In essence, the presence of a rash, lymphadenopathy, diarrhea, and a high lymphocyte (activated T cell) count distinguishes Omenn syndrome from the traditional SCID patients. Although not typical, there are reports of patients with RAG1 mutations who have B cells and circulating antibodies but no T cells.

	CD25	CD122	CD124	CD127	CD132	Extra Chain	JAK 3
IL-2	+	+			+		+
IL-4			+		+		+
IL-7				+	+		+
IL-9					+	IL-9-Rα	+
IL-15		+			+	IL-15-Rα	+

TABLE 1-1 Cytokine Receptors That Share CD132, a Signaling Molecule That Associates with JAK 3

C A S E

2

RD is a 1-year-old adopted boy in your practice who has had a surprisingly high (eight) number of severe recurrent viral and fungal infections (e.g., respiratory syncytial virus, *Candida albicans*) during his first 14 months. Each of these has eventually resolved, albeit very slowly, and the fungal infections have responded to the appropriate medication. You are nevertheless concerned to find the underlying cause of his problem. Recent chest radiographs performed at a local hospital to rule out pneumonia have been returned to you by the radiologist with a note that there was an abnormality, in particular an apparent absence of a thymic shadow. The radiologist has asked if there are any other stigmata of congenital absence of a thymus. As you describe this child's history, you also mention his physical appearance (eyes widely separated, low ears, cleft palate).

QUESTIONS FOR GROUP DISCUSSION

1. Compare the types of infections that this patient has with those of the patient in Case 1.
2. What is the significance of the fact that this patient has a history of viral and fungal infections but not bacterial infections? What types of cell defects in (a) innate immunity or (b) adaptive immunity would present in this manner?
3. Why would a history of viral infections not necessarily accompany a history of infection with *Candida albicans?*
4. The chest radiograph revealed that the thymic shadow was missing. What is the function of the thymus? Review the steps that precursor lymphoid cells undergo to differentiate to CD4+ T cells or CD8+ T cells. Be sure to include the following terms in your discussion: (a) *somatic recombination,* (b) *interactive avidity,* (c) *positive selection,* (d) *negative selection,* (e) *death by neglect,* (f) *T cell receptor excision circles* (TRECs), (g) *lineage determination/gene silencing,* and (h) *T cell repertoire.* As well, be prepared to describe the phenotype of developing cells with respect to the following molecules: CD2, CD3, CD4, and CD8.
5. Given that the thymic shadow is lacking in the radiograph, it seems reasonable to investigate T cell function and T cell numbers. A commonly used test of T cell function (providing the child is not a newborn) is the skin test. What does this test measure? What common antigen is used in this test? Explain why this particular antigen is selected.
6. Another test of T cell function is T cell proliferation using mitogenic lectins. Which lectins are used to stimulate T cells? Describe the assay in general terms.
7. Explain how a congenital thymic defect could affect antibody titers to immunization antigens (e.g., tetanus).
8. What does the acronym "CATCH22" signify?
9. For many immunodeficiency disorders, bone marrow transplantation (BMT) is the treatment of choice when an appropriate donor can be identified. Why would BMT not be considered for this patient? What would you recommend?
10. Explain why a "successful" thymic graft could allow a patient's T cells to respond to mitogenic lectins but not necessarily to foreign antigens.

RECOMMENDED APPROACH

Implications/Analysis of Family History

A family history is not possible because the child has been adopted.

Implications/Analysis of Clinical History

Viral and fungal infections point us immediately to a defect in T cells (Fig. 2–1). Although a defect in phagocytes may result in increased susceptibility to fungal infections, T cells are the key players in both viral and fungal infections. (Recall that the patient in Case 1 had a clinical history of fungal, viral, and bacterial infections.)

Implications/Analysis of Laboratory Investigation

The absence of a thymic shadow indicates a defect during embryogenesis resulting in partial or complete

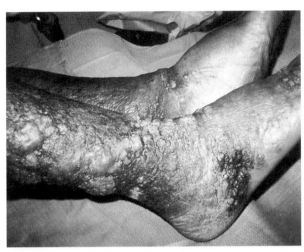

FIGURE 2–1 Cutaneous Kaposi's sarcoma lesions in HIV-infected individual. Patients with T cell deficiencies are susceptible to opportunistic infections. (From Skoner D, Urbach A, Fireman P: Slide Atlas of Pediatric Allergy and Immunology. St. Louis, Mosby, 1992.)

absence of a thymus. When the defect is very severe, T cell maturation cannot occur in the thymus. A deficiency of T cells would explain RD's clinical history. Additionally, RD's physical appearance is consistent with that of children diagnosed with this defect.

Additional Laboratory Tests

To do a complete workup, RD's physician ordered (1) a complete blood cell count (CBC) with differential, (2) a skin test for T cell function, (3) antibody titers for immunization antigens, and (4) flow cytometric analysis of T and B cells. The skin test for T cell function consists of an intracutaneous injection of two or three standardized test antigens, one of which is *C. albicans*. Antigens to which most members of the population have been exposed are selected for this test. Prior exposure to any one of the antigens activates memory T cells and results in the formation of an induration at the site of injection that is maximal 48 to 72 hours later. This is also referred to as a "delayed-type hypersensitivity reaction."

RD's blood cell count was low (see Appendix for reference value), whereas the differential showed a profound decrease in lymphocytes (normal pediatric value = 48%). Skin tests to all three antigens were negative, despite the documented infection with *Candida albicans*. A negative skin test to all three antigens is interpreted as a defect in T cell function. (When the skin test is not definitive, a test that measures polyclonal activation of peripheral blood cells with T cell mitogens [concanavalin A and phytohemagglutinin] is used to assess T cell function.) In this assay, peripheral lymphocytes are incubated with a mitogenic lectin and proliferation (DNA synthesis) is assessed by measuring the amount of ^{3}H-thymidine that is incorporated into the cells. Results of RD's tests to detect the presence of serum antibodies specific for antigens used in pediatric immunization, DPT (diphtheria toxoid, pertussis, and tetanus toxoid), were all below normal. This is not surprising in that antibody responses to protein antigens require both cognate interaction with T cells as well as T cell–derived cytokines.

Flow cytometry can be used to assess the ratio and absolute cell number of cells (e.g., T and B cells). When this technique is used, fluorophore-labeled monoclonal antibodies, specific for proteins on the various cell types, are required. To analyze the lymphocyte subsets, antibodies to T cell proteins (anti-CD3, anti-CD4, anti-CD8) and to B cell proteins (CD19) are used. In RD's case the differential had indicated a significant decrease in the percentage of lymphocytes. Flow cytometric analysis used to determine the ratio of circulating B cells to T cells indicated a profound decrease of circulating T cells (normal ratio of B cells/T cells is 5%-24%/57%-84%). The absolute number of T cells was less than 100 cells/mm^3, suggesting that RD's problems were due to an inherited defect that led to a deficiency in the number of T cells. The prototypical T cell immunodeficiency disorder is DiGeorge syndrome.

A diagnosis of DiGeorge syndrome was confirmed after fluorescence *in situ* hybridization (FISH) analysis of blood smears. For this test, a fluorochrome-labeled single-stranded DNA probe is hybridized to denatured metaphase chromosome (single-stranded) smears on a glass slide. Hybridization with the labeled DNA probe is detected by fluorescence microscopy. The absence of hybridization indicates a deletion. For this syndrome, the deletion was on chromosome 22.

DIAGNOSIS

Based on the molecular cytogenetic analysis (FISH), RD was diagnosed with congenital thymic aplasia, also referred to as DiGeorge syndrome.

THERAPY

Depending on the severity of the defect, pharmacologic intervention may suffice during infections. However, more severe cases require transplantation of functional components of fetal/postnatal allogeneic thymic tissue slices placed into both quadriceps muscles or under a renal capsule. Because thymic aplasia is the result of abnormal development of the third and fourth pharyngeal pouches during embryogenesis, patients also have hypoplasia (or aplasia) of the parathyroids.

Allogeneic Thymus

In thymic fragment transplantation, the major histocompatibility complex (MHC) proteins that are expressed on the allogeneic thymic epithelium are a major factor in the selection of thymocytes (i.e., developing T cells) that will be positively selected for export to the periphery (or death). Consequently, antigen recognition in the periphery will occur only when antigenic peptides are presented to T cells within the groove of the MHC proteins that are the same as those that were present on the thymic epithelium (self-MHC/self peptide) during T cell maturation/education.

Therefore, the question arises, "How can T cells educated on an allogeneic thymus (allo-MHC) recognize self MHC-antigenic peptide in the periphery?" What is surprising is that 1 year after transplantation, even non–MHC-matched patients have been reported to have developed antigen-specific proliferative responses. Recognition of antigenic peptide/MHC complexes on host cells by T cells that have been educated in a thymus expressing a different MHC (allo-MHC) is inconsistent with current dogma.

The presence of T cells that have matured in the allogeneic thymus can be assessed by detecting T cell receptor rearrangement excision circles (TRECs, see later) in circulating T cells. T cell proliferative responses after stimulation with a T cell mitogen do not involve MHC recognition, and so one would predict that T cells isolated from these patients would proliferate when so stimulated. This is, in fact, what has been observed in several of the patients receiving a thymic transplant.

In addition to the thymic aplasia, patients with DiGeorge syndrome may lack parathyroid glands. These patients require regular therapy with an active form of vitamin D. In some cases patients are prescribed calcitriol, which is the active form of vitamin D required to increase calcium and phosphorus in the bloodstream. In the normal individual, precursor vitamin D is ingested with food and absorbed throughout the body, including the skin, where it is modified by sunlight radiation. Subsequent modifications in the

liver and the kidney generate calcitriol. Calcitriol enhances absorption of calcium and phosphate from the gastrointestinal tract.

ETIOLOGY: DiGEORGE SYNDROME (CONGENITAL THYMIC APLASIA)

DiGeorge syndrome results from defective embryogenesis leading to a reduced and defective (or absent) thymus and other organs derived from the third and fourth pharyngeal pouches. These patients are hypocalcemic and exhibit distinctive physical features, including widely separated eyes, low ears, and a cleft palate. The acronym CATCH22 (*c*ardiac defect, *a*bnormal facial features, *t*hymic hypoplasia, *c*left palate, *h*ypocalcemia, and chromosome *22*) is often used to refer to the collection of symptoms that characterize this disorder. Not all children have congenital heart disease, although this disorder is the second most common cause of congenital heart disease. In virtually all cases of congenital thymic aplasia there is a microdeletion in one copy of chromosome 22.

Because the thymus is the organ of differentiation for all T cells (see later) these individuals have few or no circulating T cells and have increased susceptibility to viral, fungal, and intracellular bacterial infections. Patients with reduced or partial thymus function have low T cell numbers and improve with age, perhaps owing to an extrathymic maturation site.

T CELL DEVELOPMENT IN THE THYMUS

Role of the Thymus

The rationale for transplanting a thymic tissue fragment into patients with DiGeorge syndrome is to provide an organ of differentiation for precursor T cells generated in the bone marrow (Fig. 2–2). To understand the complexities associated with this therapeutic intervention, it is important to know something about how T cells recognize antigenic peptides and the role of the thymus in selecting antigen-specific T cell receptors (TCRs). Each TCR chain consists of a variable and a constant region. Although most T cell clones express T cell receptors constructed with the same constant regions, each clone expresses receptors with a unique variable region. The key event in the construction of a unique TCR variable region is somatic recombination.

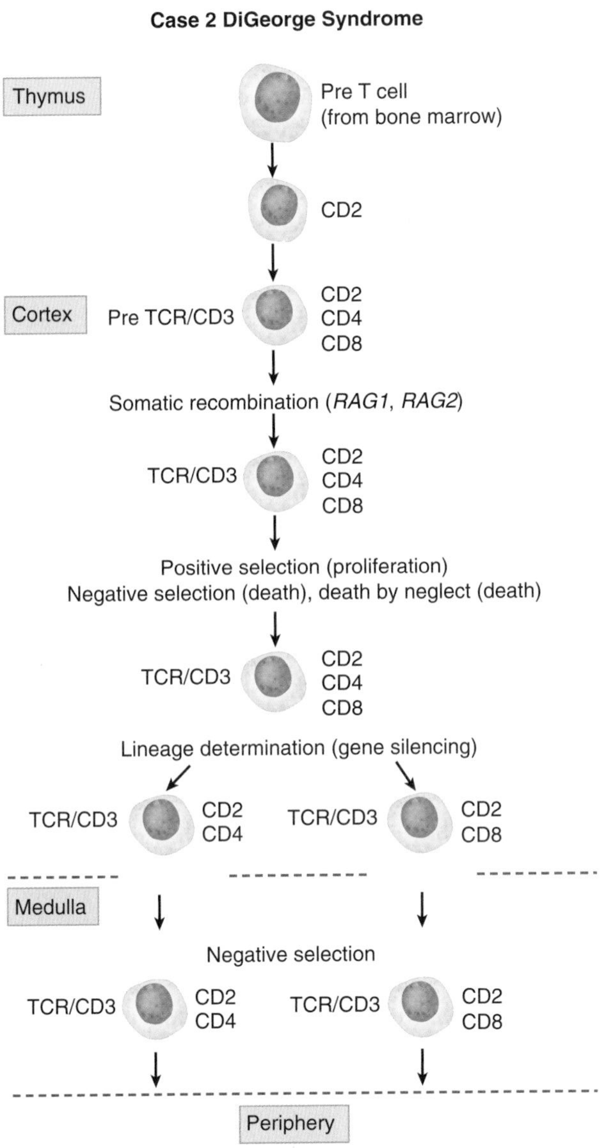

Case 2 DiGeorge Syndrome

FIGURE 2–2 Defects in thymus development lead to Di-George syndrome. The absence of a thymus leads to a deficiency in T cells and associated immune dysfunction in T cell–mediated responses.

Somatic Recombination Determines the Variable Regions of TCRs

Variable regions are constructed during somatic recombination from segments termed variable (V), diversity (D), and joining (J). More specifically, the TCRα variable regions are composed of a "V" and a "J" segment (VJ), whereas the TCRβ regions are composed of "V," "D," and "J" segments (VDJ). During the somatic recombination process, which is initiated by the action of recombinase activation genes 1 and 2 (RAG1 and RAG2), intervening DNA segments that existed between the selected V, D, or J segments are excised, forming circular episomes called TRECs. In any given individual, somatic recombination and diversification can create a repertoire of 10^{12} to 10^{15} different TCRs, each potentially giving rise to a unique T cell clone.

Selection of TCRs in the Thymus

The random selection of V, D, and J gene segments again leads to the generation of T cells expressing TCRs that may be autoreactive or TCRs that are unable to activate T cells. Consequently, those T cells must be deleted during the screening process in the thymus. The fate of the thymocyte (life or death) depends on the interactive avidity between the developing T cell (thymocyte) and the thymic epithelium. Interactive avidity includes the (1) intrinsic affinity of the TCR for self antigen/MHC complex, (2) density of TCRs, (3) density of self antigen/MHC complexes on the thymic epithelium, and (4) density of antagonistic peptide complexes (i.e., cell/cell molecular interactions that repel one another).

In addition to these factors there is a contribution resulting from the interaction of a variety of accessory molecules and adhesion molecules as they interact with their counterpart on the thymic epithelium (cognate ligand). Insignificant interactive avidity with the thymic epithelial cell results in death from neglect. If recognition exceeds a predetermined threshold, thymocytes are clonally eliminated or functionally inactivated by an active process termed *negative selection*. Finally, positive selection and preferential expansion of T cells occurs when the interactive avidity of recognition is intermediate (i.e., between the two extremes noted). Following the screening process in the thymic cortex, lineage determination/gene silencing occurs, a phenomenon in which gene silencing of either the CD4 or the CD8 gene occurs. As a result, each T cell expresses either CD4 or CD8, which determines both function and antigen recognition by class I or class II MHC. A more finely tuned process of negative selection occurs in the medulla.

John, a 12-month-old boy with severe gram-positive bacterial pneumonia, has been referred to the local pediatric hospital by the family's general practitioner. In addition to the fact that this is his fourth such infection in 6 months, he has had recurrent diarrhea (Giardia lamblia) and his tonsils/adenoids are barely detectable. As well, John is below the norm for height and weight. He has received the recommended DTaP (diphtheria, tetanus toxoids, and acellular pertussis) pediatric immunizations (see Fig. 45–1). John has three healthy sisters aged 3, 5, and 7 years. The family lost a boy at 10 months of age to bacterial pneumonia 8 years ago. Blood test results show low total serum immunoglobulin levels, few B cells, but normal numbers and functioning of T cells. All tests for macrophage/neutrophil function and number are normal. Medical and family histories, as well as blood test results, were included in the file that the family physician sent to the hospital. How would you proceed?

QUESTIONS FOR GROUP DISCUSSION

1. Explain why the fact that only male members of this family have been affected with this or a similar disorder is significant.
2. Defects in some cell lineages can be ruled out based on the fact that disease susceptibility is limited to bacteria but not viruses or fungi. Explain.
3. Susceptibility to bacterial infections is increased in patients with particular defects in complement. How can an overall defect in complement activation be detected?
4. Myeloid cell numbers and function are normal. What immunodeficiency disorder can be ruled out if a nitroblue tetrazolium test is normal? (See Case 6.)
5. Serum levels, response to immunization antigen, and B cell numbers and function are all below normal, suggesting that John's problem is a defect in B cells. What B cell marker is used to determine B cell numbers using flow cytometry? When is this marker expressed during B cell maturation in the bone marrow?
6. B cell numbers are low, suggesting that the defect is an early block in B cell differentiation (so-called differentiation arrest). What is the classic immunodeficiency disorder resulting from a differentiation arrest in the early stage of B cell development?
7. What is known to date about the genetic defect in Bruton's agammaglobulinemia?
8. How might Bruton's agammaglobulinemia be treated?
9. Why is it unlikely that this patient has transient hypogammaglobulinemia of infancy?

10. Explain how a defect in CD4+ T cell maturation could cause this disorder.

RECOMMENDED APPROACH

Implications/Analysis of Family History

John has three sisters, but they have not presented with severe and recurrent gram-positive bacterial infections (Fig. 3–1). On the other hand, the family has lost a boy to bacterial pneumonia, suggesting that this is an X-linked recessive immunodeficiency disorder. That is, the gene that is missing or mutated is present on the X chromosome. Because females have two X chromosomes, a gene mutation on one chromosome will not manifest as an immunodeficiency disorder when there is a normal copy of that gene on the other chromosome. Nonetheless, the female remains a carrier and can pass the defective gene to her offspring. Females who inherit two defective genes will also present with the disorder. In contrast, males have only one X chromosome and if a gene on that chromosome is mutated, the child will develop the associated disorder. Although identification of males with a similar disorder helps in the diagnosis, the absence of other affected male infants does not rule out a diagnosis of an X-linked disorder.

Implications/Analysis of Clinical History

John's problems with infections did not begin until he was several months of age, suggesting that prior to this he was protected against infection by maternally transmitted IgG antibodies. Because IgG antibodies have a

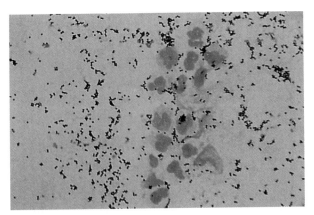

FIGURE 3–1 *Staphylococcus aureus.* Gram stain of pus from patient with a wound infected with *S. aureus.* Note the gram-positive cocci and the pink-colored pus cells. (Gram stain, ×1000.) (From Hart CA, Shears P: Color Atlas of Medical Microbiology, 2nd ed. St. Louis, Mosby, 2004.)

half-life of about 3 weeks, the maternal IgG antibodies that have crossed the placenta will protect the infant for the first few months of life.

Implications/Analysis of Laboratory Investigation

The blood workup (complete blood cell count and differential) indicated a decrease in lymphocyte count. John has not presented with any viral or fungal infections so the decrease in lymphocyte count is unlikely to be caused by a defect in T cell numbers or function. Bacterial infections could also be caused by a complement or B cell dysfunction. Because there is a decrease in lymphocyte numbers but not in myeloid cells (neutrophils, monocytes), it is likely that John has a B cell defect.

Quantitative assessment of serum immunoglobulin using either nephelometry (see Case 5) or enzyme-linked immunosorbent assay (ELISA) (see Case 7) indicated that serum immunoglobulin levels were below normal (normal pediatric level: see Appendix). B cell numbers, assessed by flow cytometry using fluorescently labeled anti-CD19 antibodies, were also below normal. CD19 is a B cell marker that is initially expressed during the pro–B cell stage and continues to be expressed at all stages of B cell development, including the mature B cell. A CD19+ B cell count of less than 100 mg/dL is suggestive of a primary immunodeficiency: X-linked agammaglobulinemia (XLA).

John's response to vaccination antigens (tetanus and diphtheria toxoids) was measured using an ELISA to assess B cell function. The antibody titers were below the level of detection. Polyclonal activation of peripheral blood B cells with a B cell polyclonal activator was also below normal.

Although bacterial infections can also result from defects in the complement system, the low B cell numbers, low serum IgG, undetectable titers to immunization antigens, and defect in B cell function suggest that this is not a complement dysfunction. However, a complement defect could be ruled out by measuring the overall activation of both the classical (CH50) and alternative (AH50) pathways (see Case 11).

Additional Laboratory Tests

John has few B cells and low serum immunoglobulin levels, which is suggestive of an early block in B cell differentiation (so-called differentiation arrest) and is a relatively classic presentation of XLA (Bruton's hypo- [or agamma-] globulinemia). A block at a later stage in B cell differentiation would have higher circulating B cell numbers. Molecular testing for mutations in the Btk kinase, the defect in XLA, would confirm the diagnosis.

DIAGNOSIS

John was diagnosed with X-linked agammaglobulinemia (Bruton's hypo- or agammaglobulinemia).

THERAPY

Gamma Globulin Therapy

Conventional treatment involves the *life-long* replacement of the defective components (i.e., serum immunoglobulin replacement). Passive immunization with monthly intravenous injections of pooled gamma globulins (~500 mg/kg administered over ~4 hours) that contain IgG against a broad spectrum of bacteria, viruses, and parasites is recommended. Because many of these patients are IgA deficient the immune globulin selected must not contain any IgA, to avoid possible anaphylaxis (see Case 5).

Bone Marrow Transplant

In the absence of human leukocyte antigen (HLA)-matched bone marrow, transplantation is not typically considered, given the risk-benefit costs. However, successful bone marrow transplantation has been reported for a number of children.

ETIOLOGY: X-LINKED AGAMMAGLOBULINEMIA

In XLA, mutations in the X chromosome gene encoding the Btk tyrosine kinase (Bruton's agammaglobulinemia kinase) are present in all patients. The initial B cell development block occurs at the pro-B cell to pre-B cell transition. Because this kinase plays a key role in signaling pathways that regulate activation, differentiation, and proliferation of B cells, these mutations lead to a profound dysfunction in B cell numbers and function. Molecular genetic testing may allow identification of carriers of the Btk gene and hence provide the basis for early diagnosis of XLA.

TRANSIENT HYPOGAMMAGLOBULINEMIA OF INFANCY

In all infants, signs of hypogammaglobulinemia occur around 6 months of age when passively transferred maternal antibodies have been degraded. The serum immunoglobulin level at this time is approximately 350 mg/dL, so it is not surprising that most infants experience many respiratory tract infections around this age. Transient hypogammaglobulinemia of infancy, also referred to as hypogammaglobulinemia of early childhood, presents as many of the same infections as described for John, including recurrent gastroenteritis, otitis media, and respiratory tract infections. Additionally, IgG serum levels are depressed or undetectable. In contrast to patients with XLA, however, IgM serum levels are normal, as is the B cell count. Some studies have shown that, at least in some patients, *in vitro* stimulation of B cells in response to direct B cell activation results in the production of IgG. In these same patients, there is a deficiency in the number and function of CD4+ T cells, suggesting that the defect in this disorder results from a maturational delay in T cell development. T cells are required for B cell activation and isotype switching.

Richard is a 12-month-old infant with a severe gram-negative kidney infection (pyelonephritis). This is his third such infection in 6 months, although investigation of the urogenital system for congenital defects (e.g., ureteral valvular defects) revealed no abnormality. The mother insists that "something" must be wrong because he has had recurrent sinopulmonary infections and repeated episodes of diarrhea. Richard has three healthy sisters aged 1, 3, and 4 years. An uncle died at 10 years of age with bacterial pneumonia. Despite the fact that he had received childhood immunizations, blood tests performed at a hospital elsewhere revealed low serum IgG, IgA, and IgE levels but high serum levels of IgM. B and T cell numbers were normal, as was the function of T cells. There was no evidence for defective neutrophil functioning. How would you proceed?

QUESTIONS FOR GROUP DISCUSSION

1. Explain why X-linked congenital disorders would be high on the list of considerations in this case.
2. Explain how the serum immunoglobulin profile in this case differs from that in the patient in Case 3 (X-linked agammaglobulinemia).
3. A deficiency of all antibody isotypes but an increase in IgM indicates that normal plasma cell differentiation is occurring but that class (isotype) switching is not occurring. Explain the role of T cells in isotype switching.
4. Explain why each of the following can now be ruled out as presumptive diagnoses:
   (a) severe combined immunodeficiency
   (b) DiGeorge syndrome
   (c) X-linked agammaglobulinemia
   (d) complement defect
   (e) NK cell defect
5. If you are unable to rule out the disorders in question 4, what tests would you order to help you rule out the clinical conditions?
6. CD40 ligand (CD154) is upregulated when T cells are activated. This molecule plays an important role in antigen-induced B cell differentiation. Explain.
7. Compare and contrast the clinical presentation of hyper IgM syndrome and transient hypogammaglobulinemia of infancy.
8. Patients with this disorder have increased bacterial and some fungal infections. How could you rule out a disorder in which there is a defect in the phagocytic enzyme complex NADPH oxidase?
9. Explain why knockout mice for inducible co-stimulator gene (ICOS) also show profound defects in isotype switching.

10. Explain the role of CD28 and CD152 (formerly CTLA-4) in T cell activation and downregulation of T cell activation, respectively. Note that both these molecules bind CD80 and CD86 on antigen-presenting cells.

RECOMMENDED APPROACH

Implications/Analysis of Family History

Richard's clinical history combined with a number of healthy sisters and evidence for the death of an uncle from bacterial pneumonia is highly suggestive of an X-linked congenital defect in immune functioning.

Implications/Analysis of Clinical History

A clinical history that includes chronic sinusitis and recurrent diarrhea caused by protozoa or bacteria, as well as hospitalization with bacterial pneumonia in a male infant suggests an X-linked immunodeficiency disorder. Defects in B cells, phagocytes, or complement could lead to some of these symptoms. However, sinopulmonary infections are highly suggestive of a deficiency in IgA. Therefore, laboratory investigations should focus initially on total serum immunoglobulin levels and levels of various antibody subclasses.

Implications/Analysis of Laboratory Investigation

Richard's initial blood work consisting of a complete blood cell count and differential was normal so this is

A

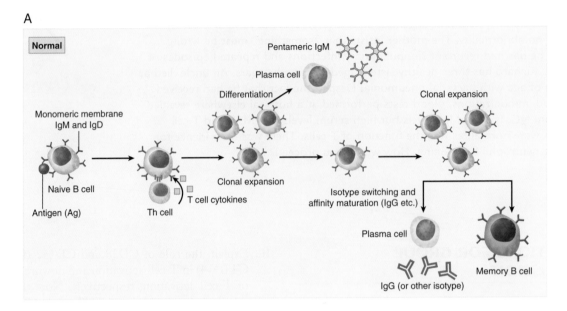

B

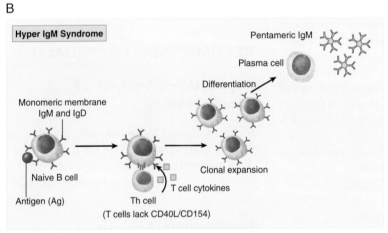

FIGURE 4–1   B cell activation in response to T cell–independent antigen. **A,** B cell activation to T cell–independent antigens requires cognate interaction with T cells, as well as T cell cytokines. This leads to isotype switching, differentiation to plasma cells, or memory cells. A required signal for isotype switching is CD40 (on B cells) with CD154 (on T cells). **B,** T cells do not express CD154, and so isotype switching does not occur (hyper IgM syndrome). (*A,* Modified with permission from Gorczynski R, Stanley J: Clinical Immunology. Austin, Landes, 1999.)

not a problem in T cell or B cell development (see Case 1). Serum immunoglobulin measures (see Case 3) indicated little to no IgG, IgA, or IgE, but IgM was present in higher concentrations than the normal reference value, suggesting that there is a problem in isotype switching. The normal numbers of B cells and the high concentrations of IgM rule out X-linked (Bruton's) agammaglobulinemia (XLA) as a possible diagnosis.

B cell activation leading to isotype switching requires T cell–derived cytokines as well as cognate interaction with activated T cells (Fig. 4–1A). As such,

a deficiency or defect in T cells could account for the observed levels of IgG, IgA, and IgE. However, we are told that T cell function is normal. In light of normal T cell function, the molecular interactions between B and T cells should be investigated.

Additional Laboratory Tests

Flow cytometric analysis of cell surface markers on T and B cells revealed normal expression of CD40 on B cells but no detectable expression of CD154 (CD40 ligand) on activated T cells.

DIAGNOSIS

The lack of CD154 expression on activated T cells is a strong indication that Richard has X-linked hyper IgM syndrome because CD40-CD154 interaction is required for isotype switching of activated B cells (see Fig. 4–1B). On the basis of the clinical history and laboratory investigations it is possible to rule out XLA as a cause of these infections. In XLA there are few B cells and even IgM is deficient. Transient hypogammaglobulinemia of infancy is also ruled out because in this disorder IgM levels are normal. Additionally, there is published evidence for a maturational defect in CD4+ Th1 cells. Both cognate (T-B cell) interaction and T cell–derived cytokines are required for isotype switching in B cells.

THERAPY

Conventional treatment in hyper IgM syndrome involves pharmacologic treatment of infections as they arise. In addition, life-long replacement of the defective components (i.e., serum immunoglobulin isotype replacement) is required. The latter is a costly proposition and not without its own risks (inadvertent transmission of disease, e.g., hepatitis C, HIV). Bone marrow transplantation might be a suitable alternative if rejection could be controlled (see Transplantation Immunology, Section V).

ETIOLOGY: HYPER IGM SYNDROME

The X-linked variant of hyper IgM syndrome (hyper IgM type I) is caused by a mutation or defect in CD154 (formerly known as CD40 ligand) that is expressed on activated T cells, primarily CD4+ T cells. Patients with this syndrome have increased infections from bacteria, protozoa, and some fungi (e.g., *Giardia, Campylobacter, Cryptosporidium,* and *Pneumocystis jiroveci* [formerly *P. carinii*]). Delayed expression of CD154 may explain the clinical presentation of infants diagnosed with transient hypogammaglobulinemia of infancy.

Several mutations and deletions in the gene encoding CD154 have been identified. Some mutations, which still allow expression of CD154, may prevent CD154 binding to CD40 or only allow binding with low affinity. Several of these mutations affect the tertiary or quaternary structure of the molecule. Without sequencing of the CD154 gene product, or detailed assessment of CD154 mRNA expression/stability, it is often difficult to define unequivocally the precise nature of a CD154 defect in hyper IgM syndrome.

Role of CD28 and CD152

CD80 and CD86 (formerly known as B7-1 and B7-2) are expressed on antigen-presenting cells, including dendritic cells, macrophages, and B cells (see Fig. 4–2A). They are both ligands for CD28, which is constitutively expressed on T cells, and CD152 (formerly CTLA-4), which is induced after T cell activation. It has long been recognized that T cell activation requires at least two signals, the first being delivered via the T cell antigen receptor and the second via CD28, whose interaction with CD80/86 triggers a signal transduction cascade that results in the stabilization of mRNA for IL-2, a growth factor for T cells. CD152 is induced on activated T cells and probably plays a more important role in downregulating the T cell response after binding to the same ligands CD80 and CD86. Because CD80 and CD86 have a higher affinity for CD152, the inhibitory signal plays the dominant role once CD152 is expressed on the cell surface.

Inducible Co-stimulator and CD154 Expression

Studies with knockout mice for the ICOS (inducible co-stimulator) gene also show profound defects in isotype switching after B cell activation. ICOS is expressed only on the surface of activated T cells and has been shown to upregulate CD154 on T cells following ICOS-B7h interaction (Fig. 4–2B). B7h is constitutively expressed on naive B cells and is a newly discovered member of the B7 (CD80/86) family. This defect in isotype switching is reversed when anti-CD40 antibodies are used to stimulate CD40 directly (instead of binding CD154). Cytokine secretion is also affected in the ICOS knockout mice. T cells from such animals show increased production of IL-2 and interferon gamma (IFNγ) but a decrease in IL-4 and IL-10 after immune stimulation. IL-4 is required for isotype switching to IgE. *Note:* The reader should beware of some potential confusion caused by redundant nomenclature. B7h (the ligand for ICOS) has also been named B7RP-1, GL-50, ICOSL, and LICOS. The inducible co-stimulator (ICOS) is also known as activation-inducible lymphocyte immunomodulator (AILIM).

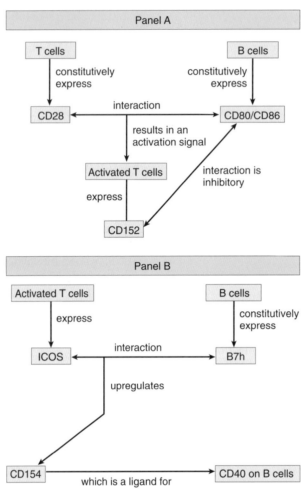

FIGURE 4–2 Interaction of T cells and B cells. **A,** Interaction of CD80/86 (B cells) with CD28 leads to T cell activation, whereas interaction with CD152 downregulates activated T cells. **B,** ICOS-B7h interaction upregulates CD154, which is a ligand for CD40. Activated cells express the inducible co-stimulator (ICOS), which is a ligand for B7h on B cells. This interaction leads to the upregulation of CD154 (CD40L) on T cells, which is a ligand for CD40 on B cells.

Autosomal Recessive Forms of Hyper IgM

Although hyper IgM type I is the most common form of this disorder, autosomal recessive forms have been identified. The autosomal recessive forms of this disease, hyper IgM types II and III, are caused by mutations in the AID (activation-induced cytidine deaminase) gene and CD40, respectively. Both class switch recombination and somatic hypermutation (somatic mutation) require the action of the AID enzyme, which deaminates cytidine to uridine. More recently, a recessive mutation in the gene encoding uracil-DNA-glycosylase (UNG), an enzyme in the base-excision repair pathway for removal of uracils

occurring in DNA, has been identified as also causing hyper IgM syndrome.

It is becoming increasingly clear that mutations can occur in several genes that encode proteins acting at different stages of class switching and that all such mutations can produce similar clinical manifestations (phenotype), although the genotypes are distinct. One model that has been put forth by Durandy and Honjo (see Further Reading) is that AID deaminates cytosine in the immunoglobulin switch region (DNA), thereby forming uracil. However, the uracil, which should only be present in RNA, must be removed and this is mediated by UNG. As such, mutations in either AID or UNG enzymes would lead to the same clinical picture.

Bill was apparently well for most of his infant life, although he seemed to both his parents to have had an excess of upper respiratory tract infections and diarrhea (*Giardia lamblia*) compared with his friends. He had received all childhood immunizations without any notable negative side effects. At the age of 9 he developed an extremely severe case of sinusitis that responded well to antibiotics but caused even his family physician to wonder if there was something else going on. He was small for his age. There were no other siblings, but close attention to the family tree revealed that both an aunt and an uncle had also suffered from recurrent sinopulmonary infections and, in one case, a severe gastrointestinal infection. The aunt was still alive. Unfortunately the uncle had developed leukemia several years earlier and had died unexpectedly while receiving a blood transfusion at a small village hospital where he lived. A cousin had been diagnosed with common variable immunodeficiency (CVID) at age 30. Analysis of serum immunoglobulins using rate nephelometry, a technique that measures the amount of light scatter occurring as a beam of light encounters immune complexes in a dilute solution, showed IgG and IgM levels were normal but IgA levels were not detectable. IgG titers to childhood vaccines were in the normal range. A complete blood cell count with differential showed normal values.

QUESTIONS FOR GROUP DISCUSSION

1. This patient has had a number of infections in regions where mucous membranes play a protective role. What antibody isotype predominates at these sites?

2. The patient has received all childhood immunizations. How can this be used to assess B cell function?

3. Rate nephelometry is a technique used to quantitate serum immunoglobulin. What would you expect this test to reveal in this patient?

4. On the basis of the nephelometry results, the patient was diagnosed with selective IgA deficiency. Explain therefore the significance of a family history in which one relative died while receiving a blood transfusion while another was diagnosed with common variable immunodeficiency.

5. Explain in basic terms the principle underlying rate nephelometry.

6. Some patients with selective IgA deficiency have a normal total IgG level but yet have a deficiency of IgG2 or IgG4. Explain how this is possible.

7. Explain why intravenous administration of immunoglobulin (IVIG) is not an option for patients with selective IgA deficiency.

8. Explain why patients with selective IgA deficiency are at risk for an acute transfusion reaction if the serum contains some serum IgA.

9. How can transfusion reactions be avoided in patients with selective IgA deficiency?

10. ICOS (inducible co-stimulator) is found on activated, but not resting, T cells. On what cells is the counter molecule for ICOS expressed? What defects are noted in mice in whom the gene for ICOS or its counter molecule has been "knocked out"?

RECOMMENDED APPROACH

Implication/Analysis of Family History

Bill's relatives have had similar clinical presentations, suggesting that Bill's condition is the result of an inherited disorder. Because both males and females have presented with similar symptoms, Bill could have an autosomal recessive disorder.

Implication/Analysis of Clinical History

Consider first the types of infections that are reported: upper respiratory tract infections, sinusitis, and giardiasis. All of these infections are occurring in regions lined with mucous membranes where secretory IgA normally has a role in neutralizing pathogens that cause these infections (see Fig. 3–1). Already we should be considering that a defect in IgA is a possibility. This is further supported by the fact that an uncle had died during a blood transfusion (see later). As well, a cousin had been diagnosed with common variable immunodeficiency, a disorder that is more common among relatives of individuals with selective IgA deficiency than one would find in the general population.

Implication/Analysis of Laboratory Investigation

B cell function was normal, as determined by measuring antibody responses to vaccines (DPT: diphtheria, pertussis, tetanus toxoid) administered during childhood immunization. In major centers, quantitative measures of serum IgG, IgA, and IgM are determined using rate nephelometry, a technique that measures the amount of light scatter occurring as a beam of light encounters immune complexes in a dilute solution. This technique is a modification of the precipitin reaction (radial immunodiffusion) that was used for so many years to quantitate serum immunoglobulins. In rate nephelometry, the solution contains excess antibodies (anti-immunoglobulin for a particular isotype) and so when serum antibodies are added, immune complexes form readily. As the number of immune complexes increases, so does the amount of light scatter.

Additional Laboratory Tests

In some patients with IgA deficiency there is an accompanying defect in IgG antibody subclasses IgG2 or IgG4. Because some patients with a defect in IgG2 or IgG4 have elevated levels of IgG1 and IgG3, giving a normal total IgG level, rate nephelometry should be used to measure the subclass distribution. About 80%

of total serum is IgG, with normal subclass distribution being IgG1, 67%; IgG2, 20% to 25%; IgG3, 5% to 10%; and IgG4, 5%.

Individuals with a deficiency in IgG2 do not produce antibodies in response to some encapsulated bacteria (e.g., *Haemophilus influenzae* type b), and so assessment of the antibody response to this vaccine would provide some insight into the patient's IgG2 status. In this case, Bill's clinical history did not include infections with encapsulated bacteria. His antibody response to childhood vaccines was normal, as was the distribution of IgG subclasses. Patients with serum levels below 7 mg/dL, in the presence of normal IgG and IgM, are considered to have IgA deficiency. Some patients have low levels of IgA, whereas others have a total absence of IgA.

DIAGNOSIS

Bill was diagnosed with selective IgA deficiency.

THERAPY

Secretory IgA is the predominant antibody at mucosal surfaces; therefore, patients present primarily with sinopulmonary and gastrointestinal infections (Fig. 5–1). In general, it is only necessary to treat the

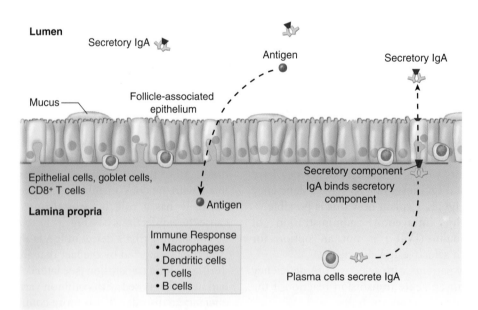

FIGURE 5–1   Synthesis and transportation of IgA to the lumen. IgA is synthesized in the lamina propria, binds to secretory component, and is transported to the lumen through epithelial cells. A portion of the secretory component remains attached to the IgA.

recurrent infections. Any other "heroic" measure to replace missing IgA is not warranted (cost/safety issues). Insufflation (intranasal) IgA preparations have been considered as therapy for upper respiratory tract sinus infections.

ETIOLOGY: SELECTIVE IgA DEFICIENCY

Selective IgA deficiency is the most common of the primary immunodeficiency disorders. This disorder has a genetic component in that family members and related individuals present with similar clinical symptoms. Although the cause of the defect is unknown, B cells are unable to switch isotypes to IgA production. Most patients are asymptomatic.

Anaphylaxis

Individuals who also have an IgG2 deficiency and present with recurring infections from encapsulated bacteria (e.g., *Streptococcus pneumoniae*) may benefit from gamma globulin prophylaxis. However, gamma globulin preparations carry minute amounts of IgA, so individuals who become sensitized to IgA and have anti-IgA antibodies are at risk for anaphylaxis on re-exposure to administered IgA.

Acute Transfusion Reaction

An acute transfusion reaction is also a risk for individuals with anti-IgA antibodies who receive a transfusion of blood containing some serum IgA. This is the most likely cause of Bill's uncle's death. Acute transfusion reactions occur within minutes of initiation of transfusion, reflecting effector molecules released from memory immune cells "armed" to detect the presence of molecules already recognized as being foreign. Patients typically become flushed and agitated and complain of a pain in the abdomen or chest. To avoid transfusion reactions or to avoid sensitizing IgA-deficient patients with IgA, it is recommended to transfuse red blood cells that have been washed to remove donor serum IgA

Associated Disorder

Common Variable Immunodeficiency

For individuals with IgA deficiency it is not uncommon to have a relative develop CVID as an adult. A diagnosis of CVID requires a deficiency in at least two antibody isotypes (e.g., IgG < 4 g/L; IgA < 0.5 g/dL; IgM decreased or absent). Although the cause of CVID is not known, studies of various patient populations have demonstrated different defects, including defects in B cell maturation, T cell abnormalities, and even defects in inducible co-stimulator (ICOS). ICOS is expressed on activated, but not resting, T cells. It binds to its counter molecule ICOS ligand (B7h) on B cells and provides important signals involved in ongoing B cell growth and differentiation.

About 10% of individuals diagnosed with CVID have a homozygous loss of ICOS on T cells, suggesting that ICOS-B7h interaction plays a role in class switching in activated B cells. Knockout mice for either ICOS or B7h have normal T and B cell subpopulations but defective germinal centers after antigen activation and decreased antibody production.

C A S E

6

Jason, a 6-year-old boy who lives on a farm, has convinced his parents that he should be allowed to take care of the chicks that are in the hay loft area of the barn. He is intrigued with this brood of chicks and spends hours just lying down in the hay to watch them or dragging hay over to their nest. When he is not in the barn, Jason is "helping" his mother with the new garden. After several weeks of this regimen, Jason started having difficulty breathing and seemed to "always be coughing." The parents took him to their family physician, who had already treated Jason for a severe diaper rash *(Candida albicans)* when he was an infant and over the past few years for numerous severe bacterial infections.

The physician ordered several tests, including a complete blood cell count and differential, total serum immunoglobulins, immunization antigen titer, T cell function test, and a bronchoalveolar lavage to use for culture. The white blood cell count showed a mild leukocytosis, but the differential indicated a normal percentage of each cell type. Total IgG was normal for the pediatric population (see Appendix), as was the antibody titer to immunization antigens. T cell function was normal. An inquiry into Jason's family revealed that he had three older sisters and two brothers, none of whom had presented with clinical symptoms analogous to those for which Jason's parents had sought medical attention. How would you proceed?

QUESTIONS FOR GROUP DISCUSSION

1. Fungal infections (e.g., *Candida albicans*) occur frequently in patients with T cell disorders. However, laboratory tests indicated that this patient's T cell number and function were normal. What other cell type plays an important role in the elimination of fungal infections?

2. This patient has a history of both fungal and bacterial infections. Therefore, which cell type should you consider investigating with respect to cell number and function?

3. The phagocyte plays an important role in the innate immune system using as its armamentarium lysosomal enzymes, reactive oxygen intermediates (ROIs), and nitric oxide. ROIs are generated during the respiratory burst. Which enzyme complex is required to trigger the sequence of events that generates the ROIs?

4. Describe the laboratory tests used to determine if the NADPH oxidase enzymatic complex is functional.

5. Culture of the bronchoalveolar lavage fluid revealed that Jason was infected with *Aspergillus fumigatus*, a fungus that is widely distributed in nature, including garden soil and hay lofts. Despite this, aspergillosis is not common. Explain.

6. In a normally functioning immune system, T cells enhance the phagocytic ability of phagocytes. Explain.

7. Recently, prophylactic administration of the cytokine interferon gamma (IFNγ) has gained

popularity as a therapeutic intervention to treat patients with a defect in a component of the NADPH oxidase complex. Explain. What is the source of IFNγ in an intact immune system?

8. Describe some of the effects of IFNγ, other than effects described in question 7.

9. Describe the rationale for bone marrow transplantation and gene therapy.

10. Explain the role of NRAMP-1 in host defense.

RECOMMENDED APPROACH

Implications/Analysis of Family History

An inquiry into Jason's family revealed that he had three older sisters and two brothers, none of whom had presented with clinical symptoms analogous to those for which Jason's parents had sought medical attention.

Implications/Analysis of Clinical History

Whereas bacterial infections can be commonly seen in complement and cell-trafficking abnormalities, susceptibility to fungal infections should trigger a concern to investigate a defect in phagocyte or T cell function.

Implications/Results of Laboratory Investigation

Laboratory tests revealed a mild elevation in white blood cell count, normal differential, normal serum immunoglobulins, and normal B cell and T cell function tests. These tests rule out obvious B cell and T cell development disorders (see Cases 2 and 3). It is reasonable to conclude that Jason's infections are not due to defects in adaptive immunity. As well, because the complete blood cell count and differential were normal, a deficiency in development of cell population(s) in the innate immune system can also be ruled out.

Culture indicated an infection with *Aspergillus fumigatus*. Infection is generally acquired from breathing in *Aspergillus* conidia (spores), which are widely distributed in nature, including hay lofts and garden soil. In immunocompromised individuals these infections can give rise to aspergillosis (Fig. 6–1). Individuals with normal numbers and function of phagocytes and CD4+ T cells can usually overcome these infections

Given that T cell numbers and function are normal, as are the myeloid cell numbers, we need to consider the possibility that a functional defect in the innate immune system is the cause of the infections.

Additional Laboratory Tests

Destruction of pathogens by the phagocyte is mediated by the armamentarium in the phagosome, and

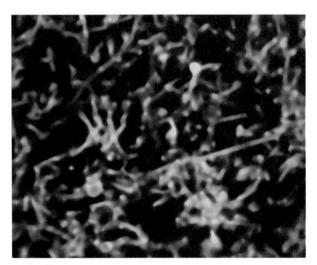

FIGURE 6–1 Aspergillosis in lung of patient with chronic granulomatous disease. Slide is viewed by fluorescence microscopy, showing yellow branching hyphae typical of *Aspergillus*. (*Note:* unlike *Candida*, *Aspergillus* lacks budding yeasts.) (Acridine orange fluorescence, ×400.)

this includes reactive oxygen intermediates, lysosomal enzymes, and nitric oxide. Although any one of these can be defective, the most prominent defects that alter intracellular killing of pathogens by phagocytes are those that result in mutations of the proteins that compose the NADPH oxidase system. Activation of this enzyme complex induces a respiratory burst (an increase in oxygen consumption), so named because oxygen is used by the cell to generate reactive oxygen intermediates (ROIs: e.g., superoxide anion, hydroxyl ion, hydroxyl radical, and hydrogen peroxide).

Nitroblue Tetrazolium Test

Classically, the overall function of the NADPH oxidase complex has been determined using the nitroblue tetrazolium (NBT) dye reduction test. NBT is a yellow dye that becomes insoluble and turns purple (chemical reaction) resulting from the presence of NADPH oxidase activity. In this test, a droplet of the patient's blood is placed onto a slide along with a neutrophil activator and NBT. The patient's cells take up the dye, and if NADPH oxidase is functioning normally the dye is reduced, causing it to change to dark blue/purple.

Flow Cytometry

More recently, flow cytometry has been used to assess the respiratory burst. In this approach, phagocytes take up dihydro-rhodamine-123, a dye that does not fluoresce in resting cells. On activation of NADPH oxidase, the dye emits a fluorescence that is detected using flow cytometry. One of the advantages of this more recent approach is that it has been easier to quantitate this assay than the NBT assay. Analysis of NADPH oxidase in Jason's phagocytes indicated that the NADPH oxidase system was defective.

DIAGNOSIS

Jason was diagnosed with chronic granulomatous disease. Because some NADPH oxidase defects are X linked, the flow cytometry test for NADPH oxidase activity was extended to Jason's mother, sisters, and brothers. Only his 12-year-old brother showed evidence for defective NADPH oxidase function. Interestingly, blood cells from his mother and one sister showed mixed populations of neutrophils, with about 50% exhibiting a normal respiratory burst and 50%

not doing so. Females carry two X chromosomes, one of which is randomly inactivated in all cells. Therefore, females who are carriers but do not express the disease have a mutated gene on only one X chromosome. A normal gene is expressed in about half the cells and a defective gene in the other half. Thus "functionally normal" females (carriers) are, in fact, genetic mosaics.

THERAPY

Administration of antibiotics to combat bacterial infections and potent antifungal agents (e.g., oral itraconazole) represent the mainstay of treatment. Prophylactic administration of IFNγ has gained popularity as a therapeutic intervention.

Interferon γ

In one study of chronic granulomatous disease (CGD) patients with a defect in p47phox, 70% of patients treated with IFNγ had enhanced production of ROIs. However, this response itself has not been seen uniformly. Such conflicting reports may represent patient populations that have different subunit defects or different mutations in any particular subunit. Some mutations might cause total inactivation of NADPH oxidase activity, whereas other mutations may cause a decrease in activity that can be rescued with high concentrations of IFNγ. Despite the conflicting reports regarding increases in ROIs after IFNγ treatment, a reduction in the number of bacterial infections is generally observed consistently, suggesting that IFNγ is also stimulating other intracellular antimicrobial defense mechanisms. In normal individuals, IFNγ induces transcription of gp91 PHOX and enhances production of ROIs.

Other Effects of IFNγ Treatment

IFNγ induces transcription of inducible nitric oxide synthase, an enzyme that catalyzes the conversion of L-arginine ($+O_2$) to L-citrulline and nitric oxide. Nitric oxide is toxic to many pathogens. Other systems activated by IFNγ include, but are not limited to, IDO (indoleamine 2,3 dioxygenase oxidase) and NRAMP (natural resistance associated macrophage protein).

IDO is a key enzyme required for the catabolism of tryptophan, an amino acid that is required for the protein synthesis. NRAMP1 is a membrane protein and, as such, is present on the phagosome membrane because the phagosome is formed when membrane pseudopods extend around the pathogen. This strategic location of NRAMP1 allows it to transport metal ions from the phagosome to the cytosol. The removal of metal ions from the phagosome is a host defense mechanism because the phagosome milieu contains metal ions required by some bacteria present in that vacuole. These bacteria have metal ion transporters that take up metal ions from this milieu and incorporate them into metalloenzymes. This host defense mechanism is believed to be particularly important in patients infected with *Mycobacterium* species because these metal ions are essential for their survival.

Bone Marrow Transplant

In more severe cases of CGD, bone marrow transplantation to replace hematopoietic cells has been performed when a suitable donor has been available. However, bone marrow transplantation carries a high mortality risk.

Gene Therapy

In the future, treatment may rely on gene therapy in which a corrected version of the defective NADPH oxidase subunit is cloned into the patient's cells. As an example, one recent clinical trial performed in association with the NIAID's Laboratory of Host Defenses, described five adult patients with a defect in p47phox who were treated using a gene therapy approach.

These patients were first treated with the cytokine granulocyte-macrophage colony-stimulating factor (GM-CSF), a growth factor for CD34+ stem cells (precursors of hematopoietic cells), in order to expand the CD34+ stem cell pool. CD34+ peripheral blood stem cells were then isolated from the patients and transduced *ex vivo* with a retroviral vector containing a DNA encoding the NADPH oxidase subunit, p47phox. The transduced cells were then infused back into the patients. In all five patients, functionally active (NADPH+) neutrophils were detected in circulation, with activity peaking at about 1 month. In two patients, the transduced cells were still detectable 6 months later. No toxicity of treatment was observed.

ETIOLOGY: CHRONIC GRANULOMATOUS DISEASE

Chronic granulomatous disease (CGD), one of the more common immunodeficiencies that affects innate immunity, is characterized by the absence of a respiratory burst and associated ROIs due to a defective subunit in the multi-subunit NADPH oxidase enzyme complex. In the resting phagocyte, some of the subunits are distributed in the plasma membrane; others are in the cytosol. Phagocytosis triggers subunit assembly on the phagocytic vacuole, a respiratory burst, and production of ROIs (see Fig. 4–1).

Some of the genes encoding the NADPH oxidase subunits that assemble to form a complex are encoded on autosomal chromosomes. However, others (e.g., gp91 PHOX) map to the X chromosome. The gp91 PHOX is the most common mutation in patients presenting with CGD and so the majority (>80%) of affected individuals are male. This is consistent with the observation that Jason's 12-year-old brother was the only family member who had a defective NADPH

oxidase test. Although a defective NADPH oxidase leaves individuals susceptible to recurrent bacterial infections, the most frequent cause of death is chronic infection with *Aspergillus* species. Chronic infections are often complicated by the end result of chronic inflammatory processes and tissue remodeling, namely, excessive scar tissue contributing to noncompliant lung function.

When patients with a defective NADPH oxidase are infected with bacteria that are hydrogen peroxide producing but catalase negative, some bacterial destruction can still occur. Here the hydrogen peroxide produced by the bacteria in the phagocytic vacuole acts as a substrate for myeloperoxidase (a lysosomal enzyme) to generate bactericidal hypochlorite when chloride ion is present.

7

Paul is 4 years of age and suffers from recurrent gram-negative bacterial infections, all of which have eventually cleared with long-term antibiotic therapy. Although he has been hospitalized three times for pneumonia *(Chlamydia pneumoniae)*, there is no evidence for increased susceptibility to viral or fungal infections, and all of his childhood immunizations are up to date. An infectious disease specialist at a local tertiary care center was unable to establish an etiology for the problem. Further exploration of the family tree revealed that both male and female relatives had presented with a similar clinical history of recurrent infectious illnesses. Blood cell count and differential, performed on several occasions, indicated normal numbers of B cells, T cells, neutrophils, and monocytes. Serum immunoglobulin levels were also shown to be normal for all isotypes, as were antibody titers for various vaccine antigens. Other culture assays, performed to investigate cytokine production (from T cells) after stimulation with known T cell polyclonal activators, were normal. How would you proceed?

QUESTIONS FOR GROUP DISCUSSION

1. Paul's clinical history does not show an increased susceptibility to either fungal or viral infections. What type of cell defects would you consider to be unlikely?
2. What tests could you request to rule out a defect in T cell function? Describe these tests in general terms.
3. In fact, most of Paul's infections have been bacterial. In general terms, what three cells/systems would be high on your list for investigation?
4. Explain how you could rule out a deficiency in the proteins that play a role in the activation of complement.
5. Explain how you would rule out a defect in B cell number and function.
6. Results from the blood work indicated that the myeloid cell numbers were normal. Additionally, tests to measure the respiratory burst indicated that the NADPH oxidase complex was functioning normally. These tests suggest that both the phagocyte cell number and function are normal. Assuming that the complement tests were normal, as were tests for B cell numbers and function, how would you proceed? Explain, keeping in mind that Paul's clinical history has been marked by bacterial and fungal infections.
7. All the tests administered have indicated normal cell numbers and function for both the adaptive and innate immune systems. Therefore, it seems reasonable to determine if (a) the immune cells are reaching the sites of infection, (b) immune cells are recognizing the antigens, or (c) a defect in a signaling cascade is the root of Paul's problem. What tests could you request to rule out each of these possibilities?
8. Cells of the innate immune system including macrophages and dendritic cells express pattern recognition receptors (PRRs), which recognize so-called pathogen-associated molecular patterns (PAMPs) conserved among microbes. The best-studied PRRs to date are the toll-like receptors (TLRs) discovered around 1998. At least nine different TLRs have been described, each recognizing distinct ligands. How could one test for the presence of these receptors on these cells?
9. Interaction of TLRs with their cognate ligand leads to the activation of NFκB. Why is this signal so important in immunologic responses?
10. Most of Paul's infections were the result of infections with gram-negative bacteria. Which TLR receptor recognizes lipopolysaccharide, a major cell wall component of gram-negative bacteria?

RECOMMENDED APPROACH

Implications/Analysis of Family History

An analysis of Paul's family history revealed that both males and females had presented with similar symptoms, indicating that the recurrent infections are not likely caused by a defective gene encoded on the X chromosome. The familial nature of the problem, however, suggests a genetic basis for the recurrent infections.

Implications/Analysis of Clinical History

A clinical history indicating recurrent bacterial infections could indicate a dysfunction in B cells, phagocytes, or complement. The absence of recurring viral and fungal infections suggests that the cause of the infections is not likely to be NK cells or T cells.

Implications/Analysis of Laboratory Investigation

Paul's initial blood work consisting of a complete blood cell count and differential was normal, so this is not a problem in T cell or B cell development (see Case 1). As predicted, T cell numbers/function were normal, as were serum immunoglobulin levels, indicating that B cell isotype switch mechanisms are intact.

Assessment of B Cells

Although assessment of serum immunoglobulins has typically been performed using serum electrophoresis, immunoelectrophoresis, or immunofixation, most laboratories use rate nephelometry, which provides a rapid and quantitative measure (see Case 5). Whereas B cell function can be analyzed using *in vitro* assays, antibody titers after immunization with protein antigens (e.g., tetanus toxoid) and polysaccharide (e.g., *Haemophilus influenzae* type b) are used initially to determine B cell responses. If these antibody titers (and serum immunoglobulins) are low, then the more advanced *in vitro* tests are performed.

An enzyme-linked immunosorbent assay (ELISA) is commonly used to test for the presence of serum antibodies specific for a particular antigen (e.g., tetanus toxoid) that has been absorbed to wells in a plastic culture dish. Detection requires the addition of antihuman antibodies specific for the isotype of interest, as well as an indicator system to identify the positive samples.

Assessment of T Cells

A simple initial test of T cell function in older children is the delayed-type hypersensitivity (DTH) skin test, which uses a panel of antigen to which most of the population has been exposed (e.g., *Candida albicans*). In this test, the antigen is injected intradermally and the effect examined 48 hours later. Individuals with normal cell-mediated immunity who have previously been infected with this fungus (sensitized) will have an inflamed, thickened, and tender area (induration) at the injection site.

In younger children and in individuals not exposed to the panel of antigens, the T cell proliferative response to polyclonal stimulation is performed instead of the DTH test. Polyclonal activators for T cells include concanavalin A (ConA) and phytohemagglutinin (PHA). ConA and PHA, also referred to as lectins, crosslink sugar molecules on the T cells and trigger their activation, which can be detected by measuring their proliferation.

Assessment of Phagocytes

Given that the infections are primarily bacterial, and that the B cell arm of the immune system is normal, one would suspect a phagocytic or complement dysfunction. Analysis of the respiratory burst (see Case 6) to rule out chronic granulomatous disease as a possibility should be performed.

Altered Cell Trafficking

In the presence of normal cell numbers and function, recurrent infection could be caused by the inability of immune cells to get to the site of infection or the lack of antigen presentation to T cells. However, a defect in antigen presentation would also result in viral and fungal infections, ruling out defective antigen presentation as a likely explanation. Altered cell trafficking is also not high on the list of possible explanations because there is no evidence for the classic presentation of necrotic skin lesions. To rule out this disorder, you should measure the expression of CD18, the common chain in β2 integrins. (See Additional Laboratory Tests.)

Complement

Given the nature of Paul's infections, it is reasonable to test for defects in the complement system. (See Additional Laboratory Tests.)

Additional Laboratory Tests

Flow cytometric analysis for the expression of CD18, a cell surface adhesion molecule, was within the normal range, ruling out the immunodeficiency disorder leukocyte adhesion defect (see Case 8) as a possible cause of Paul's infections. Tests to assess total complement function (CH50 and AP50) were normal (see Case 11). We are faced with the fact that recurrent bacterial and fungal infections are occurring despite the presence of an intact and normal immune system and normal trafficking. Therefore, a defect in antigen recognition is one of the few remaining candidates to account for Paul's problem with infections and so we should look at antigen recognition by dendritic cells and macrophages, cells of the innate immune system.

Assessment of Toll-like Receptors

Interaction of macrophages and dendritic cells with antigen may be direct/cognate or mediated via opsonins (e.g., C3b, IgG) that bind to specific receptors on the cell surface. Direct interaction with microbes is mediated by a number of different receptors, including the pattern recognition receptors (PRRs) that recognize so-called pathogen-associated molecular patterns (PAMPs) conserved among microbes. The best-studied PRRs to date are the toll-like receptors (TLRs), discovered around 1998. At least 10 different TLRs are described, each recognizing distinct ligands, although there is a potential for even further heterogeneity from heterologous expression of components of different TLRs that form "unique" receptors at the cell surface. Given Paul's susceptibility to gram-negative bacteria, it seems reasonable to measure the expression of TLR4 because recognition of lipopolysaccharide, a major cell wall component of gram-negative bacteria, is mediated via TLR4.

Flow cytometric analysis of TLR4 expression indicated that Paul's peripheral blood cells lacked TLR4, which is consistent with the nature of his infections. If gram-positive bacteria had caused Paul's infections, expression of TLR2 would have been assessed.

DIAGNOSIS

On the basis of the just-described tests, the diagnosis was a lack of TLR4 on the cell surface.

THERAPY

Treatment is generally prophylactic (mixtures of antibiotics, including sulfonamides).

ETIOLOGY: LACK OF TLR4

The immunodeficiency seen in this case is seldom as severe as in, say, a hypogammaglobulinemic child, reflecting the redundancy both in PRRs and in the way in which effective host resistance can be established. For example, adaptive immunity can be recruited if dendritic cells are able to endocytose antigen and display antigenic-peptide/MHC on their cell surface for recognition by CD4+ T cells. Given the defect in TLR4, opsonin-mediated endocytosis of bacteria can still occur if complement fragments (e.g., C3b) are deposited on the bacterial cell surface, a phenomenon that occurs quite rapidly after activation of the alternative pathway of complement.

Role of Other TLRs

Other TLRs that play an important role in innate immunity include TLR2, which binds peptidoglycan and lipoteichoic acid of Gram-positive bacteria, and lipoproteins present in several pathogens. In contrast, TLR9 binds CpG motif of bacterial oligonucleotides. Interaction of TLRs with their cognate ligands results in the intracellular activation of NFκB and altered gene transcription (see Case 10). Many TLRs are expressed at the cell surface, whereas several (TLR7, TLR8) are apparently expressed only intracellularly (likely detecting viral targets and/or altered expression of host molecules associated with "danger"). There is speculation as to why it is necessary for dendritic cells to express, in addition, this PRR repertoire (given that general inflammation associated with infection [viral/bacterial] is thought to result in sufficient dendritic cell activation [with cytokine production] to "drive" subsequent T cell activation). One explanation may be that in addition to providing a further activation signal to dendritic cells (measured by, for instance, the increased CD40 expression on these cells engaging PRRs), the different PRRs provide some additional information about the nature of the immunologic insult recognized (e.g., bacterial/viral) and thus help "mold" the resulting protective response.

The discovery of TLRs, their cognate ligands, and signaling transduction pathways has opened the door to a myriad of possibilities for therapeutic intervention in which signaling via TLRs is either suppressed or enhanced. The suppression or downregulation of TLR4 by administering pharmacologic agents that compete for binding with lipopolysaccharide would offer hope for patients with septic shock. Alternatively, enhancing signaling via one TLR versus another could drive antigen-dependent T cell development toward a Th1 or Th2 response, depending on the needs of the patient.

8

TC is a 9-year-old child with recurrent necrotic infections on the legs and arms. Discussion with the parents to determine anomalies since birth revealed that TC's umbilical cord had persisted much longer than that of his siblings. As well, TC's wounds healed more slowly and left noticeable scars. Both parents emphasized that they were well and that no members of the extended family had presented with similar history. Swabs reveal repeated bacterial infections. A complete blood cell count with differential showed a normal number of leukocytes, although the numbers were slightly elevated. Serology showed no deficit in immunoglobulins, complement, or numbers and function of B and T cells. B cell function was based on antibody titers to childhood immunization, whereas T cell function was based on cytokine secretion by polyclonally stimulated T cells. What might be going on, and what would you do about it?

QUESTIONS FOR GROUP DISCUSSION

1. TC has had repeated bacterial infections. What immunologic cells or factors function to destroy this type of infection?

2. It is not surprising that TC's leukocyte count is slightly elevated because he has an infection. Yet, laboratory investigations revealed no defects in B cell or phagocyte number or function. Additionally, the CH50 and AP50 tests for complement were normal. How would you proceed?

3. Given the laboratory tests and the fact that the infections are localized (not systemic or multi-site), review briefly some of the immunodeficiency disorders that can be ruled out.

4. What tests could you perform to rule out defects in the phagocytic function (see Case 6) or defects in toll-like receptors (see Case 7)?

5. What is the significance of necrotic rather than pustular manifestations of infection?

6. If one of the primary components of pus is dead neutrophils, what does the presence of necrotic rather than pustular infections suggest? (*Hint:* neutrophils are circulating cells and are not normally found in tissues.)

7. Review the processes involved in getting leukocytes from the circulation to the site of infection? Include in your answer each of the following (a) selectins, (b) integrins and their counter molecules on the endothelium, (c) PECAM, (d) chemokines, (e) matrix metalloproteinases, and (f) transmigration/diapedesis.

8. Activated tissue macrophages secrete the cytokines interleukin-1 and tumor necrosis factor. What role do these cytokines play in the inflammatory response?

9. The $\beta2$ integrins are heterodimers that play an important role in the firm adhesion of circulating leukocytes to the vascular endothelium. What is the common chain of these $\beta2$ integrins? Name two of the best characterized members of the $\beta2$ integrin family and their counter molecules that are upregulated on the endothelium during an inflammatory state.

10. A defect in CD18, the common chain of $\beta2$ integrins, leads to the immunodeficiency disorder leukocyte adhesion defect (LAD). How would you test for this defect?

RECOMMENDED APPROACH

Implications/Analysis of Family History

An inquiry into TC's family history revealed that no other family members had presented with these types of infections. The absence of familial presentation does not rule out an autosomal recessive disorder because both parents would need to be carriers of the defective gene. That is, both parents could be immunologically normal but each have one defective and one normal gene for the responsible gene (e.g., CD18, see later). TC would have had to inherit the two defective genes. A new mutation, however, cannot be excluded as a cause of the disorder.

Implications/Analysis of Clinical History

We need to determine why this child has prominent lesions on the skin. These areas represent places where our natural skin defense barrier is being constantly challenged by mechanical means, yet most people do not get these infections! The prevalence of bacterial infections points to defects in B cells, phagocytes, or complement. However, the lack of systemic (blood-borne) disease, such as respiratory tract infections with *Pseudomonas aeruginosa* or *Streptococcus pneumoniae* suggests this is unlikely to be a defect in the functional activity of B cells or phagocytes. The lack of viral infections suggests that this is not likely a T cell or NK cell disorder.

Implications/Analysis of Laboratory Investigation

A complete blood cell count (CBC) is a test that determines the quantity and proportion of various components in blood and includes measures of white blood cells (leukocytes), white blood cell differential, red blood cell, platelet, hemoglobin, and hematocrit (ratio of the volume of red blood cells to the volume of whole blood). A simple blood cell count measures the total white blood cell count, whereas the CBC gives, as well, a white blood cell differential that provides information regarding percentages of granulocytes, monocytes, lymphocytes, basophils, and eosinophils in the sample. A normal white blood cell count is *very age dependent!!!* (See Appendix.)

TC's high normal white blood cell count and differential, with normal serum immunoglobulins, normal antibody titers to childhood immunization, and normal cytokine production by T cells should suggest that this is not likely to be a simple B cell and/or T cell disorder. Therefore, it is reasonable to conclude that TC's infections are not due to defects in adaptive immunity. All of the information here points toward possible defects in the innate defense mechanisms. Because the CBC/differential was normal, a deficiency in any cell population of the innate immune system can be ruled out. Normal complement CH50 and AH50 tests, which measure the overall activity of the classical and alternative pathways, respectively, ruled out complement defects (see Case 11). Results of all these laboratory tests suggest the defect does not lie in a component of any effector mechanism *per se*.

Additional Laboratory Tests

One would certainly run some tests to make sure an unusual presentation of chronic granulomatous disease (CGD) (see Case 6) or other enzymatic defect that leads to defective macrophage resistance is not missed. CGD, associated with defects in NADPH oxidase, affects all the phagocytes in the body, wher-

ever they might be, and so a CGD defect generally presents with frequent common multiple-site infections (e.g., the lung, upper respiratory tract). Although one might consider toll-like receptor (TLR) defects (see Case 7) or subtle nucleotide oligomerization (NOD) protein defects (see Case 9), the clinical presentations are not consistent with mutations in either of these proteins. Rather, laboratory results are consistent with the hypothesis that this child has normal effector cells that would combat infection appropriately if they were able to reach the site of infection. The defect sounds most likely to be one of altered cell migration, with the relevant effector cells not getting to the site of action. For leukocytes to leave the circulation and enter tissues at the site of infection, a number of adhesive interactions must take place between the leukocytes and the activated vascular endothelium (Fig. 8–1). A prominent molecule on leukocytes is CD18, which is known to be a component of several cell surface adhesion molecules (β2 integrins). CD18 flow cytometric analysis revealed that TC's leukocytes did not express detectable CD18.

DIAGNOSIS

TC was diagnosed with leukocyte adhesion deficiency-1 (LAD-1).

THERAPY

Treatment of LAD (except in severe cases, where one might consider bone marrow transplantation) is with antibiotics.

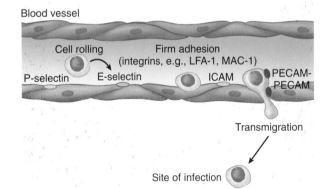

FIGURE 8–1 Defects in CD18 lead to a deficiency of β2 integrins on the leukocyte surface. Defects in CD18 lead to a defect in cell surface expression of β2 integrins in that they have CD18 as a component (e.g., LFA-1). Consequently, leukocytes are unable to marginate on the endothelium, a step required for diapedesis. (Modified with permission from Gorczynski R, Stanley J: Clinical Immunology. Austin, Landes, 1999.)

ETIOLOGY: LEUKOCYTE ADHESION DEFICIENCY-1

LAD-1 is an autosomal recessive disorder characterized by repeated bouts of skin associated bacterial infections that heal very slowly (Fig. 8–2). Skin infections result in necrotic sores, without evidence for pus. (Pus is the detritus of dead white blood cells, lymph, and the remains of dead bacteria that collects at the site of infection.) In addition to the skin, common sites of infection are the oral mucosa (e.g., gingivitis) and the respiratory tract. LAD-1 is suspected when there is a delay in umbilical cord separation.

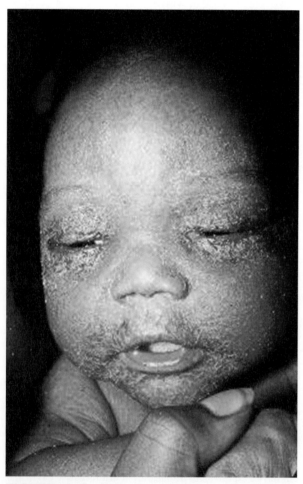

FIGURE 8–2 Child with staphylococcal scalded skin syndrome (SSSS) after release of exotoxin from disseminated staphylococcal infection. (From Fireman P, Slavin R: Atlas of Allergies, 2nd ed. St. Louis, Mosby, 1996.)

Why Do Phagocytes Not Get to the Site of Infection?

It is now known that lymphoid (and other) cells of the immune system migrate within the body using discrete receptor-ligand interactions. Adhesion molecules and their ligands expressed on leukocyte cell surface (and the surface of target cells/tissue) regulate whether cells "flow" in the circulation or become arrested at certain sites (e.g., high endothelial venules) before subsequent migration into tissues. Defective genes for these "adhesion" molecules or their ligands will result in the cells being unable to adhere or undergo transmigration (through the endothelium).

Role of CD18 in Adhesion

Transmigration of leukocytes into sites of inflammation requires sequential adhesive interactions and follows a series of stages: cell rolling (selectins), firm adhesion (integrins), and transmigation (PECAMs). CD18 is the common chain of heterodimers that constitute the β2 integrin family of molecules whose role is the "firm adhesion" of leukocytes to the vascular endothelium during an inflammatory response.

CD18 pairs with different CD11 chains to form different adhesion molecules. Two of the best characterized members of the β2 integrin family are LFA-1 and Mac-1 (CD11a-CD18 and CD11b-CD18, respectively). During an inflammatory response, integrins present on different subsets of circulating leukocytes interact with their counter molecules (intercellular adhesion molecules [ICAMs]) that are upregulated on the cytokine activated vascular endothelium. Interleukin-1 (IL-1) and tumor necrosis factor (TNF) act on the endothelium and induce the *de novo* expression of E-selectin and ICAM-1 on the vascular endothelium, as well as the upregulation of ICAM-2 expression.

OTHER DEFECTS IN CELL TRAFFICKING

LAD-2: Defects in Carbohydrates (Selectin Counter Molecules)

Carbohydrates present on circulating leukocytes are the counter molecules/ligands for E-selectin and P-selectin. P-selectin is the first selectin to be expressed on the endothelium during an inflammatory response because histamine (released from mast cells) triggers its translocation from the cytosol to the cell surface. Defects in fucose metabolism result in a deficiency of particular carbohydrates on the leukocyte cell surface. Because these carbohydrates are ligands for the E-selectin and P-selectin, cell rolling that should slow the leukocytes at the site of inflammation does not occur.

Wiskott-Aldrich Syndrome

Another interesting defect that can present in somewhat similar form is Wiskott-Aldrich syndrome. This is an X-linked disorder characterized by immunodeficiency, eczema, decreased numbers/function of platelets, increased susceptibility to infection, and decreased peripheral blood white cells (leukopenia).

The defect in this immunodeficiency disorder lies in the Wiskott-Aldrich syndrome protein (WASP), which plays an important role in normal actin polymerization in the cell. In addition to the pleiotropic changes just listed, mutations in WASP result in unstable actin polymerization and abnormal migration (motility defects) in monocytes/dendritic cells and lymphocytes, resulting in altered cell trafficking. A number of structurally defective WASP proteins have been described in various gene families.

CASE

9

Mark is 2 years of age and has already suffered from more than his share of childhood infections and prolonged episodes of diarrhea. He has been hospitalized twice for bacterial pneumonia, has had almost constant (according to his mother) viral infections, and twice has had oral thrush *(Candida albicans)*. He is under the care of an infectious disease specialist at a tertiary care center, who now believes he understands the etiology of the problem. Further exploration of the family tree revealed evidence of a distant great-grandparent who was perpetually "sick" and two cousins, Sally and Joe, who have recurrent infectious illnesses. Simple blood tests performed on many occasions have never revealed defects in the total number of B cells and T cells or neutrophils/monocytes. However, T cell subset analysis by flow cytometry indicated severe CD4+ lymphopenia and serum immunoglobulin levels, although present, were low. Antibody titers to childhood immunizations were negligible. Nitroblue tetrazolium tests indicated a normal respiratory burst after phagocytosis (see Case 6).

QUESTIONS FOR GROUP DISCUSSION

1. Based on the clinical history and laboratory tests that indicate each of the following, what immunodeficiency disorders can be ruled out?
   (a) low, but detectable, serum immunoglobulin
   (b) normal *total* numbers of T cells and B cells
   (c) normal numbers of monocytes and neutrophils
   (d) normal nitroblue tetrazolium test
2. Based on the clinical history and laboratory tests that indicate each of the following, for what immunodeficiency disorders should you request tests?
   (a) low CD4+ T cell counts
   (b) low serum immunoglobulin and negligible antibody titers to childhood immunization
3. Why is it unlikely that this patient has a defect in complement activation? Phagocyte defect?
4. Note that the infections cover all classes of infection (bacteria, fungi, viruses). What single cell type plays a crucial role in the immunologic responses to all of these infections? Explain.
5. Both phagocyte and B cell function tests were normal. How would you test for T cell function without the confounding variable of antigen presentation?
6. The tests for T cell function were normal, as were tests for cell surface markers (e.g., CD28) on T cells. This poses an interesting dilemma. Everything in the clinical history points to a T cell defect. How can you account for this seemingly improbable result?

7. T cells cannot be activated by antigen alone. Review how CD4+ T cells recognize antigen. What tests should you request now?
8. What is the role of the class II transactivator protein (CIITA) in regulating the expression of class II MHC antigens on the antigen-presenting cell surface?
9. Explain how a defect in class II MHC can result in a low CD4+ T cell count.
10. CIITA belongs to a family with a common nucleotide oligomerization domain (NOD). What is the role of NOD in proteins?

RECOMMENDED APPROACH

Implications/Analysis of Family History

An inquiry into Mark's family history revealed that two cousins (one male and one female) as well as a great-grandparent had presented with similar recurrent infections, suggesting a possible autosomal recessive inheritance for this disorder.

Implications/Analysis of Clinical History

A defect in phagocytes, leukocyte trafficking, or complement could account for the bacterial infections, but they would not, alone, account for other types of infection. A clinical history of fungal or viral infections strongly suggested a defect in T cell function.

Therefore, a defect that affects both B cells and T cells should be considered.

Implications/Analysis of Laboratory Investigation

A normal white blood cell count and differential suggests that the problem is not in cell development. Additionally, an absolute deficiency in any cell population can be ruled out. However, subset analysis of T cells revealed a paucity of CD4+ T cells, indicating that the defect was evident at the level of CD4+ but not CD8+ T cells. Although B cell numbers are normal, serum immunoglobulin levels are low, which is not surprising given the relative CD4+ lymphopenia. However, we cannot rule out a B cell functional defect. A decrease in the number of CD4+ T cells and the pattern of infections is highly suggestive of HIV infection. This would not, however, account for the familial nature of the disease.

Additional Laboratory Tests

Serologic testing using an ELISA ruled out HIV as a cause of the low CD4+ T cell count. Flow cytometric analysis of various cell surface markers on T cells did not reveal any deficiencies. Analysis of B cell markers indicated a deficiency in expression of cell surface class II MHC proteins. Class II MHC heterodimers are constitutively expressed on antigen-presenting cells, where they display antigen fragments to CD4+ T cells (Fig. 9–1; see Antigen Recognition, later). Further analysis indicated that all antigen-presenting cells lacked expression of class II MHC. Because CD4+ T cells are only activated when they recognize the class II antigen complexes and because B cell activation requires CD4+ T cell help, a deficiency of class II on antigen-presenting cells alone could explain the reduction in B cell responses. Nevertheless, this does not explain the paucity of CD4+ T cells.

In the normal thymus, immature thymocytes co-express CD4 and CD8 during development. Progression to either single positive (CD4 or CD8) T cells requires the interaction of the T cell receptor with either class I or class II MHC present on the thymic epithelium. In the absence of class II MHC expression, developing thymocytes undergo either CD4 gene silencing to produce CD8+ T cells or remain as double positive (CD4+, CD8+) T cells. Thus, absence of class II expression results in defective development of CD4+ cells (as well as the other features described).

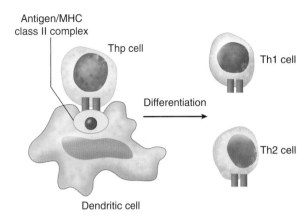

FIGURE 9–1   CD4+ T cells recognize antigen/MHC class II complexes on antigen-presenting cells. Activation of CD4+ T cells occurs after recognition of antigen/MHC class II complexes on antigen-presenting cells providing the appropriate co-stimulatory molecules are present. (Modified with permission from Gorczynski R, Stanley J: Clinical Immunology. Austin, Landes, 1999.)

DIAGNOSIS

Mark was diagnosed with bare lymphocyte syndrome (BLS), a primary immunodeficiency disorder that results from a lack of class II MHC expression.

THERAPY

Prophylactic Treatment

Pharmacologic intervention is provided for infections as they arise. Prophylactic administration of intravenous gamma globulin therapy may be a consideration.

Bone Marrow Transplant

Although there have been reports of successful bone marrow transplants in young children with BLS, bone marrow transplant for these patients does not have the same success rate as has been reported for other disorders. This is not surprising in that expression of class II MHC on antigen-presenting cells is only of immunologic benefit if CD4+ T cells are present. CD4+ T cells are generated in the thymus, after interaction with class II MHC on the thymic epithelium (see earlier). Full reconstitution would thus depend on replacement of host thymic epithelium (as well as thymic stem cells) by donor marrow.

Patients with BLS have normal numbers of circulating T cells, but most of them are CD8+. The fact that there are a few patients with low numbers of circulating CD4+ T cells may be explained from studies with mice in which mice with defects in one of the trimeric complex proteins (RFX5, see later) express very low levels of MHC class II in the thymic cortex. Because fewer than 100 patients have been identified with BLS, it is difficult to investigate these issues in patient populations.

Gene Therapy

Although it is technically possible to introduce the gene for CIITA (*ex vivo*) into antigen-presenting cells that have been removed from the patient, as discussed earlier, this would not correct the problem leading to defective CD4+ T cell development. In contrast, *in utero* gene transfer should, in theory, lead to the expression of class II MHC on the thymic epithelial cells as well as on antigen-presenting cells. However, to overcome the problem in a young infant is a challenge, because of the limitations in gene delivery to targeted tissues, particularly the thymic cortex. Furthermore, constitutive expression of class II MHC in tissues that would not normally express this heterodimer could serve as a stimulus for inappropriate immune responses, leading to autoimmunity.

ETIOLOGY: BARE LYMPHOCYTE SYNDROME

Bare lymphocyte syndrome is a primary immunodeficiency disorder that phenotypically manifests as an absence of constitutively expressed class II MHC proteins on the surface of antigen-presenting cells, as well as interferon γ (IFNγ)-inducible class II MHC expression on antigen-presenting cells and other cell types. Clinically, all patients present with a wide spectrum of microbial infections that include those caused by bacteria, fungi, viruses, and protozoa such that patients often die before they are 10 years of age. Virtually all children with BLS have chronic diarrhea (reflective of intestinal infection) and thus do not thrive. Most present with lower respiratory tract infections.

BLS is an autosomal recessive disorder in which a defect in class II MHC expression is the result of mutations in any one of the four genes that encode transacting regulatory transcription factors for class II MHC. Three of the genes encode proteins (RFX5, RFXANK, RFXAP), which form a trimeric complex that binds to the class II MHC promoter regulatory region; the fourth gene encodes CIITA, a non–DNA-binding transcriptional co-activator that controls class II MHC transcription. Irrespective of the defect, class II MHC gene expression does not occur. When the defect is in CIITA, the trimeric complex can still bind to the promoter region but gene transcription does not occur. Consequently, a mutation in any one of the four genes leads to the same clinical presentation.

Role of CIITA

Although several roles have been postulated for CIITA as a master regulator, the most simplistic is that it functions as a scaffold (via protein-protein interactions) for recruitment of other factors required for transcription of class II genes. CIITA is also required for expression of the genes that encode Ii, the invariant chain, HLA-DM and HLA-DO, which play a role in intracellular trafficking and peptide loading of class II MHC.

CIITA is constitutively expressed in antigen-presenting cells and upregulated by IFNγ. *De novo* expression of class II MHC may also occur in non–antigen-presenting cells after stimulation with IFNγ. The expression of IFNγ-induced class II MHC can be inhibited in the presence of cytokines (TGFβ, IL-4, IL-10, and IL-1β), reflecting the role that CIITA plays in an immune response. In the absence of class II MHC/peptide on the cell surface, CD4+ T cells cannot be activated. Interestingly, some pathogens (*Chlamydia* species, *Mycobacterium bovis*, cytomegalovirus, varicella-zoster virus) have acquired immunoevasive strategies that result in the inhibition of IFNγ-induced expression of CIITA and hence of class II MHC expression. Of clinical interest is the report that statins, lipid-lowering drugs, inhibit IFNγ-induced class II MHC.

CIITA and Nucleotide Oligomerization Domain Protein

CIITA is now known to belong to a family of molecules having in common a nucleotide oligomerization domain (NOD) responsible for self-self protein interactions, which are apparently essential for signaling function from these interacting molecules. The most important proteins bound by CIITA are not well characterized, although a number of nuclear factors have been shown to bind to it (including cyclic adenosine monophosphate response element binding protein

[CREB]). The mutations in CIITA that affect its role may, in fact, reflect defective NOD functioning.

Antigen Recognition

T cell receptors (TCRs) are heterodimers expressed on the cell surface in association with five invariant polypeptides collectively termed CD3. These heterodimers recognize antigenic peptides complexed with MHC proteins. Two broad classes of proteins encoded by the MHC loci are referred to as class I MHC proteins, which are expressed on all nucleated cells, and class II MHC proteins, which are constitutively present on antigen-presenting cells. T cells that express the lineage-defining molecule CD8 recognize antigenic fragments complexed with class I MHC. In contrast, T cells that express the lineage-defining molecule CD4 recognize antigenic fragments complexed with class II MHC.

CASE 10

Barry is 16 months of age and since his adoption at birth has been hospitalized on several occasions with multiple and severe gram-positive bacterial infections of the respiratory tract, skin, soft tissues, gastrointestinal tract, and even bones. On two occasions he has suffered from meningitis, and on at least one occasion he developed nearly overwhelming septicemia, with systemic spread of gram-negative bacteria. Laboratory analysis at the time of these various infections indicated that he had had infections with *Mycobacterium avium,* as well as with both gram-positive *(Streptococcus pneumoniae, Staphylococcus aureus)* and gram-negative *(Haemophilus influenzae and Pseudomonas aeruginosa)* organisms.

Interestingly, despite childhood immunization with *H. influenzae,* as well as infection with *S. pneumoniae* and *H. influenzae,* there was a dearth of specific antipolysaccharide antibodies, probably contributing to the susceptibility to encapsulated bacteria. IgM levels were elevated, with a slight diminution in IgG and IgA levels. Levels of T cells and B cells and macrophages/neutrophils were normal, as was the subset distribution of T cells and the surface expression of CD40L/CD154 (see Case 4). Analysis of phagocyte function (see Case 6) and proliferation of mitogen-stimulated T cells were at the low end of normal (see Case 2). NK cell levels were normal, with evidence for some decrease in killing function (~threefold on a cell-for-cell basis compared with normal).

Physically, Barry had multiple morphogenetic abnormalities, including dry skin, sparse hair, and abnormally shaped teeth. Notably, despite the hot summer spell, there was no evidence of sweat and when Barry cried tearing did not occur. Detailed examination of the possible defects in this child at a specialist immunogenetics clinic suggested this was an example of an X-linked hypohidrotic/anhidrotic ectodermal dysplasia syndrome with immunodeficiency (XL-EDA-ID/EDA-ID), now known to represent one of a family of similar disorders with genetic aberrancy in intracellular NFκB signaling.

QUESTIONS FOR GROUP DISCUSSION

1. Once again, we are faced with a patient who has recurrent bacterial infections. Based on previous cases, what types of defects would you initially want to consider?

2. The initial blood work indicated normal numbers of cells indicating that this problem is not one of cell development. However, analysis of serum immunoglobulin indicated a decrease in all antibody isotypes and an increase in IgM. These results are similar to those described for the patient in Case 4. What test would you perform to rule out, or confirm, that Barry has (or does not have) the same disorder?

3. On the basis of the tests in question 2, we have ruled out hyper IgM syndrome as a possible diagnosis. Because Barry has a history of infections with both gram-negative and gram-positive bacteria, what TLRs would you investigate?

4. Results of investigations of TLRs revealed that both TLR2 and TLR4 expression was normal. On consultation with an internist you learn that Barry's morphogenetic abnormalities are consistent with hypohidrotic/anhidrotic ectodermal dysplasia (HED/EDA). Over 150 distinct phenotypes have been classed as ectodermal dysplasia. What is the most common defect in this disorder?

5. Three forms of ectodermal dysplasia are known to result from defects in NFκB signaling pathway. Review the activation of NFκB. Include the following in your discussion: (a) serine kinase complex: IKKα, IKKβ, IKKγ (NEMO); (b) phosphorylation, ubiquitination, degradation; (c) IκB, NFκB dimer; and (d) translocation and transcription. What is the role of NFκB in immunity and inflammation?

6. Explain how a mutation in NEMO (see question 5) would affect the activation of NFκB.

7. More than 30 NEMO mutations have been identified and they do not necessarily lead to the same

clinical manifestation, although they all affect some components of the immune system. List some of the genes (whose proteins play a role in immunity) that are regulated by NFκB.

8. On what chromosome is NEMO encoded?

9. As a summary, name the disorder associated with each of the following NEMO mutations:
    (a) hypomorphic mutations (reduced level of activity)
    (b) NEMO stop codon mutations
    (c) Mutations that abolish NEMO function (in females)

10. How would you expect a total deletion of NEMO to present? Why is this disorder lethal in males but not females?

RECOMMENDED APPROACH

Implications/Analysis of Family History

No information is available because Barry is adopted. Therefore, we are not able to assess whether Barry's problems are due to an X-linked disorder.

Implications/Analysis of Clinical History

Barry's history of frequent infections with various bacteria suggests a major defect in complement, phagocytes, or B cell function. However, lacrimal and sweat gland defects, combined with morphogenetic abnormalities and bacterial infections, suggest that Barry's problem is not restricted to one particular cell defect.

Implications/Analysis of Laboratory Investigation

Barry's initial blood work consisting of a complete blood cell count and differential was normal so this is not a problem in T cell or B cell development. Serum immunoglobulin measures indicated little or no IgG or IgA. In contrast, IgM was present in higher concentrations than the normal reference value. The fact that there is IgM present in serum indicates that normal B cell differentiation to plasma cells is occurring so the defect is not in antigen-dependent B cell differentiation but in isotype switching.

B cell activation leading to isotype switching requires T cell–derived cytokines as well as cognate interaction with T cells. Therefore, a deficiency or defect in T cells could lead to a problem in B cell activation and isotype switching. However, we are told that T cell function is normal, as is the expression of CD40L whose defect on T cells leads to an immunodeficiency disorder characterized by an inability to isotype switch (see Case 4).

Additional Laboratory Tests

Detailed laboratory investigation led to a diagnosis of EDA-ID. Laboratory results consistent with a diagnosis of EDA-ID would include a defect in signaling via various cytokines, including interleukin [IL]-1, tumor necrosis factor [TNF], and IL-18. Because all of the receptors for these cytokines signal via NFκB (nuclear factor kappa B), mutational analysis of various proteins required for NFκB signaling would have shown a mutation in NEMO (NFκB essential modifier). NEMO is the noncatalytic component of IKK, a serine kinase complex that is required for activation of NFκB. NFκB is also a key signaling component in TLRs (see Case 7), NOD activation (see Case 9), and even for T cell and B cell receptor mediation activation.

DIAGNOSIS

Barry was diagnosed with X-linked hypohidrotic (anhidrotic) ectodermal dysplasia with immunodeficiency.

THERAPY

Therapy consists of life-long treatment of infections as they arise and treatment with gamma globulin.

ETIOLOGY: EDA-ID

Hypohidrotic (anhidrotic) ectodermal dysplasia (HED/EDA) was described first in Great Britain in about 1848. About 150 types of ectodermal dysplasias have been described, with the common feature being that the affected tissues are derived mainly from the ectoderm germ layer. Of the 150 ectodermal dysplasias, the hypohidrotic/anhidrotic form is the most common. Hypohidrotic derives from the word "hypohidrosis" and indicates a severe decrease in sweat production. The cause of HED/EDA is a mutation in ectodysplasmin, a protein that controls normal ecto-dermal growth/differentiation.

NFκB and IκB

Patients have been identified whose clinical presentation is consistent with HED/EDA but who do not have mutations in the gene encoding ectodysplasmin. Rather, these patients have a mutation in a noncatalytic component of IKK, the serine kinase complex essential for NFκB activation (Fig. 10–1). NFκB was described initially as a transcription factor required for transcription of the kappa light chain constant region in B cells, so patients with mutations in IKK would express immunoglobulins with lambda light chains. NFκB is now known to be a family of transcription factors composed of homo-heterodimers made up of the structurally related (and evolutionarily conserved) proteins, NFκB1 (p50) and NFκB2 (p52), RelA/p65, RelB, and c-Rel. These proteins are constitutively expressed and are sequestered in the cytosol where they remain inactive as a result of their association with inhibitor proteins (IκB) that block sequences required for NFκB localization to the nucleus (i.e., NFκB activation).

IκB proteins block sequences required for NFκB localization to the nucleus. Therefore, IκB protein must be degraded to free the NFκB dimers so that they can translocate to the nucleus where they stimulate transcription. Degradation of IκB by the proteosome requires ubiquitination and prior phosphorylation by IKK. Various stimuli can trigger signaling events that lead to phosphorylation of IκB (by IKK). There are several IκB proteins (e.g., IκBα, IκBβ, and IκBε).

IKK

IKK, the serine kinase complex that phosphorylates IκB, consists of two catalytic subunits (IKKα, IKKβ) and a noncatalytic subunit NEMO (formerly IKKγ), which is expressed on the X chromosome. Mutations in NEMO affect the function of IKK and therefore of NFκB. The extent to which NFκB activation is diminished depends on the particular NEMO mutation and so there is variability in the observed immunologic defects from different patients with this disorder.

NEMO versus Ectodysplasmin Defects

A defect in NEMO is much more profound (than a defect in ectodysplasmin) because NFκB activation

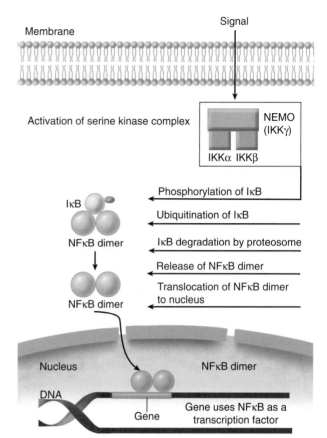

FIGURE 10–1 Mutations in *NEMO* affect transcription of genes that use NFκB as a transcription factor. Phosphorylation, ubiquitination, and degradation of IκB is required to release the NFκB dimer and allow it to translocate to the nucleus where it serves as a transcription factor for many different genes.

regulates expression of genes important for adaptive immunity, for adhesion and cell motility, for cell proliferation/apoptosis, and for cytokine and chemokine expression. In essence, activation of NFκB is required for the activation of numerous genes that play a role in immunity and inflammation. Therefore, it is thus not a surprise that interference with this pathway, and in NEMO, can have such profound defects. Patients with a mutation in the NEMO gene also present with hyper-IgM syndrome (see Case 4), an immunodeficiency disorder caused by a defect in CD40 or CD40L/CD154, because CD40 ligation itself also leads to activation of NFκB.

Severe NEMO Mutations

NEMO mutations can result in different clinical syndromes depending on the nature of the defect

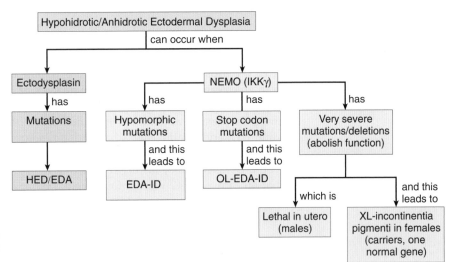

FIGURE 10–2 The mutation site in the *NEMO* gene determines the severity of the disorder.

(Fig. 10–2). EDA-ID results from hypomorphic mutations in coding regions (reduced level of activity). Documented cases of patients with defects in the NEMO stop codon exhibit similar pathologic processes but also present with osteopetrosis and lymphedema (OL-EDA-ID). In contrast, deletions or mutations that abolish NEMO function lead to incontinentia pigmenti, an X-linked dominant disorder that is lethal *in utero* for males. Females that inherit one copy of the defective gene develop symptoms similar to those of EDA as well as hyperpigmentation of the skin and central nervous system defects.

Mary is 20 months of age and has been hospitalized with a fever, irritability, and moderate dehydration. Blood work suggests a bacterial infection, with elevated neutrophils (>96%; normal: ~70%), although the chest radiograph and urinalysis are normal. Computed tomography (CT) indicated intracranial evidence for generalized edema with some compression of the ventricles. Despite the risk associated with elevated cerebrospinal fluid (CSF) pressure, a lumbar puncture was performed that showed an elevated white cell count. An analysis of the CSF by polymerase chain reaction (PCR) assay revealed the presence of *Neisseria meningitidis*. Mary has been receiving intravenous antibiotics for 30 hours, and there is some improvement in her condition. Query into the child's background indicated that Mary had been breast fed until she was 3 months of age and had been relatively healthy until this recent infection. Detailed family history reveals that a distant male cousin and an aunt both died at an early age (<2 years) of meningitis. What further tests might you order? What is the significance of the history and findings?

QUESTIONS FOR GROUP DISCUSSION

1. In several of the preceding cases, we have considered patients who presented with bacterial infections. Unlike these patients, who had recurrent infections with several gram-negative and/or gram-positive bacteria, Mary has only presented with infection with *Neisseria meningitidis*. Why is a phagocyte or B cell defect unlikely?

2. The family history revealed that both males and females had presented with this type of infection. What does this indicate? Explain the term *autosomal recessive*.

3. We have learned in previous cases that bacterial infections are often indicative of a B cell, phagocyte, or complement disorder. Explain how an overall test of complement activity using CH50 and AH50 can be used to determine if there is a problem with activation of the (a) classical pathway, (b) alternative pathway, or (c) terminal pathway of complement?

4. Explain how (a) the classical pathway of complement and (b) the alternative pathway are activated.

5. List the biologic activities of the proteolytic fragments generated from the activation of (a) the classical pathway and (b) the alternative pathway of complement.

6. How would deficiencies in the early components of the classical pathway of complement present clinically?

7. Describe the two types of meningococcal vaccines available and the (a) limitations of each and (b) advantages of each.

8. Why is a defect in the C3 component of complement so devastating?

9. Describe the role of properdin and the significance of the fact that the gene that encodes this protein is expressed on the X chromosome.

10. Describe the role of each of the following complement regulatory proteins: (a) decay accelerating factor, (b) S-protein, (c) CD59, (d) homologous restriction factor, and (e) C1 inhibitor protein.

RECOMMENDED APPROACH

Implications/Analysis of Family History

An inquiry into Mary's family history revealed that a distant male cousin and an aunt had both died of meningitis at an early age (<2 years). An inherited disorder is suspected when genetically linked individuals present with the same type of clinical history. Autosomal recessive defects are suspected when both males and females are affected.

Implications/Analysis of Clinical History

Both innate and adaptive immunity play a role in the elimination of bacterial pathogens, with phagocytes, complement, and B cells being the key players. Because there is no indication of prior bacterial infections, it is unlikely that there is a defect in phagocyte function or in B cells, particularly when one considers Mary's age. That is, the protection conferred by the mother's antibodies *in utero* ceases around 6 months of age. Furthermore, the only cell abnormality was an increase—not decrease—in neutrophils.

Implications/Analysis of Laboratory Investigation

The white blood cell count and differential indicated an increase in the number of circulating neutrophils, which is consistent with a bacterial infection (see Case 6). Results of the CT scan and lumbar puncture, combined with the PCR, indicated that Mary has neisserial meningitis. PCR is now used instead of culture in major laboratories because it is more accurate, even if the patient has already been taking antibiotics. Considering the family history and the severity of this infection, an investigation into possible autosomal recessive disorders was pursued.

Additional Laboratory Tests

Deficiencies in the complement terminal pathway proteins that compose the membrane attack complex (C5 to C9) or deficiencies in the components of the alternative pathway (e.g., Factor B and properdin) present most commonly as infections with *Neisseria meningitidis*. Therefore, laboratory investigation should now focus on analysis of the complement pathway (Fig. 11–1).

Rather than testing for individual complement components, an overall assessment of the alternative, classical, and terminal pathways is achieved by measuring the ability of the patient's serum (complement)

to lyse sheep red blood cells using the CH50 and AH50 tests. A CH50 test is defined as the amount of the patient's serum that will lyse 50% of sheep red blood cells coated with antibody. The AH50 is similar to the CH50; however, the sheep red blood cells are not coated with antibody. In effect, the CH50 measures classical pathway and terminal components whereas the AH50 measures the alternative pathway and terminal components.

If the CH50 is normal, but the AH50 is abnormal, the defect lies in the alternative pathway components. In contrast, if both the CH50 and AH50 are abnormal, it is likely that there is a deficiency in one of the terminal pathway components. In Mary's case, both the CH50 and AH50 were abnormal, indicating a defect in one of the terminal pathway components. Nephelometry can be used to identify the particular component that is deficient. However, in the absence of gene therapy, which may be a possibility in the future, information regarding the particular terminal pathway component would not alter the treatment and so is not usually performed.

DIAGNOSIS

Mary was diagnosed with meningococcal meningitis associated with a complement deficiency in one of the

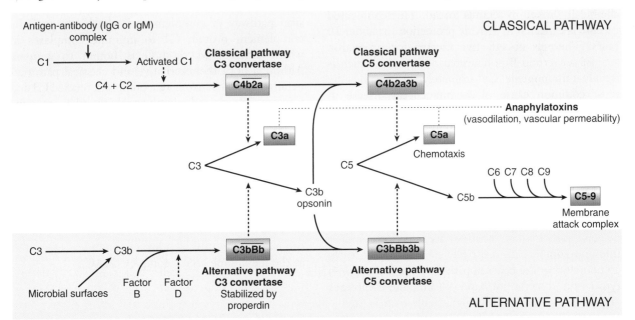

FIGURE 11–1 Overview of complement activation. Defects in the early components of the classical pathway are associated with autoimmune complex diseases, whereas defects in the terminal pathway components present as recurrent neisserial (bacterial) infections. Defects in C3 result in more infections than other defects because they affect both the alternative and the classical pathway. (From Kumar V, Cotran R, Robbins S: Robbins Basic Pathology, 7th ed. Philadelphia, Saunders, 2002; Modified from Abbas A, Lichtman A, Pober J: Cellular and Molecular Immunology, 3rd ed. Philadelphia, Saunders, 1995.)

components of the terminal pathway. *Neisseria meningitidis*, a gram-negative bacterium, is surrounded by a polysaccharide capsule whose composition defines the serogroup of the pathogen. Five serogroups (A, B, C, Y, and W-135) cause most of the infections in North America. Patients with deficiencies in the terminal complement pathway are susceptible to infections with all *Neisseria* species.

THERAPY

Aggressive antibiotic therapy was provided. Immunization, although highly recommended for this patient population, will provide protection only if the vaccine contains the same polysaccharide capsule serotype as that of the infecting pathogen. There are two types of meningococcal vaccines available, a polysaccharide vaccine and a conjugate vaccine. The polysaccharide vaccine (e.g., Menomune, Mencevax) consists of purified meningococcal polysaccharide from serogroups A, C, Y, and W135 but is only effective when administered to individuals older than 2 years of age. Protection is relatively short term—2 to 3 years. In contrast, the conjugate vaccine (e.g., NeisVac-C, Menjugate) is effective even when administered to children 6 weeks of age, but it consists solely of meningococcal polysaccharide serotype C capsule chemically linked to tetanus toxoid. This conjugated vaccine is expected to provide protection for about 10 years. There is no effective vaccine for protection against serogroup B polysaccharide capsule, which is weakly immunogenic. Unfortunately, serotype B is the most common cause of meningococcal disease in young children and there is no cross-reacting protection from vaccines for other polysaccharide capsule serotypes.

OTHER COMPLEMENT DEFECTS

Complement deficiencies do not present as physical defects, rather they manifest as infections and/or immune complex diseases. Deficiencies in the early components of the classical pathway (C1, C2, and C4) typically lead to the formation of immune complexes and so are generally indistinguishable from systemic lupus erythematosus (SLE). In contrast, defects in C3 are associated with susceptibility to all bacterial infections because degradation products of C3 function as opsonins to facilitate phagocytosis. Additionally, both the alternative and the classical pathway are affected.

As mentioned earlier, defects in the terminal pathway components and the alternative pathway are associated with infections with *Neisseria* species. Most of the complement defects have an autosomal mode of inheritance. One exception is properdin, which is encoded on the X-chromosome.

OVERVIEW OF COMPLEMENT

The complement system is a family of proteins whose proteolytically derived fragments facilitate elimination of microorganisms, alter vascular permeability, and participate in the inflammatory response. Complement proteins are synthesized mainly by the liver; however, some of these proteins are also synthesized by macrophages and fibroblasts. Activation of complement occurs via either the classical or the alternative pathway, which converge to a common or terminal pathway.

Activation

The initiating stimulus for activation of the alternative pathway is the deposition of spontaneously generated C3b fragments onto a microbial cell surface. In contrast, the initiating stimulus for activation of the classical pathway of complement is the binding of the complement protein C1 to immune complexes in which either IgM or IgG is bound to antigen. Although both the alternative and classical pathways generate distinct enzymatic complexes, termed C3 and C5 convertases, that hydrolyze the complement components C3 and C5, respectively, the proteolytic products of these convertases are independent of the particular pathway that is activated.

Many cells have receptors for the proteolytically derived complement fragments and this dictates which cells respond to complement activation. Osmotic lysis of cells or microbes, however, requires that the components of the terminal pathway insert into the target cell membrane forming a protein complex referred to as the membrane attack complex (MAC).

REGULATORY PROTEINS

Complement activity and deleterious complement effects on autologous cells are minimized by a variety of soluble, or membrane-bound, proteins. These natural regulatory molecules are important physiologically for homeostasis of the complement cascades. Some of these proteins are associated exclusively with one complement activation pathway or another, whereas others are protective in a more general way. Regulatory proteins that regulate both pathways include (a) decay-accelerating factor that inhibits formation of both C3 convertases; (b) S-protein, CD59, and homologous restriction factor, all of which inhibit formation of the membrane attack complex of the terminal pathway; and (c) the C1 inhibitor protein that prevents spontaneous activation of the classical pathway of complement. The role of the complement system in host defense is underscored when one considers the clinical consequences of microbial evasion strategies and genetic complement deficiencies.

George, a frequent visitor to your emergency department, is generally in a state of total intoxication. He is 55 years old and has lived on the streets for as long as you can remember. In winter he stays overnight in a local shelter. When you see him tonight he looks quite ill and has obviously lost a significant amount of weight compared with when you saw him last (~2 to 3 months ago). He admits he has chronic night sweats and a persistent cough with some whitish-yellow sputum. He has no history of diabetes, and indeed his blood sugar, even now, is within the normal range of 5 to 8 mmol/dL. He is unaware of any obvious acute presentation of a febrile illness and admits to a general lethargy over the past 2 to 4 weeks. There is no history of travel out of the city (including to local farms). He is currently afebrile but certainly does not look well. Blood work is unremarkable, with the exception of a modest increase in neutrophils. His chest radiograph shows significant consolidation in the lower lobes and evidence of an infectious process (inflammation) in the upper zones also (Fig. 12-1). In room air, his oxygen saturation is only 89% (normal 97% to 100%), and he is not a cigarette smoker.

QUESTIONS FOR GROUP DISCUSSION

1. Malignancies, autoimmunity, or a chronic infection could all present with the complex of symptoms described in this case. To focus our investigations on the most probable cause of George's symptoms, we need to eliminate the "unlikely" causes based on the given negatives. What diseases or disorders does each of the following negatives diminish as a likely cause for his symptoms?
   (a) nonsmoker
   (b) no evidence of intravenous drug use
   (c) no evidence of travel
   (d) no evidence of homosexual behavior
   (e) no evidence of previous transfusions
2. How would you rule out the disease/disorders that you listed in question 1?
3. George is afebrile so it is unlikely that he has an acute infection. List three to four chronic infections that could present in this manner. Explain how each can be ruled out.
4. Describe the Mantoux test and explain why it is referred to as a delayed-type hypersensitivity reaction. Explain why a positive control is necessary. What antigen would you use as a positive control? Describe the confirmatory test that you would use in cases in which the patient has a positive Mantoux test.
5. The emergence of drug-resistant strains of *Mycobacterium tuberculosis* presents a dilemma for you as a physician when treating patients with George's history. Explain.
6. Tuberculosis is a chronic disease resulting from infection with *M. tuberculosis*. Discuss how most infections are acquired. What populations are, therefore, most at risk for infection?
7. *M. tuberculosis* has evolved evasive strategies to hinder the immune system. One evasive strategy allows it to thrive in the phagocytic vacuole. Describe the role of lysosomal enzymes, reactive nitrogen intermediates, and nitric oxide in host defense (see Case 6).
8. Explain the role of NRAMP1 in host phagocyte host defense. Discuss how the reduced expression of NRAMP1 could facilitate growth of *M. tuberculosis*.
9. Explain why immunosuppression can lead to reactivation of this infection.
10. Discuss the immunoevasive strategies that *M. tuberculosis* has evolved to resist destruction in the phagosome.

RECOMMENDED APPROACH

Implications/Analysis of Family History

No mention has been made of family history, presumably because there was nothing remarkable. George is often in close proximity with people who are "at risk" for certain community-acquired infections (e.g., tuberculosis) simply because he is living in hostels.

Implications/Analysis of Clinical History

Malignancy, autoimmunity, or a chronic infection could help explain this symptomatology.

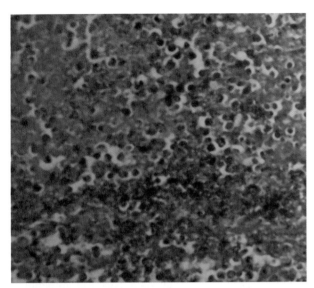

FIGURE 12–1 Tuberculosis infection in lung with acid-fast bacilli seen in alveolar wash sample.

The weight loss/night sweats and cough would be consistent with a malignancy such as a lymphoma. It is unlikely that he has an HIV infection because there is no evidence of intravenous drug use, homosexual behavior, or previous transfusions. You should, however, confirm that these are not considerations.

George is afebrile right now so it is unlikely that he has a fulminant (acute) infection, but a chronic infection is a possibility. The fact that George is a nonsmoker should "steer you away" from a lung malignancy, although the primary pathology certainly seems to be in the lungs. A vasculitic type process in the lungs, such as occurs in autoimmune disorders, might present in this fashion. However, there are no obvious precipitants (e.g., drug-antibody complexes) for such a reaction. The emphasis on "no travel" excludes infections that are unique to "hot spots" or specific locales, such as aspergillosis resulting from contact with moldy hay in farming areas or blastomycosis resulting from inhalation of the *Ajellomyces dermatitidis* (formerly *Blastomyces dermatitidis*) conidia (spores) present in soil in the Mississippi Valley area of the United States.

Implications/Analysis of Laboratory Investigation

Several of the tentative assumptions just described can be ruled out on the basis of the laboratory investiga-

tions. The fact that the blood sugar value is normal rules out diabetes, whereas a normal blood cell count and differential rules out a lymphoma and acute viral or bacterial infection. An abnormal chest radiograph in the absence of overt fever, along with hypoxia (poor oxygenation), is suggestive of a chronic infection with slower-growing organisms.

Additional Laboratory Tests

Indigent elderly alcoholics represent a population at risk for numerous chronic infectious diseases, one of the more important of which is tuberculosis (TB). A Mantoux test should be given to check for an immune response to *M. tuberculosis*, the causative agent of TB. Chronic viremias (e.g., hepatitis B/C and HIV) could present this way and can be ruled out using ELISAs to detect antibodies specific for the various antigens. In this case, George had a positive reaction to the Mantoux test.

A Mantoux (tuberculin) test, consisting of purified protein derivative (PPD) isolated from cultures of *M. tuberculosis*, is injected intradermally to assess prior exposure to *M. tuberculosis*. A positive test manifests as a local area of cytokine (IFNγ)-induced erythema and induration reaching a maximum at 24 to 48 hours. Unlike edema there is no pitting when pressure is applied to this region. This reaction is referred to as a delayed-type hypersensitivity reaction (DTH). As a word of caution, a negative Mantoux test could indicate that the individual is immunosuppressed and has not generated an immune response to the infection. Therefore, a positive control using *Candida* antigen should be administered in the "other" arm. Virtually everyone has been exposed to *Candida*, which is the rationale for using this antigen as a positive control. To confirm infection with *M. tuberculosis*, an acid-fast smear of George's sputum and a polymerase chain reaction (PCR) assay to detect the presence of the *M. tuberculosis* was performed. Both tests were positive.

DIAGNOSIS

The diagnosis was tuberculosis resulting from infection with *M. tuberculosis*.

THERAPY

Therapy consists of a multi-drug regimen for 6 to 12 months determined by susceptibility testing of initial isolates. Of concern is the fact that drug-resistant tuberculosis is increasing in prevalence. Unfortunately, patient noncompliance contributes to the emergence of drug-resistant strains of *M. tuberculosis*. Given this reality, two questions arise: Should George's therapy be supervised? What should you do in the face of noncompliance, which will surely be the case with this patient? Some of these issues may not be relevant in the future in that a phase 1 clinical trial to test the efficacy of a recombinant tuberculosis vaccine with 20 volunteers will begin in the United States this year.

ETIOLOGY: TUBERCULOSIS

Tuberculosis is a chronic disease resulting from infection with *M. tuberculosis* (see Fig. 12–1). Most infections are acquired by inhalation of airborne droplets containing the organism. Phagocytosis by alveolar macrophages is the first line of cellular defense.

Host Response

Phagocytes play a central role in host defense to *M. tuberculosis*. Recognition may be indirect (opsonin mediated) or direct (e.g., TLR-2 and TLR-4; see Case 7). Phagocytosis of *M. tuberculosis* by alveolar macrophages results in the formation of a phagosome, a vesicle that is normally the site of microbial destruction (see Case 6). Included in the host defense armamentarium are lysosomal enzymes, reactive oxygen intermediates, and nitric oxide. *M. tuberculosis* has evolved immunoevasive strategies, however (see later), that allow it to thrive in the phagosome.

As well as the products just listed, phagocytes express a "natural resistance associated macrophage protein 1" (NRAMP1) that may play a role in phagocyte host defense. This protein is an integral membrane protein that becomes part of the phagosome during phagocytosis and as such functions as a divalent-metal efflux pump at the phagosomal membrane. In so doing, NRAMP1 limits the availability of some divalent cations required for survival of bacteria within the phagosome. Studies in West Africa to examine susceptibility to tuberculosis have shown that reduced expression of NRAMP1 increased susceptibility.

Infection by *M. tuberculosis*

M. tuberculosis bacteria that thrive within the phagosome will ultimately cause lysis of the macrophage, resulting in the production of cytokines and a number of chemical mediators (chemokines) whose actions result in the attraction of monocytes and other leukocytes to the region. Recruited monocytes differentiate to macrophages that phagocytose *M. tuberculosis*, and the process is repeated. The bacteria continue to thrive until activated CD4+ T cells (secreting type 1 cytokines and chemokines) arrive at the site of inflammation. Interferon gamma (IFNγ), a type 1 cytokine, enhances the activity of NADPH oxidase and the inducible nitric oxide synthase (iNOS). Tumor necrosis factor (TNF), another type 1 cytokine, functions as a second signal for activation of iNOS and NADPH oxidase during some bacterial infections. The net effect of T cell–derived cytokines is the reduction of bacterial growth and formation of granulomas that may contain the infection to this site for years, but necrosis of tissue, as a result of the inflammatory reaction, may lead to dissemination even years later.

Often the disease will be dormant until the host becomes immunosuppressed (decrease in CD4+ T cell–derived type 1 cytokines), at which time the disease is reactivated. When the infection is not successfully contained, large numbers of organisms may escape into the bloodstream resulting in miliary tuberculosis, the most serious manifestation of this infection.

Immunoevasive Strategies

M. tuberculosis has evolved several evasive strategies to avoid the host immune attack. One such strategy includes an ability to inhibit fusion of lysosomes with the phagosome, thereby excluding the lysosomal contents from the site of microbial destruction. Furthermore, *Mycobacterium* species secrete proteins that "mop up" (scavenge) reactive oxygen intermediates generated after activation of NADPH oxidase and the accompanying respiratory burst. Consequently, the macrophages are deprived of much of the armamentarium required to destroy these bacteria, which proliferate and cause the destruction of the alveolar macrophages.

You have been Anthony's general practitioner since childhood. Other than the usual run of minor childhood disorders, there has been nothing of note in his medical history. Both parents and a younger sibling are well. He is currently 22 years of age and is home for the summer, on vacation from college. Anthony had called your office, requesting a complete physical examination, and, as a precursor to that visit, you have ordered a series of routine tests, including serum blood cell counts and electrolyte determinations, chest radiograph, and urinalysis. The day before the appointment the laboratory results become available and show, somewhat surprisingly to you, a marked increase in some liver enzymes (transaminases) and an elevated bilirubin level. Physical examination of this young man when he did come in revealed, not surprisingly, a mild jaundice, with some tenderness at the liver edge. There were no other significant abnormalities, although you also note some healing bruises and pinpricks in the forearm. He seems to be sniffing a lot, as though he has a perpetual postnasal drip, and he seems to be somewhat more edgy in your presence than usual. How are you going to open up a conversation? What do you want to address? Do you have significant concerns?

C A S E
13

QUESTIONS FOR GROUP DISCUSSION

1. Given the conglomeration of findings, how are you going to open up a conversation to address the overriding concern of drug use/abuse?
2. Cocaine may explain the sniffles and edginess, but resolving track marks and liver disease should alert you to intravenous drug use. As such, you should request serologic tests to determine if this patient has been exposed to a number of infections. For which infectious agents would you request an antibody titer?
3. At early stages of infection, serologic tests often provide false-negative results. Explain why this is so, and how one would confirm these results and the principle underlying the confirmatory tests.
4. Anthony's confirmatory test was positive for HIV. Draw a schematic illustrating HIV infection of a CD4+ T cell. See Figure 13-2. Identify gp120, gp41, CD4, and the chemokine receptor. Also, explain the term "facilitated HIV infection in trans." (*Hint:* What is the role of DC-SIGN in HIV infection?)
5. When Anthony was informed that he was HIV positive, he asked his physician if he could begin highly active retroviral therapy (HAART). What is the underlying principle of the drugs that constitute HAART? Explain why antiretroviral therapy (HAART) is effective by illustrating the steps these drugs target during productive viral infection of a cell.
6. As Anthony's physician, you realize that you have to convince him that there are limitations to

HAART. Discuss the advantages and disadvantages of HAART.
7. In addition to the advantages and disadvantages of HAART, you also explain to your patient that the "hit hard, hit early" slogan does not represent the current recommendations regarding when to commence therapy. What are the generally accepted guidelines for commencing HAART therapy?
8. HIV has evolved a number of viral evasive strategies. Describe several of these and explain how these contribute to viral persistence in a normal individual such that individuals develop acquired immunodeficiency syndrome (AIDS).
9. Interleukin (IL)-2 is a growth factor for T cells. Therefore, it seems reasonable to consider IL-2 as a therapeutic agent to expand the population of CD4+ T cells, which are the primary target of HIV infection. However, clinical trials have shown that IL-2 therapy can actually lead to an increase in viral load. Despite this, some advocates of IL-2 therapy argue that therapy with this cytokine in the presence of HAART is a good idea. Explain.
10. Describe the various approaches in attempts to develop an effective HIV vaccine and explain why an effective HIV vaccine is not likely in the immediate future.

RECOMMENDED APPROACH

Implication/Analysis of Family History

There is nothing remarkable about the family history and because you have been Anthony's physician since childhood you are more concerned about recent lifestyle changes now that he is attending college.

Implications/Analysis of Clinical History

You should be concerned about the conglomeration of findings and need to find out if they are all symptomatic of the same problem. An overriding concern here is drug use/abuse. Cocaine may explain the sniffles and edginess, but the evidence for resolving track marks and liver disease should alert you to intravenous drug use. Anthony admits to intravenous drug use, although he claims it was a short period (less than 2 weeks) and that he has not had heroin for more than a month. Unfortunately it seems as though there was at least one episode of shared needle use. Further questioning reveals a recent history of fever (lasted >10 days ~2 weeks ago) but no cough and no hematuria. There is no candidiasis. He casually mentions that he had diarrhea for days after he got home, attributing that to eating at a pretty run-down roadside café when he was driving home for the holidays.

Implications/Analysis of Laboratory Investigation

Based on the clinical history, physical examination (track marks on the arm, healing bruises, jaundice), and laboratory test results (elevated liver enzymes) you should be concerned about hepatitis and HIV infection. These infections are increased, depending on the setting in which intravenous drug use is occurring.

Additional Laboratory Tests

A complete blood cell count with differential was requested, along with enzyme-linked immunosorbent assays (ELISAs) to detect anti-hepatitis (A/B/C) antibodies. Additionally, a repeat liver enzyme assessment was ordered. The white blood cell count and differential was normal, and there was no evidence of anti–hepatitis B or anti–hepatitis C antibodies. However, there was evidence for hepatitis A seroconversion (anti-hepatitis A antibodies). Repeat blood work suggested the liver tests were normalizing. HIV serology was negative. At this stage you are a little more relieved.

Recognizing, however, that in the early stages of infection there are significant false-negative results in viral diagnostic tests that are based on antibody detection, you order more sensitive tests (viral load using nucleic acid amplification, e.g., polymerase chain reaction) for HIV and both hepatitis B and C. In most individuals the viral load (number of viral particles in circulation) is highest just before seroconversion. The viral load analysis for HIV comes back positive.

DIAGNOSIS

On the basis of the nucleic acid amplification tests, Anthony is informed that he is infected with HIV, the causative agent of acquired immunodeficiency disease (AIDS). Anthony's CD4+ T cell count will need to be monitored. As the number of CD4+ T cells decreases, the number of opportunistic infections increases (Fig. 13–1).

THERAPY

Highly active antiretroviral therapy (HAART) is the treatment of choice for HIV-infected patients. This drug regimen includes two antinucleoside analogue inhibitors and a protease inhibitor or a non-nucleoside

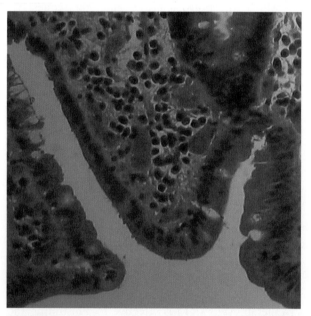

FIGURE 13–1 Section of duodenum from HIV-infected patient with opportunistic infection by *Cryptosporidium*. Note small spherical bodies (schizonts) on the surface epithelium, weakly staining with hematoxylin and eosin (×400). The lamina propria is heavily infiltrated with plasma cells.

reverse transcriptase inhibitor. Even though the use of HAART is not a controversial issue, the "when" to initiate therapy is highly debated. This controversy follows the realization that the "hit hard, hit early" slogan of the mid 1990s does not lead to the eradication of the virus in patients despite long term, and early, drug therapy. HIV is detectable in latent infected cells even after prolonged therapy, and so the approach to drug therapy has had to be modified.

Advantages and Disadvantages of HAART

There are advantages and disadvantages to HAART. In patients receiving HAART, plasma HIV RNA levels fall to below the level of detection within 2 to 6 months. There is an increase in CD4+ T cell count and therefore delayed progression to AIDS. As well, in some cases HAART is accompanied by enlargement of the thymus. Whether this enlargement is due to regeneration of the thymus and active thymopoiesis or from the migration of peripheral blood cells into the thymus is currently being addressed using *in vivo* TREC (T cell receptor excision circles) assay of thymic function (see Case 2). On the down side, hepatotoxicity is a serious consideration, as is the development of viral variants that are resistant to the drugs. Additionally, HAART therapy does not eliminate HIV from resting memory CD4$^+$ T cells carrying an integrated copy of the viral genome. Therefore, on discontinuation of HAART, viral load measures (plasma HIV-1 RNA) become significant when the latently infected cells are activated even by stimulatory molecules normally present in lymphoid tissues.

Patient Compliance with Treatment

The emergence of variants that are resistant to the ongoing drug therapy is substantially increased by the lack of patient adherence. In some cases this may reflect a regimen too complicated for the patient, a very large number of pills, or poor tolerance to the medication. In other cases, the patient's desire for such intense treatment is not sufficient to merit adherence to therapy.

When to Begin Therapy

The question still remains as to when to begin therapy. Issues at stake are whether viral load or CD4+ T cell count should be used as a guideline for initiating therapy. Even those that advocate using CD4+ T cell count as the marker for therapy do not agree as to what that CD4+ T cell number should be. Those that believe that therapy should be initiated when the CD4+ T cell count falls below 200 cells/μL support their argument by emphasizing the reduced time for toxicity, enhanced quality of life before therapy, and a decrease in potential for viral resistance.

On the other hand, those that believe that therapy should be initiated when CD4+ T cell count is 350 cells/μL argue that initiating therapy at this time prevents irreversible immune damage, minimizes the spread of HIV to more restricted sites (e.g., central nervous system), and minimizes the potential for development of more virulent HIV. The initiation of HAART when the CD4+ T cell count is less than 350 cells/μL, or sooner if the HIV RNA load is higher than 5000 copies/mL, is another option that is under consideration. Once drug therapy is initiated, patient adherence and viral load should be monitored regularly.

Role of Cytokines in Therapy

Although HAART is changing the course of HIV infections, the reality is that the toxicity of the drugs and the emergence of drug-resistant escape mutants indicate that immunologic therapies should be pursued. Furthermore, the realization that discontinuation of therapy results in a rebound of viral burden emphasizes the need for immunologic forms of therapy.

Clinical trials have focused on those cytokines that would restore the patient's cells (e.g., granulocyte-macrophage colony-stimulating factor [GM-CSF] for myeloid cells; IL-2, a growth factor for T cells; IL-12, to enhance polarization of T cell development toward CD4+ Th1 cells). Whereas larger randomized trials have been initiated for some of the therapies, others have been shown to actually cause an increase in plasma viral load. *In vitro* studies have shown that latently infected cells are activated and induce viral replication in the presence of some cytokines (e.g., IL-2, IL-6, and tumor necrosis factor-α).

Those who advocate the use of IL-2 as therapy to increase the number of CD4+ T cells in conjunction with HAART suggest that the IL-2 would activate latent cells with the net effect being their eradication, while the patient is protected by HAART. Implicit assumptions in this approach are that the virus strains are not resistant to HAART and that all the latent cells are CD4+ T cells. Recall that some cells that do not express CD4 can be infected after binding to galactosyl ceramide.

Another cytokine, IL-15, has been recommended for immunotherapy, based on the advantage that it does not enhance HIV replication but does play an important role in NK cell and CD8+ T cell cytotoxicity, CD4+ Th1 cell development, and activation of dendritic cells, monocytes, and neutrophils.

Vaccines

A number of pharmaceutical firms (e.g., VaxGen, Aventis Pasteur, Wyeth, Chiron, GlaxoSmithKline) are presently engaged in human trials for an HIV vaccine using various vectors and vaccine strategies. Ideally, a vaccine stimulates the immune system such that sterilizing immunity results (i.e., exposure to the virus fails to establish an ongoing infection in the immunized host). At this time, however, a vaccine that slows down or inhibits HIV replication would be beneficial to the millions of people infected with HIV.

Recombinant Protein Vaccines

From a historical point of view, it is not surprising that the early attempts at vaccine development used a recombinant form of the HIV envelope protein, gp120. After all, a recombinant vaccine for hepatitis B has been very effective. The ineffectiveness of the HIV vaccines is due, in part, to the fact that the neutralizing antibodies formed were specific for laboratory strains of HIV. In other vaccines, several anti-HIV antibodies developed, but these were not neutralizing. In general, neutralizing antibodies are not generated until late in the course of the HIV infection.

Recombinant Viruses and DNA Vectors

It also became evident early on that an effective vaccine would need to generate anti-HIV specific cytotoxic CD8+ T cells. Traditionally, this has been achieved by using attenuated viruses as vaccines (e.g., measles, mumps, rubella), but the risks associated with reversion to wild-type virus eliminate this as an option for HIV. Rather, recombinant DNA techniques have been used to insert HIV genes in the genome of nonlethal viruses from which genes relevant for viral production have been removed (e.g., canary poxvirus,

adeno-associated virus). Because the principal function of these modified viruses is to ensure that HIV genes enter the cell cytosol, this can also be accomplished using microparticles containing HIV nucleic acids.

Once the genetic material is in the cell, it can be transcribed and translated into proteins. The proteins generated are hydrolyzed by the proteasome and the fragments translocated to the endoplasmic reticulum where they encounter class I MHC molecules and form complexes that are subsequently expressed on the surface of the cell. CD8+ T cells that recognize the complexes will be activated if the appropriate co-stimulatory molecules are also present. Unfortunately, these vaccines have not been particularly effective in generating either strong cytotoxic T cell or antibody responses. A modified approach, the "prime, boost" approach, has been used in attempts to enhance the response. In this approach, the vector is administered in the initial vaccine and this is followed by a protein injection weeks later.

Antigen-Pulsed Dendritic Cells

Several studies have shown that HIV-positive patients have fewer dendritic cells and that these cells have a reduced capacity to activate T cells. In the absence of antigen presentation, T cells cannot be activated, and so it has been suggested that this is one of the reasons why the immune system cannot clear HIV infection. To address this issue in an animal model, cytokine-treated (GM-CSF, IL-4) dendritic cells were pulsed with inactivated simian immunodeficiency virus and then injected into rhesus monkeys. Reports from this study are impressive; however, whether this approach would be efficacious or feasible for human vaccines is the focus of several investigations.

Vaccine Failures: "Original Antigenic Sin"

Despite the vast amount of research and various clinical trials, an effective vaccine is not likely in the near future. One of the reasons for this is the high frequency of mutations that escape detection by activated cytotoxic T cells and by anti-HIV antibodies.

Because mutations can occur early in the course of the disease, the activated cytotoxic T cells are no longer effective, yet immune response to escape mutants is much weaker than that to the primary HIV isolate ("original antigenic sin"). Antibody responses to the initial epitopes have also been reported to dominate. In addition to a blunted response to the escape mutants, the decrease in CD4+ T cells hampers cytotoxic T cell development (and antibody responses) because both require cognate interaction with, and cytokines derived from, CD4+ T cells.

ETIOLOGY OF AIDS: HUMAN IMMUNODEFICIENCY VIRUS

The human immunodeficiency virus type 1 (HIV) is the causative agent of AIDS, a disease in which the patient's CD4+ T cell count is so drastically reduced that the patient becomes susceptible to numerous opportunistic infections. Transmission occurs from one person to another via infected body fluids (e.g., semen, blood). Retroviruses are enveloped single-stranded RNA viruses, whose genome encodes several proteins, including reverse transcriptase that reverse transcribes the RNA to double-stranded DNA. Activation of the infected cell is required for integration (random) of the double-stranded DNA into the

genome. This double-stranded viral DNA is integrated into the host chromosome, where it can remain in a latent phase for years as a provirus until the cell is activated to replicate. Because the HIV provirus is integrated into the host chromosome, all the progeny of the infected cells will also have the provirus in their genome.

Cell Infection

Cell Surface Receptors

Productive infection requires that HIV binds to both a primary receptor, CD4, and a co-receptor CCR5 or CXCR4 on the target cell. CCR5 and CXCR4 are chemokine receptors that are targeted by different HIV strains (Fig. 13–2). CCR5 is used primarily by macrophage (M) tropic strains, whereas CXCR4 is used primarily by T cell (T) tropic strains. HIV interacts first with the primary receptor, CD4, via its envelope glycoprotein, gp120. Binding to CD4 creates a complex that allows gp120 to bind to CCR5 or CXCR4. After this binding, gp41, which is a fusion

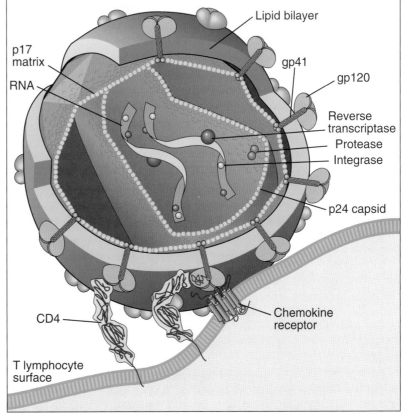

FIGURE 13–2 Structure of human immunodeficiency virus-1 (HIV-1). An HIV virion is shown interacting with a CD4+ T cell. HIV interacts first with the primary receptor, CD4, via its envelope glycoprotein, gp120. Binding to CD4 creates a complex that allows gp120 to bind to CCR5 or CXCR4. Following this binding, gp41, which is a fusion protein, enters the cell membrane to initiate fusion of the viral envelope and subsequent delivery of the viral proteins and genome into the cell. (From Abbas A, Lichtman A: Cellular and Molecular Immunology, 5th ed. Philadelphia, Saunders, 2003; Modified from front cover, The New Face of AIDS. Science 272:1841–2102, 1996. © Terese Winslow.)

protein, enters the cell membrane to initiate fusion of the viral envelope and subsequent delivery of the viral proteins and genome into the cell. Under some circumstances, HIV can infect cells that do not express CD4 (e.g., endothelial cells, microglial cells) by binding galactosyl ceramide.

"Facilitated Infection In Trans": Role of DC-SIGN

In context of HIV infection, the term *facilitated infection in trans* refers to the transfer of HIV from a dendritic cell surface molecule, DC-SIGN (dendritic cell–specific ICAM-3 grabbing nonintegrin), to CD4 on a target cell. In an emerging model, dendritic cells play an important role in the establishment of primary HIV infection by capturing viral particles in peripheral mucosal tissues and transporting them to the secondary lymphoid tissues.

In this model, capture occurs when DC-SIGN, a lectin, on dendritic cells binds HIV gp120 with high affinity, internalizes the complex into an acidic compartment, and recycles back to the surface where the HIV can be transferred to CD4+ T cells. Although studies indicate that internalization into an acidic compartment is essential for subsequent in trans infection, the strategies employed to evade degradation in the endocytic vacuole have not been determined.

Productive infection of CD4+ T cells, however, requires that T cells be activated. T cell activation occurs when antigen-specific receptors interact with complexes of class II MHC-antigen peptide on the surface of antigen-presenting cells. Therefore, antigen processing of HIV must also occur. The simplest explanation that would allow both events to occur is that DC-SIGN complexes are internalized via endocytic vesicles that escape fusion with lysosomes, while HIV particles internalized after binding to primitive pattern receptors are handled via the well-described pathway of antigen processing and cell surface expression with class II MHC.

Interaction of dendritic cells with CD4+ T cells in secondary lymphoid tissues via antigen-specific T cell receptors, co-stimulatory molecules, and adhesive molecules would bring the DC-SIGN-HIV complexes into close proximity to CD4, thereby facilitating infection (i.e., facilitated infection in trans) of the T cells.

DC-SIGN was first identified as a molecule that bound intercellular adhesive molecules (ICAM)-2 and -3 with greater affinity than leukocyte function antigen (LFA)-1, the previously known receptor for these adhesive molecules. ICAM-2 is expressed on both resting and activated vascular endothelium, as well as resting T cells. ICAM-3 is expressed also on resting T cells, as well as other leukocytes.

HIV Evasive Strategies

The failure of the immune system to eradicate HIV infection in previously healthy individuals is testament to the various immune strategies that are employed by the virus. The effectiveness of these immune evasive strategies is underscored when one considers that, despite the millions of people infected worldwide, there is not a single documented case of infection being eradicated by the immune system. This is unique in the world of viruses where, despite epidemics that kill millions of people (e.g., influenza viruses), a substantial number of the population can eliminate the infection. This holds true, even for devastating Ebola virus infections.

An understanding of the evasive strategies used by HIV may be critical for the development of therapeutic interventions. Mutagenesis, inhibition of class I MHC expression, and inhibition/downregulation of CD4 expression are well documented HIV strategies that either allow HIV to thwart the immune system or allow it to persist and replicate more effectively.

Mutagenesis of Viral Proteins

Retroviruses have an RNA genome that is converted to double-stranded DNA by the action of viral reverse transcriptase, a polymerase that has no proofreading activity, and so this leads to a very high error rate during this process. Existing antibodies do not recognize these "new" antigens, and activated T cells do not recognize the antigenic peptides that are displayed with MHC on the cell surface. In some cases, the mutated peptides cannot associate with existing MHC alleles, or they bind MHC with very low affinity, thereby reducing the stability of the MHC-peptide complex. Responses to the mutated viruses are typically blunted. In the absence of MHC-peptide recognition, T cell activation does not occur.

Downregulation of Class I Expression

Downregulation of class I MHC expression is a relatively common viral evasive strategy, but the mechanisms by which this is achieved vary from virus to virus. In HIV, downregulation of class I MHC is attributed to the action of the HIV regulatory protein, Nef, because its presence, or absence, in the HIV genome affects expression of class I MHC on the cell surface, a requirement for activation of cytotoxic T cells. At least two different mechanisms have been reported to explain this effect; the first is that Nef increases the endocytosis of surface class I MHC; the other is that Nef redirects class I MHC from the Golgi to the cytosol, or sequesters the complex in the Golgi. Irrespective of the mechanism, a decrease in the class I MHC-HIV peptides expressed on the infected cell surface will hinder recognition and targeting by cytotoxic T cells. Interestingly, the amount of class I MHC expressed on a cell surface has been shown to depend on the particular Nef allele encoded by a particular viral variant.

Downregulation of CD4

Nef has also been reported to play a role in the enhanced endocytosis of cell surface CD4 and rerouting from the Golgi apparatus, which results in decreased cell surface expression. How a reduction in CD4 expression benefits the virus is speculative because HIV (via gp120) must bind to CD4 to gain entry into the cell. What has been postulated is that a decrease in CD4 would reduce further HIV entry and hence avoid superinfection, which would be cytopathic to the cell. Alternatively, a reduction in CD4 cell surface expression reduces the likelihood of syncytia formation (by syncytium-inducing viruses), a phenomenon in which the gp120 embedded in the host cell membrane binds to other cells expressing CD4 such that cell fusion results. Syncytia can consist of four to five T cells that are effectively eliminated from immune responses.

Blocking Apoptosis of Infected Cells

Cells infected with HIV will ultimately undergo apoptosis, but productive infection and viral persistence necessitates that apoptosis be delayed at least until viral assembly and budding from the cell has occurred. In addition to its role in downregulating CD4 and class I MHC molecules, the Nef protein has been shown to prevent apoptosis of infected cells via interaction with cytosolic kinases.

FURTHER READING

Andrews T, Sullivan KE: Infections in patients with inherited defects in phagocyte function. Clin Microbiol Rev 16:597, 2003.

Aradhya S: A recurrent deletion in the ubiquitously expressed NEMO (IKK gamma) gene accounts for the vast majority of incontinentia pigmenti mutations. Hum Mol Genet 1:2171, 2001.

Arakawa H, Hauschild J, Buerstedde JM: Requirement of the activation-induced deaminase (AID) gene for immunoglobulin gene conversion. Science 295:1301, 2002.

Babgdong L, et al: *In vivo* analysis of Nef function. Curr HIV Res 1:41, 2003.

Badley AD, et al: Mechanisms of HIV-associated lymphocyte apoptosis. Blood 96:2951, 2000.

Baldini A: DiGeorge syndrome: An update. Curr Opin Cardiol 19:201, 2004.

Bartsch O, et al: DiGeorge/velocardiofacial syndrome: FISH studies of chromosomes 22q11 and 10p14, and clinical reports on the proximal 22q11 deletions. Am J Med Genet 117A:1, 2003.

Bellamy R, et al: Variations in the NRAMP1 gene and susceptibility to tuberculosis in Western Africa. N Engl J Med 338:640, 1998.

Bhushan A, Covey LR: CD40:CD40L interactions in X-linked and non X-linked hyper IgM syndrome. Immunol Res 24:311, 2001.

Caamano J, Hunter CA: NFκB family of transcription factors: Central regulators of innate and adaptive immune functions. Clin Microbiol Rev 15:414, 2002.

Carrol ED, et al: Anhidrotic ectodermal dysplasia and immunodeficiency—the role of NEMO. Arch Dis Child 88:340, 2003.

Casper-Bauguil S, et al: Mildly oxidized low density lipoproteins decrease early production of interleukin 2 and nuclear factor κB binding to DNA in activated T-lymphocytes. Biochem J 337:269, 1999.

Chinen J, Puck JM: Successes and risks of gene therapy in primary immunodeficiency diseases. J Allergy Clin Immunol 113:595, 2004.

Clark-Curtiss JE, Haydel SE: Molecular genetics of *Mycobacterium tuberculosis* pathogenesis. Ann Rev Microbiol 57:517, 2003.

Collins KL, et al: HIV-1 Nef protein protects infected primary cells against killing by cytotoxic T lymphocytes. Nature 391:397, 1998.

Collins KL: How HIV evades CTL recognition. Curr HIV Res 1:31, 2003.

Cooper MA, Pommering TL, Koranyi K: Primary immunodeficiencies. Am Fam Physician 68:2001, 2003.

Cosma CL, Sherman DR, Ramakrishnan L: The secret lives of the pathogenic mycobacteria. Ann Rev Microbiol 57:641, 2003.

Cox GM, et al: Superoxide dismutase influences the virulence of *Cryptococcus neoformans* by affecting growth within macrophages. Infect Immun 71:173, 2003.

Davenport MP, et al: Cell turnover and cell tropism in HIV infection. Trends Microbiol 10:275, 2002.

Doffinger R, et al: X linked anhidrotic ectodermal dysplasia with immunodeficiency is caused by impaired NF-kappa B signaling. Nat Genet 27:277, 2001.

Durandy A, Honjo T: Human genetic defects in class switching recombination (hyper IgM syndrome). Curr Opin Immunol 12:543, 2003.

Edwards E, Razvi S, Cunningham-Rundles C: IgA deficiency: Clinical correlates and responses to pneumococcal vaccine. Clin Immunol 111:93, 2004.

Engel BC, Kohn DB, Podsakoff GM: Update on gene therapy of inherited immune deficiencies. Curr Opin Mol Ther 5:503, 2003.

Fallarino F, et al: Modulation of tryptophan catabolism by regulatory T cells. Nat Immunol 4:1206, 2003.

Farhoudi A, et al: Two related cases of primary complement deficiency. Immunol Invest 32:313, 2003.

Forbes JR, Gros P: Iron, manganese, and cobalt transport by Nramp1 (Slc11a1) and Nramp2 (Slc11a2) expressed at the plasma membrane. Blood 102:1884, 2003.

Futatani T, et al: Deficient expression of Bruton's tyrosine kinase in monocytes from X-linked agammaglobulinemia as evaluated by a flow cytometric analysis and its clinical application to carrier detection. Blood 91:595, 1998.

Garcia-Perex MA, et al: Mutations of CD40L in two patients with hyper-IgM syndrome. Immunobiology 207:285, 2003.

Gaspar HB, Conley ME: Immunodeficiency review: Early B cell defects. Clin & Exper Immunol 119:303, 2000.

Grimbacher B, et al: Homozygous loss of ICOS is associated with adult-onset common variable immunodeficiency. Nat Immunol 4:261, 2003.

Hacein-Bey-Abina S, et al: Sustained correction of X-linked severe combined immunodeficiency by ex vivo gene therapy. N Engl J Med 346:1185, 2002.

Hidalgo A, et al: Insights into leukocyte adhesion deficiency type 2 from a novel mutation in the GDP-fucose transporter gene. Blood 101:1705, 2003.

Illoh OC: Current applications of flow cytometry in the diagnosis of primary immunodeficiency diseases. Arch Pathol Lab Med 128:23, 2004.

Inohara N, Nuflez G: NODS: Intracellular proteins involved in inflammation and apoptosis. Nat Rev Immunol 3:371, 2003.

Krysztof M, Rieth W: Promoter specific functions of CIITA and MHC class II enhanceosome in transcriptional activation. EMBO J 21:1379, 2002.

Ku CL, et al: NEMO mutations in 2 unrelated boys with severe infections and conical teeth. Pediatrics 115:e615, 2005.

Kwak B, Mulhaupt F, Mach F: Statins as a newly recognized type of immunomodulator. Nat Med 6:1399, 2000.

Li Q, Verma IM: NFκB regulation in the immune system. Nat Rev Immunol 2:725, 2002.

Lu W, et al: Therapeutic dendritic-cell vaccine for simian AIDS. Nat Med 9:27, 2003.

Markert ML, et al: Complete DiGeorge syndrome: Development of rash, lymphadenopathy, and oligoclonal T cells in 5 cases. J Allergy Clin Immunol 113:734, 2004.

Markert ML, et al: Thymus transplantation in complete DiGeorge syndrome: Immunologic and safety evaluations in 12 patients. Blood 102:1121, 2003.

Mastroianni CM, et al: Teaching tired T cell to fight HIV: Time to test IL-15 for immunotherapy? Trends Immunol 25:121, 2004.

McAdam AJ, et al: ICOS is critical for CD40-mediated antibody switching. Nature 409:102, 2001.

Nelson M: Metal ion transporters and homeostasis. EMBO J 18:4361, 1999.

Orange JS, Geha RS: Finding NEMO: Genetic disorders of NFκB activation. J Clin Invest 112:983, 2002.

Pienaar S, et al: X-linked Hyper IgM (HIGM1) in an African kindred: The first report from South Africa. BMC Pediatr 3:12, 2003.

Puck J: Primary immunodeficiency diseases. JAMA 278:1835, 1997.

Reisner Y: ICOS: a new important player in BMT. Blood 105:3006, 2005.

Reith W, Mach B: The bare lymphocyte syndrome and the regulation of MHC expression. Ann Rev Immunol 19:331, 2001.

Ryuta N, et al: X-linked ectodermal dysplasia and immunodeficiency caused by reversion mosaicism of NEMO reveals a critical role for NEMO in human T cell development and/or survival. Blood 103:4565, 2004.

Sabroe I, et al: Toll-like receptors in health and disease: Complex questions remain. J Immunol 171:1630, 2003.

Sempowski GD, Haynes BF: Immune reconstitution in patients with HIV infection. Ann Rev Med 53:269, 2002.

Simonte SJ, Cunningham-Rundles C: Update on primary immunodeficiency: Defects of lymphocytes. Clin Immunol 109:109, 2003.

Smahi A, et al: The NFκB signaling pathway in human diseases: from incontinentia pigmenti to ectodermal dysplasias and immune-deficiency syndromes. Hum Mol Genet 11:2371, 2002.

Spearman P: HIV vaccine development: Lessons from the past and promise for the future. Curr HIV Res 1:101, 2003.

Speth C, et al: The role of complement in invasive fungal infections. Mycoses 47:93, 2004.

Su SV, Gurney KB, Lee B: Sugar and spice: Viral envelope-DC-SIGN interactions in HIV pathogenesis. Curr HIV Res 1:87, 2003.

Takada H, et al: Female agammaglobulinemia due to the Bruton tyrosine kinase deficiency caused by extremely skewed X-chromosome inactivation. Blood 103:185, 2004.

Takeda K, Kaiho T, Akira S: Toll-like receptors. Annu Rev Immunol 21:335, 2003.

Vasselon T, Detmers PA: Toll receptors: A central element in innate immune responses. Infect Immun 70:1033, 2002.

Villa A, et al: V(D)J recombination defects in lymphocytes due to RAG mutations: Severe immunodeficiency with a spectrum of clinical presentations. Blood 97:81-88, 2001.

Volberding PA: Initiating HIV therapy: Timing is critical, controversial. Postgrad Med 115:15, 2004.

Walport MJ: Complement at the interface between innate and adaptive immunity: I. N Engl J Med 344:1058, 2001.

Walport MJ: Complement at the interface between innate and adaptive immunity: II. N Engl J Med 344:1140, 2001.

Wehrle-Haller B, Imhof BA: Integrin-dependent pathologies. J Pathol 4:481, 2004.

Wen L, Atkinson JP, Gicias PC: Clinical and laboratory evaluation of complement deficiency. J Allergy Clin Immunol 113:585, 2004.

Winkelstein JA, et al: The X-linked hyper-IgM syndrome: Clinical and immunologic features of 79 patients. Medicine (Baltimore) 82:373, 2003.

Wolf D, et al: HIV Nef associated PAK and PI3-kinases stimulate Akt-independent Bad-phosphorylation to induce anti-apoptotic signals. Nat Med 7:1217, 2001.

Yang OO: CTL ontogeny and viral escape: Implications for HIV-1 vaccine design. Trends Immunol 25:138, 2004.

SECTION II

Hypersensitivity Reactions

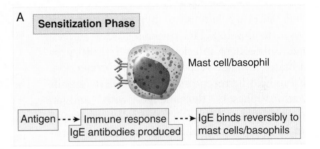

A **Sensitization Phase**

Mast cell/basophil

Antigen ---→ Immune response / IgE antibodies produced ---→ IgE binds reversibly to mast cells/basophils

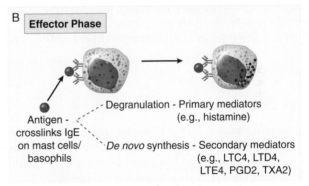

B **Effector Phase**

Antigen - crosslinks IgE on mast cells/basophils

Degranulation - Primary mediators (e.g., histamine)

De novo synthesis - Secondary mediators (e.g., LTC4, LTD4, LTE4, PGD2, TXA2)

If, as used to be claimed, all of medicine could be understood in the context of a genuine understanding of tuberculosis, then we would equally argue that clinical immunology *in toto* could be described in terms of cases in hypersensitivity disorders. From the immediate reactivity (type I) brought about by signaling following direct cross-linking of IgE on the cell surface to the more subtle reactions that follow the development of sustained T cell mediated immunity (type IV), pathology can in all cases be understood from attention to the nature of the immunization process, the recall that follows from secondary exposure to the offending pathogen/antigen, and the signaling cascades inherent in each phase.

Some of these reactions will be familiar to the reader—the typical wheal and erythema from a bee sting or a peanut allergy, for instance, and the wheezes and airway hyperreactivity of the asthmatic. Less obvious to many will be the discussion that considers the evidence that a case of infertility (case 18) may similarly represent a manifestation of a hypersensitivity disorder. Following a brief summary of the classical Gell and Coombs' classification of hypersensitivity reactions, the reader is invited to browse the cases that follow in any order, each of which will highlight important information concerning the individual types of immune hypersensitivity disorder.

Hypersensitivity reactions are classified as one of four types: type I—immediate (IgE), type II—antibody mediated (IgM/IgG binds to cell surface), type III—IgM/IgG binds to immune complexes, and type IV—T cell mediated. Regardless of the immune mechanisms involved, hypersensitivity reactions can be divided into two phases: a sensitization phase and an effector phase. The observed clinical pathology is associated with the effector phase of hypersensitivity reactions.

TYPE I HYPERSENSITIVITY REACTIONS

Individuals showing immediate hypersensitivity are predisposed to develop Th2 responses after antigen challenge. Subsequent interleukin (IL)-4/IL-10 production biases immune responses to IgE production; this IgE binds to Fc receptors on mast cells/basophils (sensitization phase). Rechallenge with antigen leads to crosslinking of IgE on the cell surface and mediator release (effector phase). The mediators produced (e.g., histamine, prostaglandins, leukotrienes) increase vascular permeability, smooth muscle contraction, and vasodilatation. Commonly used tests to delineate those individuals showing immediate hypersensitivity are skin tests and radioimmunosorbent tests (RAST).

Clinical Examples

Clinical manifestations run the gamut from (least serious to most serious) allergic rhinitis (a local irritant), to asthma (with airway compromise and wheezing), to anaphylaxis (life-threatening with systemic symptoms and shock).

Therapy and Prophylaxis

Therapy and prophylaxis for type I hypersensitivity reactions include epinephrine (immediate relief of serious symptoms); corticosteroids (delayed relief of symptoms (4 to 8 hours); and antihistamines (H1 antagonists) or mast cell membrane stabilizers (to stop histamine release, e.g., cromoglycate). A more controversial therapy involves use of desensitization. In this case we use deliberate injection of antigen in an attempt to bolster Th1 immunity, IgG production, and thus competition with IgE for antigen.

TYPE II HYPERSENSITIVITY REACTIONS (ANTIBODY MEDIATED)

Type II hypersensitivity reactions are those in which cell surface antigens are the target for antibody production and subsequent pathology. In the sensitization phase, antigen (a cell surface antigen or hapten, e.g., cell-bound drug/hapten) induces an immunoglobulin response; the immunoglobulin is then bound via the Fab region to the target cell (which expresses the antigen/hapten). In the effector phase, destruction of cells with immunoglobulin bound (and exposed Fc) occurs by complement fixation, opsonin production (C3b, C4b) and lysis/phagocytosis, or a mechanism involving antibody-dependent cell-mediated cytotoxicity (ADCC) by cells with Fc receptors (e.g., natural killer [NK] cells).

Clinical Examples

Clinical manifestations of type II hypersensitivity reactions include transfusion reactions occurring as a result of ABO incompatibility, Rh (rhesus antigen) incompatibility, or some autoimmune disorders (Goodpasture's syndrome).

Transfusion Reactions

Transfusion reactions occur when individuals with blood group type O (who can only receive blood from other type O individuals) are transfused with blood from an individual who is type AB, A, or B. In such a case, the anti-A and/or anti-B isohemagglutinins (IgM antibodies) present in the type O recipient target the donor red blood cells (transfusion reaction).

Blood type O individuals serve as universal donors because their red blood cells do not express either the A or the B antigens and so they cannot be targeted by hemagglutinins. Although blood type O individuals have anti-A and anti-B hemagglutinins, so little serum is transferred from donor to recipient that the small amount of isohemagglutinins present does not induce a transfusion reaction in the recipient. However, often to circumvent this possibility, only washed red blood cells (expressing no A or B antigens) are used for transfer. This is particularly important if the recipient is deficient in IgA (Selective IgA Deficiency; see Case 5).

Rh Incompatibility

Rh incompatibility of newborns occurs when Rh– mothers (approximately 15% of the population) carry Rh+ fetuses. In this case, anti-Rh antibodies generated in a mother immunized (unintentionally) with the Rh antigen result in devastating disease in the offspring (see Case 16). Consequently, there is concern whenever any prenatal bleeding occurs, or at birth. Therefore, we use anti-Rh immunoglobulin (RhoGam) to prevent immunization of the mother.

Autoimmune Diseases

In many autoimmune diseases, autoantibodies are generated that are specific for a cell surface antigen. These autoantibody/cell surface antigen complexes trigger type II hypersensitivity reactions, which leads to the pathology observed (e.g., Goodpasture's syndrome, diabetes).

TYPE III HYPERSENSITIVITY REACTIONS

In type III hypersensitivity reactions, persistent (chronic) antigen exposure floods the immune system with immunoglobulins along with the sensitizing antigen, resulting in high levels of immune complex formation (sensitization phase). The normal clearance mechanisms are overextended, and complexes are deposited in various sites, including blood vessel walls, basement membranes of endothelia, and so on. Subsequent complement activation occurs, and the complement cascade triggers increased vessel permeability and chemotaxis of neutrophils and macrophages (effector phase). In addition, phagocytosis of immune complexes activates the respiratory burst, with production of reactive oxygen species, cytokine secretion, and procoagulant activity.

Clinical Examples

Clinical manifestations of type III hypersensitivity reactions include systemic lupus erythematosus (SLE), serum sickness, and the Arthus reaction.

Systemic Lupus Erythematosus

In SLE, immune complexes are deposited in the kidney and capillary wall basement membrane. Often basement membrane deposition occurs in the central nervous system with resultant pathology. Immune complex deposition in the joints leads to arthritic symptoms.

Serum Sickness

Serum sickness (a systemic disorder) can follow passive immunization for postexposure therapy, such as antivenom toxin given after snake bites. The infusion of heterologous horse serum triggers an immune response because the proteins (e.g., sheep/horse) are foreign. If the foreign protein is not cleared from the system by the time antibodies are generated (7 to 10 days), immune complexes form in the circulation and deposit in various tissues. Immune complex deposition in the renal glomeruli or the synovial membranes in joints leads to glomerulonephritis and arthritis, respectively.

Arthus Reaction

The Arthus reaction (a localized immune complex disorder) occurs following intradermal or subcutaneous immunization after a previous sensitization immunization. In this case we often observe localized vasculitis/necrosis.

TYPE IV HYPERSENSITIVITY REACTIONS

Type IV hypersensitivity reactions are caused by T cell–mediated immune reactions. Again a sensitization phase generates primed T cells after antigen/antigen-presenting cell interaction. Antigens (e.g., haptens in contact sensitivity) can even be taken up by dendritic cells in skin, which migrate to draining lymph nodes to sensitize T cells. When the individual is re-exposed to antigen, a memory response is generated and cytokines are released from primed T cells. These cytokines alter endothelial permeability and can often directly stimulate other cell types (e.g., macrophages) to produce inflammatory mediators.

Clinical Examples
Granuloma Formation

Chronic antigen stimulation occurs during infection with *Mycobacterium leprae* or *M. tuberculosis*. A granulomatous inflammation is observed from stimulation by mycobacteria that escape destruction within the phagocytic vacuole.

Delayed-Type Hypersensitivity Reaction

Acute antigen stimulation (the delayed-type hypersensitivity reaction) is the basis for the Mantoux reaction to test for exposure to *M. tuberculosis*. Individuals are skin tested with purified protein derivative (PPD), the soluble antigen of *M. tuberculosis*, and we look for cytokine-induced erythema/induration at 48 hours.

Contact Hypersensitivity

Contact hypersensitivity (e.g., poison ivy) represents an epidermal sensitivity to antigen that again is cytokine mediated (from antigen-specific T cells).

Cellular Cytotoxicity

In cellular cytotoxicity, CD8+ T cells and NK cells are activated. These play an important role in viral immunity.

Josh is a 19-year-old man who has been rushed to your emergency department from a local Italian restaurant, where he had become acutely "ill" while eating. On arrival he is pale, cool, and clammy and has a low blood pressure. There is no medic-alert bracelet to be seen. Putting your stethoscope to his chest you find he has wheezes throughout his lung fields but very poor air intake. A friend who is with him says this has never happened before, and, to his knowledge, no one in Josh's family has ever been like this. What are your thoughts on how to proceed?

QUESTIONS FOR GROUP DISCUSSION

1. Describe specific conditions/circumstances that could lead to vasodilation and the patient's symptoms as described.
2. Someone who is pale, cool, and clammy is not perfusing his peripheral tissue with blood. Explain how/why this happens in (a) trauma cases and (b) immunologic reactions in which biologic vasodilators are released.
3. Explain why vasodilatation is followed by sweating.
4. A deficiency in one of the complement regulatory proteins might present in this spontaneous manner. Name the protein and explain why a deficiency would lead to the symptoms observed.
5. Shellfish and nuts are two of the most potent mediators of food allergies. However, reactions as described in this case depend on re-exposure to a previously sensitized individual. Explain.
6. Ingestion of shellfish/nuts in a previously sensitized individual can lead to anaphylactic shock. There are a number of drugs you need to consider giving at this time, each acting in a slightly different manner and with different times of onset. What are they? Describe their mode of action and how long it takes for the effect to take place.
7. Note that food allergies will often present as nausea, stomach cramps, and diarrhea. Explain.
8. How would you determine the immediate precipitant of this reaction?
9. Individuals with allergies to shellfish/nuts and insect stings should carry three things. List these and provide a rationale for each.
10. Many allergic reactions are inconvenient but not life threatening. How do these types of allergic reactions manifest clinically?

RECOMMENDED APPROACH

Implications/Analysis of Family History

Other than the fact that his friend is unaware of any other family member presenting with similar conditions, we have no information regarding family history. A first time presentation in a 19-year-old, with no apparent family history, suggests that an inherited immune defect is unlikely (e.g., anaphylatoxins of the complement cascade). The absence of the medic-alert bracelet signifies that this is not a condition that has been previously diagnosed.

Implications/Analysis of Clinical History

Pale, cool, and clammy are the cardinal signs of impending shock and indicate that the patient is not perfusing the peripheral tissues with blood, hence pale and cool skin. A number of conditions can induce these symptoms, particularly blood loss during trauma, as the peripheral vasculature constricts to conserve remaining blood flow to the central key organs (e.g., brain/heart). However, even in the absence of severe blood loss, release of inflammatory mediators that induce vasodilatation and increase vascular (capillary) permeability can lead to a reduction in blood volume and cessation of blood flow to the periphery, with a concomitant drop in blood pressure (see Etiology). The low blood pressure triggers an increase in sympathetic nervous system activity and release of catecholamines from the adrenal medulla.

A number of nontrauma conditions can manifest in this manner. For example, patients experiencing septic shock as a result of gram-negative bacterial infection, dehydration, or heart damage may also present with similar symptoms. Josh's illness, however, occurred suddenly while eating at an Italian restaurant, and this should steer us away from these causes. The acute presentation of Josh's symptoms while eating is a strong indication that something this patient ate is most likely the precipitating factor. Ingested toxins (poisons) or a protein to which Josh had been previously sensitized are both in the realm of possibilities because these stimuli can induce the observed clinical "picture."

Italian restaurants (and other exotic restaurants) are environments where nuts and shellfish are commonly on the menu. These are *two of the most potent mediators of food allergies*. Reaction depends on re-exposure of a previously sensitized individual, so your patient must have (at least once) eaten similar foods without a response (see Etiology). Drug or food allergies present like this more commonly than do toxins or poisons.

In addition to the signs of impending shock, Josh is wheezing and has poor air intake, suggesting the bronchi and bronchioles of the respiratory "tree" are constricting, which is consistent with an allergen-induced anaphylaxis.

Implications/Analysis of Laboratory Investigation

Up to this point, no laboratory tests have been requested, first, because we have been dealing with a life-threatening situation, and, second, because this is essentially a clinical diagnosis (made based on history and physical examination).

Additional Laboratory Tests

In situ/vivo Tests

At some stage you need to try to figure out the immediate precipitant of this reaction, with a focus on food allergies. In general, patients with suspected food allergies are screened with "skin prick tests." In this test, a result is interpreted as positive if the allergen used to prick the skin leads to the formation of a wheal that is 3 mm (or greater) than that produced by the control substance. For this test, and any other "*in vivo*" measures, the patient must not take antihistamines or other antiallergy drugs for a period of time before the administration of the test. The gold standard test for food allergies, however, is the double-blind, placebo-controlled test in which suspect foods, based on the patient's history, are presented to the patient in a hospital setting by a physician experienced in the treatment of anaphylaxis.

In vitro tests

In Josh's case, where anaphylaxis has occurred, it is more judicious to test for the presence of serum anti-IgE antibodies specific for peanut or shellfish proteins because these are the most potent food allergens. In general, in this test a patient's serum sample is allowed to bind specific antigens. The antigen-antibody complexes that form are detected with fluorescence or radiolabled anti-IgE antibodies. Pharmacia Diagnostics AB offers this test under the common name, Pharmacia CAP System Specific IgE RIA/FEIA. A limitation to this test is that it does not detect most of the IgE antibodies because they are bound to mast cells/basophils. Therefore, a negative result may be a "false negative." Only a positive result is of value in determining an allergy to that particular food when using this test. Once a particular food has been identified, the patient must totally avoid that food and related food groups.

DIAGNOSIS

Josh's symptoms are consistent with an immune-mediated anaphylactic shock reaction. This could progress to a total respiratory arrest in minutes, so urgent action/therapy is needed!

THERAPY

Epinephrine and antihistamines, along with corticosteroids, are important first-line treatments. As well, an intravenous line should be inserted to provide the patient with saline solution. There are a number of drugs you need to consider giving, each acting in slightly different manner, and with different times of onset.

Pharmacologic Intervention

Epinephrine

Epinephrine needs to be given first! Subcutaneous administration of epinephrine produces an immediate response (seconds to minutes). It is the treatment of choice because it stimulates α-, β1-, and β2-adrenergic receptors. Stimulation of β2-adrenergic receptors leads to an increase in cyclic adenosine monophosphate and relaxation of smooth muscles surrounding the bronchi and bronchioles, which results in bronchodilation (eliminates wheezing). Additionally, β2 agonists enhance clearance of mucus and inhibit the release of inflammatory mediators from mast cells/basophils. Stimulation of α-adrenergic receptors constricts blood vessels and increases heart rate and blood pressure. The action of epinephrine lasts for 30 to 90 minutes.

Antihistamines

Histamine mediates its effects via cognate receptors located on the surface of cells. At least four (H1-H4) different types of histamine receptors have been identified, but histamine binding to H1 receptors is responsible for the allergic and anaphylactic responses. When antihistamines bind to H1 receptors, histamine binding is prevented and this counters the action of histamine. The time to action of antihistamines is 5 to 30 minutes and effects last 2 to 4 hours. Often someone demonstrating symptoms of a food allergy or peptic ulcer will benefit from H2 blocker therapy, as well as an H1 blocker (directed to gastrointestinal tract receptors).

Corticosteroids

Corticosteroids (e.g., prednisone) are potent anti-inflammatory agents whose direct mode of action is unclear. Their effect begins in 4 to 8 hours, and lasts up to 24 hours. There is a well-described "second peak" of inflammatory mediator release occurring some 6 to 8 hours after the first response, presumably caused by persistent sensitizing antigen that re-stimulates the system as the inherent regulation (from within, or without [e.g., epinephrine]) wanes. Corticosteroids "on board" from an early time will begin to be effective just at the time this problem "rears its ugly head."

Long-Term Care

Many allergic reactions are inconvenient but not life threatening. Welts after insect bites (local histamine release to insect saliva) and orbital edema on exposure to cat/animal dander are two such examples (Fig. 14-1). Other allergies kill people! These life-threatening allergies include some food allergies (nuts/shellfish) and some allergies to insect stings (yellow jackets). Therefore, Josh should be advised to carry an epinephrine-containing pen (Epi-Pen) to deliver immediate epinephrine in the event of re-exposure, as well as diphenhydramine (Benadryl) (to

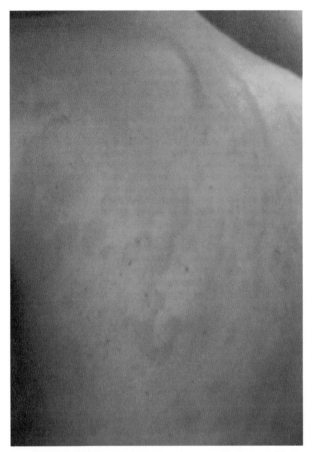

FIGURE 14–1 Typical wheal and erythema of allergic urticaria in a patient with peanut allergy.

be taken after epinephrine, as the patient is en route to the hospital). A medic-alert bracelet (in case a patient is ever unable to communicate significant medical history to caregivers) is essential.

Note that it would be well to advise this person that allergies tend to generalize over time. For example, if Josh's reaction was in response to peanuts (or peanut oil), he may, over time, be unable to tolerate any nuts. A shrimp allergy will often generalize to all shellfish (lobster, oysters, crab). The forewarning of this generalization may be merely the stomach cramps and diarrhea, but a patient may be unlucky and the only warning may be a full-blown systemic anaphylactic reaction carrying the risk of death.

IMMUNE-MEDIATED ANAPHYLAXIS

Immune-mediated anaphylaxis is the effector phase, or clinical manifestation, of a type I hypersensitivity reaction. These reactions are, as the term implies, an

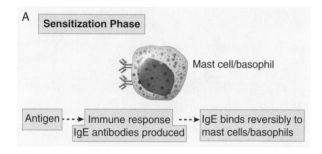

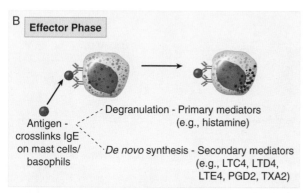

FIGURE 14–2 Sensitization (**A**) and effector (**B**) phases of type I hypersensitivity reactions. **A,** In the initial response to the allergen, IgE antibodies are generated, but by this time the allergen has long been removed from the system, so there is no antigen available to bind the newly generated IgE. Consequently, IgE antibodies bind to Fcε receptors present on mast cells and basophils. **B,** The effector phase is initiated when allergens (e.g., food allergen) enter the circulation and crosslink two IgE antibodies bound via their Fc regions to Fcε receptors on mast cells or basophils, which leads to the release of primary mediators and, subsequently, secondary mediators of inflammation. (Modified with permission from Gorczynski R, Stanley J: Clinical Immunology. Austin, Landes, 1999.)

exaggerated (hyper) response to an allergen and occur only after a sensitization phase in which IgE antibodies are produced. In Josh's case, it appears that the allergen is a protein, perhaps found in peanut oil or in shellfish.

Sensitization Phase

In the initial response to the allergen, IgE antibodies do not appear for at least 7 to 10 days after protein ingestion because of the length of time required for B cells to undergo antigen-induced differentiation and isotype switching to IgE. By this time, the allergen has long been removed from the system, so there is no antigen available to bind the newly generated IgE. Consequently, IgE antibodies bind to Fcε receptors present on mast cells and basophils (Fig. 14–2A).

Although circulating IgE antibodies have a very short half-life, antibodies bound to mast cells can persist for months. Because these IgE antibodies are bound via their Fc regions, the antigen-binding sites are readily available to bind the allergen should it enter the system again. An absolute requirement for a type I hypersensitivity reaction is the localization of IgE antibodies on mast cells and basophils, and so the effector phase/clinical manifestation cannot occur in the absence of previous exposure to the allergen.

Effector Phase

In cases of food allergies, there is a breakdown in oral tolerance such that allergen-specific IgE antibodies are generated and bind to mast cells/basophils. The effector phase is initiated when allergens (e.g., food allergen) enter the circulation and crosslink two IgE antibodies bound via their Fc regions to Fcε receptors on mast cells or basophils (see Fig. 14–2B). When the allergen crosslinks the IgE antibodies on these cells, tyrosine kinases are activated and numerous proteins are phosphorylated, including phospholipase Cγ1 and Cγ2. It is thought that this phosphorylation event triggers phospholipase C activation because inositol phospholipids are degraded and calcium is released from intracellular stores. Following these signal transduction events, mast cells degranulate, causing the release of histamine, proteases, and chemotactic factors. Crosslinking of IgE on the surface of mast cells/basophils also leads to the activation of phospholipase A_2. In some cases, this manifests as allergic urticaria.

Mast Cell–Derived Inflammatory Mediators

Inflammatory products released from mast cell/basophil granules are referred to as primary mediators (e.g., histamine). In addition to degranulation, crosslinking of IgE on the surface of mast cells/basophils leads to the activation of phospholipase A_2 and release of arachidonic acid from membrane lipids. Different products are derived from arachidonic acid, depending on the enzyme that oxygenates this fatty acid. Thromboxane A_2 (TXA_2) and prostaglandin D_2 (PGD_2) are produced when cyclooxygenase acts on arachidonic acid, but the action of lipoxygenase on this fatty acid leads to the generation of leukotrienes (LTC4, LTD4, and LTE4). Inflammatory products that are generated in this manner are referred to as secondary mediators.

Histamine Release from Mast Cells and Basophils

For the most part, mast cell/basophil degranulation occurs in response to cross linking of IgE or following binding of the complement anaphylatoxins (C3a, C4a, C5a) to cognate receptors. However, some compounds can stimulate histamine release from mast cells/basophils directly (e.g., wasp venom, bradykinin, intravenous injection of morphine). Ingestion of scombroid fish (e.g., tuna) infected with bacteria that have a high histidine content can produce symptoms similar to those discussed previously. These bacteria decarboxylate histidine to form histamine, which is a major cause of the just-described clinical presentation.

Role of Histamine in Vasodilation

Irrespective of the trigger for histamine release, a series of inflammatory events ensue after binding of histamine to H1 or H2 receptors on smooth muscles and glands. (H3 receptors are expressed on histaminergic neurons; H4 receptors are present on peripheral blood cells, spleen, and thymus.) In the cardiovascular system, histamine binds to both H1 receptors on vascular endothelial cells and H2 receptors on vascular smooth muscle cells. Although both of these signals leads to vasodilatation of small blood vessels, the responses vary in a number of ways, including the duration of response, which is more sustained after binding to H2 receptors.

Role of Histamine in Increased Vascular Permeability

Histamine binding to H1 receptors on arterioles leads to vasodilatation, but binding to H1 receptors on postcapillary venules leads to contraction of the endothelial cells and a widening of the interendothelial spaces such that the basement membrane is exposed. Because the basement membrane is permeable to serum, this leads to an increase in vascular permeability and edema. Laryngeal edema may cause obstruction of the upper airways.

Role of Histamine in the Gut

Contraction of the gut is mediated via stimulation of H1 receptors. It should not be surprising, therefore, that food allergy will often present as nausea, stomach cramps, and diarrhea, because histamine release in the gastrointestinal tract stimulates smooth muscle H1 receptors to cause contractions in the intestinal wall. Other mediators are also released that (transiently) alter membrane fluid exchanges and cause the watery diarrhea. (Acid secretion by parietal cells in the stomach is mediated by H2 receptors.)

Role of Histamine in Bronchi

Histamine binding to H1 receptors on smooth muscle that surrounds the bronchi and bronchioles leads to bronchoconstriction and difficulty in breathing.

Role of Leukotrienes and Prostaglandins

Leukotrienes and prostaglandins (inflammatory mediators) bind to their respective receptors on smooth muscle cells. LTE4, LTD4, and LTC4 are potent bronchoconstrictors and induce mucus secretion when they bind to recCysLT1 (receptor). Their action on the vasculature leads to an increase in vascular permeability. Thromboxane A_2 (TXA_2) is a potent vasoconstrictor and mediates its effects after binding to TXA_2 receptors. PGD_2/receptor interaction leads to increased mucus secretion and bronchoconstriction. Pulmonary obstruction is accentuated by hypersecretion of mucus. Both the leukotrienes and PGD_2 are more potent bronchoconstrictors than histamine.

A 23-year-old woman, LL, is seen in your office complaining of flu-like symptoms that had persisted for several weeks. A physician at a local walk-in clinic gave her an antibiotic 2 weeks ago. She does not remember the name of it, but she finished the course of medications 3 days before coming to your office. She has noticed progressive pain in her hands and feet, and this morning on arising she noticed tender small bluish red spots on her fingertips. Your routine physical examination reveals nothing else of note. She is not a smoker, and she is currently afebrile. You order routine blood work and are called by the laboratory director when he noted the results indicated that she was profoundly anemic (see Appendix for reference values). At this stage you need to consider possible explanations for these findings; how might you investigate further?

QUESTIONS FOR GROUP DISCUSSION

1. LL is profoundly anemic. Explain why (a) newly discovered lung cancer and (b) iron deficiency would not be high on your list of considerations given the information provided.
2. Under what conditions can young females "normally" become iron deficient?
3. This young woman's condition appears to be linked with an infection and the administration of antibiotics. Describe the mechanism by which a drug (antibiotic) can lead to hemolytic anemia.
4. The classic tests to detect the presence of anti-drug antibodies are the direct and indirect Coombs' tests. Compare and contrast these two tests.
5. The results of both Coombs' tests were negative. Yet, as LL's physician you are convinced that the cause of her anemia is related to her recent infection and so you request an assay for cold agglutinins. Provide the rationale for this approach.
6. The cross-reacting IgM antibodies described in question 5 are referred to as "cold agglutinins." Explain why they are so named.
7. Describe the etiology of cold agglutinin disease and why it manifests as small bluish red spots on fingertips (or outer extremities).
8. What would you recommend for therapy?

RECOMMENDED APPROACH

Implications/Analysis of Family History

No family history is provided.

Implications/Analysis of Clinical History

A prolonged infection that does not resolve with antibiotics could indicate an infection with a drug-resistant strain of bacteria. However, this would not explain the progressive pain in her hands and feet nor the tender small bluish red spots on her fingertips.

Implications/Analysis of Laboratory Investigation

A hemoglobin count of 86 g/L is of concern, and it is important to get to the root of the problem. A number of conditions can manifest as severe anemia, one of the most common being iron deficiency in young women who bleed heavily during menstruation. However, there is nothing in the clinical history to indicate this. Furthermore, this would not be associated with an infection.

A drug-induced hemolytic anemia would certainly be high on the list of possibilities here in that she has just completed a course of antibiotic medication. In drug-induced anemia, red cells bind a drug (non-specifically) and act as a "carrier" for presentation of a hapten (the drug) to the immune system. Anti-drug antibodies are generated and bind to the drug on the red blood cell surface. The resulting immune complexes engage the classical complement pathway, resulting in red cell lysis and anemia.

Additional Laboratory Tests

Further laboratory investigation using the direct and indirect Coombs' tests can be used to confirm (or rule

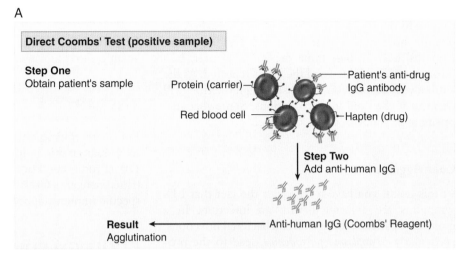

A

Direct Coombs' Test (positive sample)

Step One
Obtain patient's sample

Protein (carrier)
Red blood cell

Patient's anti-drug
IgG antibody
Hapten (drug)

Step Two
Add anti-human IgG

Anti-human IgG (Coombs' Reagent)

Result
Agglutination

FIGURE 15–1 Testing for a type II hypersensitivity reaction. **A,** In the direct Coombs' test, IgG antibodies that are bound to red blood cells are identified using anti-Fcγ antibodies generated in another species. When the anti-Fcγ antibodies crosslink anti-drug IgG antibodies, agglutination is observed and the sample is "positive." **B,** In the indirect Coombs' test we are testing for the presence of circulating anti-drug IgG antibodies in serum. Therefore, an additional step is required before agglutination can be observed. This step is the incubation of LL's serum with the red blood cells, (to which the drug has bound) to allow LL's anti-drug antibodies (if present) to bind to the red blood cell complex. Thereafter, the test is the same as that described for the direct Coombs' test.

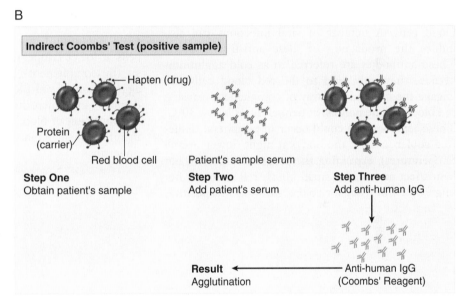

B

Indirect Coombs' Test (positive sample)

Hapten (drug)

Protein
(carrier)
Red blood cell

Step One
Obtain patient's sample

Patient's sample serum

Step Two
Add patient's serum

Step Three
Add anti-human IgG

Result
Agglutination

Anti-human IgG
(Coombs' Reagent)

out) drug-induced anemia as the cause of LL's clinical presentation.

Coombs' Tests

In the direct and indirect Coombs' tests, a positive result is the visible manifestation of agglutination, resulting from aggregation and sedimentation of particulate antigen-antibody complexes (Fig. 15–1). In this case, the direct Coombs' test was used to determine whether anti-drug IgG antibodies had formed and attached to drug/red blood cell complexes (Fig. 15–1A). The bound IgG antibodies are identified

using anti-Fcγ antibodies generated in another species. When the anti-Fcγ antibodies crosslink anti-drug IgG antibodies, agglutination is observed and the sample is "positive."

Indirect Coombs' Tests

In contrast, in the indirect Coombs' test we are testing for the presence of circulating anti-drug IgG antibodies in serum (see Fig. 15–1B). Therefore, an additional step is required before agglutination can be observed. This step is the incubation of LL's serum with the red blood cells (to which we are assuming the drug has bound) to allow LL's anti-drug antibodies (if present) to bind to the red blood cell complex. Thereafter, the test is the same as that described for the direct Coombs' test. To determine the antibody titer, LL's serum is serially diluted and the test is repeated. As the antibody concentration increases, agglutination will occur at higher and higher dilutions. Somewhat surprisingly to you, this test is negative!

Cold Agglutinins

At this point, you have to consider the fact that LL's symptoms are coincident with an infection. In a number of patients, some viral and bacterial infections, particularly *Mycoplasma pneumoniae*, lead to the production of IgM antibodies that cross react with glycophorin (Ii), a protein present on the surface of red blood cells. A number of viral infections can also induce the production of these anti-Ii antibodies. These antibodies are referred to as cold agglutinins because they only bind to the red blood cells and engage the classical pathway of complement (causing red blood cell hemolysis) at temperatures below 30°C. These temperatures could occur in peripheral tissues (the cooler parts of the body) at night (lower overall temperatures), explaining the progressive pain in her hands/feet and tender small bluish red spots on her fingertips. The assay for cold agglutinins was positive.

DIAGNOSIS

LL was diagnosed with autoimmune hemolytic anemia, also known as cold agglutinin disease.

THERAPY

For acute cold agglutinin disease, a good (conservative) treatment is simply to keep the periphery warm! For chronic conditions, pharmacologic intervention (rituximab: anti-CD20 antibody) may be an option for specific immunosuppression.

ETIOLOGY: COLD AGGLUTININ DISEASE

Cold agglutinins preferentially bind to red blood cells at lower temperatures with subsequent hemolysis (by complement), phagocytosis, or often simply aggregation of red blood cells, resulting in capillary damage and microthrombi. The net effect is the accumulation of blood in the extravascular space that manifests as small bluish red spots (as appeared on LL's fingertips).

DF is a 25-year-old woman, pregnant for the third time. She is known to have blood group A, Rh negative (Rh−) red cells. Her husband is also type A but Rh positive (Rh+). Their first-born child, a boy, was healthy but during the second pregnancy DF was noted to have an indirect Coombs' titer of 1:32 in her serum. This fetus was followed closely, and a healthy baby girl was induced (vaginal delivery) at 36 weeks of gestation. DF received RhoGam after this delivery. It is now 3 years later and DF is pregnant again. You are monitoring her indirect Coombs' antibody titer and find it to be 1:32 at 12 weeks and 1:48 at 18 weeks. Amniotic fluid was obtained beginning at 22 weeks of gestation and every 2 weeks thereafter. The amniotic fluid was shown to have increasing amounts of bilirubin (a pigment derived from a breakdown of heme), suggesting hemolysis of fetal red cells. At 28 weeks of gestation, a blood sample obtained from the umbilical vein revealed a hematocrit of 6.2% (normal 45%), confirming profound anemia in the fetus.

QUESTIONS FOR GROUP DISCUSSION

1. The significant point in this case is that the mother is Rh− and the father is Rh+. What is the Rh antigen? What percent of the population is Rh+? What is the potential problem for a fetus whose mother is Rh− and the father is Rh+?

2. Why is the risk of hemolytic disease of the newborn lower during a first pregnancy than for subsequent pregnancies? Include in your discussion how the mother could become sensitized to the Rh antigen during a first pregnancy? At the time of delivery?

3. Explain how maternal anti-Rh antibodies serve as a stimulus for complement-mediated hemolysis of fetal red blood cells. Describe the possible mechanism by which red blood cells would be destroyed after binding of IgG.

4. RhoGam is given to Rh− mothers if there is evidence of bleeding during pregnancy and especially at birth. What is RhoGam?

5. Explain (a) the "older" idea of how RhoGam prevents sensitization of the mother during placental bleeding or during the birthing process and (b) conventional wisdom as to how RhoGam works.

6. Define *hematocrit* and describe how it is determined. Under what circumstances would the fetal hematocrit continue to drop despite the administration of red blood cells into the umbilical vein?

7. Explain why the fetus was transfused with Rh− packed red blood cells when we already know that the fetus's red blood cells are Rh+.

8. Explain how ABO incompatibility could reduce the likelihood of an Rh− mother being sensitized to the Rh antigen when carrying a child.

9. What test can be used to determine if the mother has circulating anti-Rh antibodies? At what antibody titer is the fetus considered to be at risk for hemolytic disease?

10. Explain how the serum of an Rh− mother who is pregnant with an Rh+ child gives a negative indirect Coombs' test but agglutinates Rh+ cell in saline (see Case 15).

RECOMMENDED APPROACH

Implications/Analysis of Family History

The Rh antigen incompatibility between DF and her husband is of significance here because she is pregnant. The Rh antigen, so named because it was first identified on rhesus monkey erythrocytes (red blood cells), is expressed by about 85% of humans. When an Rh− individual becomes exposed (sensitized) to red blood cells expressing the Rh antigens, an immune response is generated because this is a foreign antigen. IgM and IgG anti-Rh antibodies are formed. This is of concern when an Rh− female is pregnant because IgG antibodies cross the placenta (see Etiology).

Differences in red blood cell antigens are more common in the ABO classification. ABO refers to the blood group cell surface glycolipids (antigens) used to classify red blood cells into four major groups: (1) red blood cells with A glycolipids, (2) with B glycolipids, (3) with both A and B glycolipids, and (4) red blood cells that do not express these antigens. Individuals are classed as A, B, or AB positive. Individuals who do not express either the A or B antigens are designated as having "O" blood type. In this case both DF and her husband were "A" positive, and so there was no incompatibility.

Implications/Analysis of Clinical History

This couple's first child was healthy, and there is no indication of any problem associated with the Rh incompatibility. During DF's second pregnancy, careful monitoring of antibody titers for anti-Rh antibodies indicated that DF had been sensitized to red blood cells expressing the Rh antigen and had generated anti-Rh IgG antibodies, but her antibody titer was relatively low. Antibody titer refers to the highest dilution of the serum that still induces agglutination of particles coated with the Rh antigen (see Implications/Analysis of Laboratory Investigation). After this delivery, DF was given RhoGam, an IgG anti-Rh antibody preparation. The mechanism by which it mediates its effects is not clear (see Etiology).

Implications/Analysis of Laboratory Investigation

Direct Coombs' Test

The direct Coombs' test is used to detect the presence of maternal anti-Rh IgG antibodies that have bound to the fetal red blood cells (see Case 15). The subsequent addition of anti-Fcγ antibodies, generated in another species, manifests in agglutination when (maternal) IgG antibodies are bound to the fetal red blood cells. This test is used when testing newborns for the presence of maternal IgG antibodies bound directly to the Rh antigen on their red blood cells.

Indirect Coombs' Test

In contrast, in the indirect Coombs' test we are testing for the presence of circulating anti-Rh IgG antibodies in serum (see Case 15). Therefore, an additional step is required. Red blood cells may be obtained from any source, the criteria (in this case) being that they express the Rh antigen. The mother's serum is then allowed to react with these (allo or xeno) red blood cells, which will bind anti-Rh antibodies (if) present in the mother's serum. Thereafter, the test is the same as that described for the direct Coombs' test. Anti-IgG antibodies are added and the sample is considered positive for anti-Rh antibodies if agglutination manifests (see Case 15).

Bilirubin

The amniotic fluid was monitored for the presence of bilirubin, which would indicate that fetal red blood cells are being lysed. Bilirubin, a pigment derived from the breakdown of heme (following phagocytosis of red blood cells) is released into plasma (or in this case into the amniotic fluid) where it can be detected. Red blood cells are packed with hemoglobin, a tetrameric protein synthesized by nucleated precursors (while in the bone marrow). A heme prosthetic group, to which an iron atom is incorporated, is covalently attached to each hemoglobin subunit. Hemoglobin is able to carry oxygen to the tissues because oxygen binds reversibly to the iron. The presence of bilirubin in the amniotic fluid, therefore, is an indication that fetal red blood cells are being destroyed.

Hematocrit

Under these conditions there is concern that the fetus might be anemic and so a blood sample was obtained from the umbilical vein to determine the volume of packed red blood cells in a given unit of blood (hematocrit). A hematocrit of 6.2% (normal 45%) indicated profound anemia in the fetus.

Additional Laboratory Tests

Therapy was initiated (see Therapy) and the hematocrit monitored at 31, 34, and 35 weeks of gestation. The fetus was examined at weekly intervals for the appearance of hydrops (fetal subcutaneous tissue edema), caused by altered oncotic pressure differences (serum vs. interstitial fluid) after hemolysis, with consistently negative results. To determine when the fetus was sufficiently mature to sustain extrauterine life without difficulty, measures of surfactant were taken regularly. Infants born prematurely may have a risk of respiratory distress syndrome if they lack surfactant in alveoli. In the absence of surfactant the alveoli collapse during expiration.

DIAGNOSIS

The fetus was determined to have profound anemia.

THERAPY

Because the fetus was profoundly anemic, 85 mL of type O, Rh– packed red blood cells were transfused into the umbilical vein. At 31 weeks of gestation another sample of blood was obtained from the umbilical vein and tests indicated that the hematocrit was only 19%, indicating that the fetus's red blood cells were still being destroyed. The fetus was transfused with an additional 65 mL of type O, Rh– packed red blood cells. At 34 weeks of gestation the hematocrit of a blood sample from the umbilical vein was 22%, resulting in an order for a further 70 mL of type O Rh– packed red blood cells to be transfused into the umbilical vein. At 35 weeks of gestation all measures indicated that the fetus was sufficiently mature (especially pulmonary/cardiac) to sustain extrauterine life without difficulty. Accordingly, labor was induced and a normal female child was delivered. The hematocrit in the umbilical vein blood at this time was 30%. The infant did well thereafter, and no further therapeutic measures were necessary.

HEMOLYTIC DISEASE OF THE FETUS

The rhesus incompatibility between an Rh– mother and an Rh+ offspring (the latter inherited Rh+ from the father) results in the production of anti-Rh antibodies when the mother is exposed to Rh+ red blood cells. This generally happens during birth in the first pregnancy but may occur before that if there is placental bleeding. The anti-Rh antibodies, so formed, bind any Rh+ red blood cells and this can cause red blood cell hemolysis in subsequent fetuses when IgG antibodies cross the placenta.

We generally assume (if this cannot be measured ahead of time) that every pregnant woman is Rh– and carrying an Rh+ child. Under these circumstances RhoGam is given as a precaution for any bleeding during pregnancy, and especially at birth. RhoGam is given to prevent sensitization and production of anti-Rh antibodies by the mother. This is *not* necessary if we *know* the mother is Rh+!

Mode of Action: RhoGam

RhoGam consists of an IgG anti-Rh antibody preparation. The mechanism by which it mediates its effects is not clear. It was previously believed that RhoGam "mopped up" or masked Rh antigen so the immune system never saw this antigen as a foreign determinant. In fact the amount of RhoGam given is *not* probably adequate for this to be the case. Conventional wisdom suggests instead that the immune complex formed

(Rh:anti-Rh) is preferentially tolerogenic and induces regulatory cells of some kind.

Destruction of Red Blood Cells

The formation of antigen-antibody complexes on the surface of red blood cells would suggest that their destruction is the result of complement activation. Recall, however, that activation of complement requires the strategic location of two IgG antibodies so that C1q can simultaneously bind two Fc regions, a requirement for complement activation. It has been suggested that Rh antigens are so sparsely scattered at the red cell surface that IgG molecules bound to the Rh antigens are too far apart to fix C1q for complement-mediated hemolysis to occur. In consequence, it is thought that red blood cells (coated with anti-Rh IgG antibodies) adhere tightly to Fcγ receptors on macrophages present in the red pulp of the spleen and Kupffer cells of the liver. This results in FcR opsonin-mediated phagocytosis and destruction. Consistent with this hypothesis, most IgG antibody to the Rh antigen is of the IgG3 or IgG1 subclass, the IgG subclasses that bind most tightly to the high-affinity Fcγ receptor (CD64) present on macrophages and neutrophils.

Anti-Rh Antibody Titers

As a rough "rule of thumb" the amount of RhoGam we give passively (and safely, even if there is a Rh+ fetus present) is estimated to result in a maternal titer in the indirect Coombs' test of less than 1:4. Thus, we acknowledge that such a titer of Rh antibody cannot cause significant hemolysis in the fetus. If the maternal titer is greater than 1:4, she has been alloimmunized by her fetus and the fetus is in need of careful monitoring. Note that the transfusion *must* be of Rh– red blood cells!

Effect of IgM Anti-Rh Antibodies on a Coombs' test

Consider a scenario in which the serum of an Rh– woman, who is pregnant, gives a negative indirect Coombs' test but agglutinates Rh+ cells suspended in saline. The most likely explanation for this phenomenon is that she has IgM anti-Rh antibodies that, being pentameric, are very effective in agglutinating Rh+ cells in saline, unlike IgG anti-Rh antibodies.

However, because IgM antibodies do not cross the placenta they are unlikely to cause a problem with the pregnancy. It would be wise to monitor her anti-Rh antibodies to ensure she does not (later) develop a positive indirect Coombs' test, signifying the presence of IgG antibodies.

Effect of ABO Incompatibility on Rh Alloimmunization

Note that ABO incompatibility between mother and father can itself modulate immunization to Rh determinants. Why? In the presence of ABO incompatibility, the mother would already have preexisting anti-A or anti-B IgM antibodies (isohemagglutinins). Therefore, when (and if) fetal blood enters the maternal circulation, IgM immune complexes would activate complement; fetal red blood cells would be quickly hemolyzed. This rapid destruction/elimination of the fetal red blood cells would decrease the likelihood of Rh alloimmunization of the mother.

Edward is 35 years old and has noted some general malaise over the past few months with some weight gain and bloating. He notices his feet, in particular, are quite swollen. When he urinates he has seen some darker tinges to the urine, even when he is clearly not passing concentrated urine (as in the morning). What has finally brought him to the doctor's office is some bright red sputum he coughed up this morning. He is not, and never has been, a smoker. He has had no recent symptoms suggestive of a respiratory disease and he is currently afebrile. His physician ordered routine blood chemistry, a complete blood cell count with differential, a Mantoux test, and a chest radiograph. Explain the rationale for requesting each of these laboratory tests.

QUESTIONS FOR GROUP DISCUSSION

1. Edward's primary concern is the red sputum, which he believes is blood. Although you would certainly want to investigate the possibility of a malignancy, you would not have this as the most likely cause. Explain.

2. Infection may be an issue, but if so it must be of a chronic nature such as cytomegalovirus or *Mycobacterium tuberculosis*. About which risk factors would you want to ask your patient to help rule out tuberculosis? What tests would you request?

3. In addition to the red-tinged sputum, you need to consider the weight gain (as per description), some peripheral edema, and blood in the urine. Which of these issues could be caused by a (a) liver-related problem? (b) kidney-related problem? Explain. How would you proceed to investigate this?

4. Blood chemistry revealed elevated potassium and creatinine levels. What potential problem is indicated by these results?

5. A 24-hour urine collection revealed that Edward is spilling a considerable amount of red blood cells and protein into the urine. What does this result indicate?

6. You have a patient with evidence for both lung and renal involvement. While the possibility exists that this unfortunate man has multiple problems, Occam's razor suggests that we try to explain both with one diagnosis. What feature(s) are common to both lungs and kidney?

7. Direct binding of autoantibodies to antigens of the basement membrane could trigger an inflammatory response that would present in the manner described in this case. Review the immunologic processes that would lead to the pathologic process observed.

8. What autoimmune disorders would you now suspect?

9. Explain how a biopsy with immunofluorescent staining could help you in your diagnosis of Goodpasture's syndrome, an autoimmune disorder in which antibody binding to the basement membrane leads to kidney problems, versus an autoimmune disorder in which antigen-antibody complexes lodge in the glomeruli and trigger an inflammatory response.

10. An enzyme-linked immunosorbent assay (ELISA) could be used to support the results of your biopsy. For what specific autoantibodies would you be testing?

RECOMMENDED APPROACH

Implications/Analysis of Family History

No information is provided regarding family history.

Implications/Analysis of Clinical History

Edward's primary concern is the red (blood-tinged?) sputum, and you certainly need to consider this along with other clinical presentations. Obviously there will be some concern over malignancy, but there are no obvious risk factors, and so other causes should be pursued first. Infection remains a possibility, but it must be of a chronic nature if this is causative. Certainly, tuberculosis might present this way, but one would expect a weight loss not a weight gain. Despite this, it is still important to ask about travel and exposure, both of which are risk factors for this disease. A chest radiograph and a Mantoux test were ordered to rule out exposure to *Mycobacterium tuberculosis*, the causative agent of tuberculosis.

The other issues that need explanation are the weight gain, bloating, some peripheral edema (swollen feet), and dark urine. The dark urine may be an indication of blood or bilirubin (a pigment derived from a breakdown of heme from red blood cells). Because bilirubin is metabolized in the liver, this may reflect a liver-related problem. However, this may also indicate a disorder of the renal filtration system because the renal glomerulus normally filters out red blood cells. Disorders of the renal filtration system, therefore, can lead to leakage of protein (causing osmotic shifts and edema) as well as to blood-tinged urine.

Implications/Analysis of Laboratory Investigation

The Mantoux test was negative and the chest radiograph was uninformative, although a sputum sample showed red blood cells and neutrophils, indicating an inflammatory response in the respiratory system. However, sputum culture to establish whether an infection was the stimulus for the inflammatory response indicated only normal lung/buccal flora.

Routine blood chemistry and a complete blood cell count will help to develop understanding of this problem. In this case, chemistry revealed elevated serum creatinine and potassium levels, both reflective of a potential problem in renal filtration. Creatinine, a protein released by muscles, is released into the blood and the rate at which it is removed is an indication of kidney function. An increase in serum creatinine and potassium values indicates that neither is being removed as efficiently as it should be (a normal process in the healthy functioning kidney), but verification requires a creatinine clearance test. The white blood cell count indicated an increase in both neutrophils and lymphocytes. In the absence of infection, an increase in both neutrophils and lymphocytes suggests that there is an ongoing immune response, as would occur in autoimmune disorders.

Additional Laboratory Tests

To examine kidney function in more detail, a 24-hour urine collection was ordered to measure creatinine clearance (which is not affected by muscle mass). In effect, this test measures the decrease in serum/blood creatinine over a period of time. When serum creatinine concentration is elevated, one would expect a low clearance rate for creatinine, as this test indicated.

Additionally, an assay of the urine collected indicated that Edward is spilling red blood cells and a considerable amount of protein into the urine (both normally filtered out at the glomerulus and returned to the circulation).

Occam's Razor

At this stage you have a patient with evidence for both lung and renal involvement. Occam's razor suggests we try to explain both with one diagnosis, rather than presume this unfortunate man has multiple problems (but remember...this can happen!). Because both the lung and kidney have a basement membrane that looks (immunologically speaking) the same, an inflammation at this membrane could produce the very pathologic process we are observing.

Biopsy and Staining

An antibody-mediated inflammatory reaction at this site will cause the pathophysiology described previously. You should request a biopsy of the relevant affected organs (lung-transbronchial biopsy; renal biopsy) and also staining of tissues (immunofluorescence assay [IFA]) to look for evidence of immunoglobulin deposition. For the IFA, the patient's serum is deposited on a normal kidney tissue section. To detect autoantibodies that have bound to the tissue, fluorescein-labeled anti-human IgG (or IgA) antibodies are added. Not only is the presence of fluorescein-labeled antibodies diagnostic, but so is the pattern of fluorescence that is observed. If the autoantibodies are bound directly to the tissue (e.g., Goodpasture's syndrome), a ribbon-like pattern is observed. In contrast, if preformed immune complexes have been deposited in the tissues (e.g., systemic lupus erythematosus [SLE], rheumatoid arthritis [RA]), the pattern will appear to be "lumpy bumpy."

Staining of Edward's tissue indicated a ribbon-like (smooth linear) deposit of antibody along the glomerular capillaries (basement membrane), which is consistent with a diagnosis of Goodpasture's disease. It is important to determine the cause of the pathology, not only because the treatment will be different but also because the longer-term prognosis and course of disease will be very different. The IFA test does not detect specific antibodies, rather it detects any IgG and IgA antibodies that are bound directly to the basement membrane.

Confirmatory Test

An ELISA can be performed to confirm that the patient's serum contains antibodies specific for the globular domain of collagen IV polypeptides, which is present in the glomerular basement membrane.

DIAGNOSIS

A diagnosis of Goodpasture's syndrome, an autoimmune disorder, was confirmed. This is another excellent example of a type II antibody-mediated hypersensitivity reaction (mediated by antibody binding direct to antigen on a cell surface, with subsequent induction of inflammation and pathology, via complement- and/or Fc-mediated events).

THERAPY

Plasmapheresis to remove the circulating anti–basement membrane antibodies, along with potent immunosuppression is the recommended therapy.

ETIOLOGY: GOODPASTURE'S SYNDROME

Goodpasture's syndrome is a rare autoimmune disorder in which autoantibodies bind to antigenic determinants in the basement membrane of the lungs (alveoli) and kidneys (glomeruli). These antigen/antibody complexes activate the classical pathway of complement and phagocytes, which results in inflammation in the glomeruli (glomerulonephritis) and bleeding in the lungs (pulmonary hemorrhage). Normally, the alveolar endothelium prevents antibody contact with the basement membrane; therefore, an increase in alveolar-capillary permeability, as occurs in a nonspecific inflammation, must occur to allow the anti–basement membranes access to the basement membrane epitopes.

18

Doris is a 25-year-old married black woman. Over the past 6 months she has noticed increasing swelling in her legs with "frothy" dark urine and she has had intermittent severe headaches, unrelated to menses. Despite her and her husband's wishes, she has been unable to conceive for 5 years and now has had three spontaneous abortions, all in the first 8 to 12 weeks of pregnancy. Query into the family history indicated that she was an adopted child. A detailed analysis of Doris's serum immunoglobulin, a complete blood cell count, and blood chemistry was ordered. Laboratory results indicated a mild increase in leukocytes, elevated IgG and serum creatinine levels, but a mild thrombocytopenia. Additionally, urinalysis indicated that she was spilling protein in her urine, along with some red cells.

QUESTIONS FOR GROUP DISCUSSION

1. What is the significance of leg swelling and urinary problems in an otherwise healthy 25-year-old? List the three facts that indicate that Doris has urinary problems.

2. Explain why a kidney infection or kidney stone is not high on your list of considerations. In the absence of these conditions, what would the spilling of protein and red blood cells into the urine suggest?

3. Noninfectious inflammation in the kidneys as a consequence of autoantibodies could trigger an inflammatory response. In some conditions, autoantibodies bind directly to cells forming immune complexes. In other conditions, autoantibodies form complexes with soluble antigens. These complexes may lodge in small vessels and trigger inflammatory processes. Explain how the inflammatory response would be triggered, irrespective of which of these two scenarios was occurring (see Case 23).

4. Despite the similarities with respect to urinalysis and elevated serum creatinine, there are differences with respect to clinical presentation in this patient and the one described in Case 17. Discuss these differences.

5. Doris has had severe intermittent headaches. Although this could be a forerunner of a central nervous system (CNS) malignancy, we should consider immunologic causes of headaches, given the apparent noninfectious inflammation in the kidney. What immunologic conditions can cause headaches?

6. Doris has had three spontaneous abortions. Are there any immunologic causes that can lead to spontaneous abortions? Explain how this would occur.

7. Given the diverse spectrum of symptoms, we could consider multiple causes or focus on a systemic autoimmune disorder. Explain how immune complex deposition could account for both the renal problems and the headaches.

8. What might you expect to see if we measured the serum C3 levels? Why? How could you use this "marker" to monitor active disease or therapy?

9. What would you expect to see if you performed a biopsy with immunofluorescence staining? Compare/contrast with what was reported in Case 17.

10. This patient has a mild thrombocytopenia. Explain the role that the indirect and the direct Coombs' tests have in determining the cause of thrombocytopenia.

RECOMMENDED APPROACH

Implications/Analysis of Family History

At 25 years of age, congenital defects are unlikely to make their first appearance. Unfortunately, because Doris is adopted we cannot trace any potential genetic susceptibility for her disease. However, we need to consider those disorders in which data indicate a significant ethnic susceptibility in black females.

Implications/Analysis of Clinical History

Peripheral Edema

Leg swelling in an otherwise healthy individual should make you wonder about renal problems (see Case 17). In the absence of infection or an obstruction (kidney stone, which generally presents with pain as severe as childbirth labor!), the peripheral edema suggests noninfectious inflammation "higher up" the urinary tract (in the kidney). Immune complex deposition in the glomeruli, with subsequent complement and neutrophil activation, triggers an inflammatory response that leads to a condition known as glomerulonephritis.

Headaches

In the absence of other causes (both non–life threatening [e.g., migraine] and otherwise [tumor]), headaches are often caused by inflammation within blood vessel walls in the central nervous system (CNS). This vasculitis (cerebritis) is again a result of immune complex deposition on basement membranes/endothelia, with complement and neutrophil activation, resulting in subsequent changes in vessel permeability with edema/release of inflammatory mediators.

Spontaneous Abortion

The spontaneous abortions could be an indication of an autoimmune disease, in which autoantibodies formed cross the placenta and interfere with fetal well-being. Antiphospholipid antibody, the so-called lupus anticoagulant (a misnomer, since it is a cause of thrombosis!) that is detected in about 15% of patients with systemic lupus erythematosus [SLE], has been shown to induce spontaneous abortion. This is presumed to reflect an increased susceptibility to thrombosis in the fetal:maternal circulation with subsequent fetal demise. Several other autoantibodies (antiplatelet, anti-leukocyte, and anti-DNA antibodies) are also formed in SLE patients. These autoantibodies lead to the formation of immune complexes, deposition in the glomeruli, and renal failure (glomerulonephritis).

Implications/Analysis of Laboratory Investigation

Urinalysis revealed that she was spilling protein in her urine, along with some red cells. The presence of protein and red blood cells in her urine would explain the "frothy," dark description.

Laboratory results also indicated an elevated serum creatinine level, which suggests that the kidneys are not clearing creatinine efficiently, and this should be followed with a 24-hour urine collection to measure the rate of clearance (see Case 17). Ineffective clearance of creatinine is consistent with immune complex–mediated damage to the kidneys.

The elevated IgG value indicates that there is an ongoing antibody response. In the absence of an infec-

tion, this is highly suggestive of an autoimmune (or malignant) disease. The mild lymphopenia and thrombocytopenia are both consistent with the presence of autoantibodies causing lysis of both normal white blood cells and platelets. There is no evidence of anemia (autoantibodies to red cells) and so a Coombs' test is not necessary (see Case 15).

Additional Laboratory Tests
Antinuclear Antibody Immunofluorescence Test

Based on the clinical presentation and laboratory investigations, a presumptive diagnosis of SLE would be reasonable. To further investigate this possibility, a request should be made for an antinuclear antibody (ANA) immunofluorescence assay. In this assay the patient's serum is incubated with human epithelioid cells, followed by the addition of antihuman Fcγ fluorescent-labeled (e.g., fluorescein isothiocyanate [FITC]) antibodies for detection. Although a negative result rules out a diagnosis of SLE, a positive result is not confirmatory in that normal patients and those with chronic inflammatory disorders may test positive for ANA (highly sensitive, moderate specificity). In this case, Doris's ANA test was positive, suggesting that she could have SLE.

Anti-DNA test

To support a positive ANA result, the anti-DNA antibody titer, which is commonly measured using an enzyme-linked immunosorbent assay (ELISA), should be determined. This test has moderate sensitivity and high specificity, and so a negative anti-DNA antibody test does not eliminate SLE as a possible diagnosis because not all SLE patients have anti-DNA antibodies. A positive anti-DNA antibody test, combined with a positive ANA, makes a diagnosis of SLE very likely. Doris's anti-DNA antibody titer was significantly high, supporting a diagnosis of SLE.

Complement C3 and C4

In active disease the levels of C3 and C4 are decreased. C3 and C4 are proteolytically cleaved when immune complexes activate the classical pathway of complement. Because C3 and C4 complement protein levels are "concordant" with disease activity, this can be used to monitor disease and its response to therapy.

Kidney Biopsy

The prognosis regarding kidney function is assessed using a renal (glomeruli) biopsy with immunofluorescence staining (Fig. 18–1). This assay detects immune complexes that have been deposited in the basement membrane and endothelia. You would expect to see bright staining that appears "lumpy and bumpy," indicating that the detected autoantibodies are part of a preformed immune complex and not simply bound to the basement membrane.

DIAGNOSIS

Doris has systemic lupus erythematosus.

THERAPY

Therapy for SLE consists of high doses of corticosteroid (intermittent cyclophosphamide for kidney disease).

ETIOLOGY: SYSTEMIC LUPUS ERYTHEMATOSUS

SLE is a multisystem/systemic disorder with manifestations in multiple organs/tissues (see Cases 22 and 31). There is a known genetic association with human leukocyte antigens (HLA) DR2/DR3. Further evidence for genetic susceptibility in SLE is the greater concordance in monozygotic (MZ) rather than dizygotic (DZ) twins (30% vs. <10%). There is also a correlation with the complement C2 and C4 genes and tumor necrosis factor (TNF) receptor genes. Presumably (in a multisystem/multigenic disorder) these genes are all implicated at different stages in either the ontogeny of immune development to antigens that are important in the etiology of the disease or in the subsequent inflammatory responses that follow.

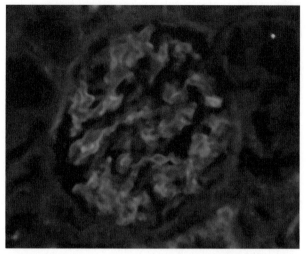

FIGURE 18–1   Lupus nephritis with immune complex deposition. Type III hypersensitivity occurs along the basement membrane of glomerular capillary loops. (Immunofluorescent staining for IgG, ×400.)

The CNS inflammation can often cause very significant CNS pathology. Seizures have been described in this scenario. Neuropsychiatric testing often reveals significant deficits (e.g., in memory, intellectual ability). These are generally not permanent if aggressive treatment of the underlying cause (i.e., SLE) is used. Presumably, the deficits reflect transient neurologic "stunning" from inflammatory processes.

Note that another autoantibody (Anti-Ro antibody), which can be passed from mother to fetus, has been described to cause transient neonatal heart block (potentially fatal fetal arrhythmia). Because the source of this autoantibody is the mother, the condition in the newborn is of a limited duration after birth. The maternal anti-Ro antibodies can be detected in the newborn, but the half life of IgG is 21 days and so the antibodies generally have disappeared by the time the infant is 6 months of age.

A married couple in your practice is planning their first pregnancy. They are both asthmatics, on regular inhalant therapy. They have both been hospitalized twice and one of them was intubated once for exacerbations. They are concerned to know the likelihood of a genetic predisposition, environmental factors, and so on, that might affect development of asthma in their child. You discuss these issues and the classic presentation and diagnosis of asthma.

QUESTIONS FOR GROUP DISCUSSION

1. In very general terms, what are the two main causes of airway obstruction in asthma (see Etiology).
2. Recent studies have attempted to unravel the complexities underlying genetic association and susceptibility to asthma using positional cloning. What is chromosomal linkage? What is the assumption in this approach?
3. Discuss the criteria that have been used to identify atopic individuals. List various gene clusters that are linked to polymorphic genes whose allelic expression is, in turn, associated with atopy in individuals.
4. What is a FEV_1? Explain its role in the diagnosis of asthma.
5. Describe the test used to measure airway hyperresponsiveness to confirm a diagnosis of asthma.
6. Explain the rationale for speculation that the presence of a dog in a family or a rural lifestyle is protective for allergic diseases.
7. Under what circumstances do high levels of IgE correlate with a particular allelic form of FcεR1-β in some Australian aborigines parasitized with helminths?
8. Explain why recent studies are focusing on the role of polymorphisms in the interleukin [IL]-4Rα component of the receptors for IL-4 and IL-13 as a contributory factor in the genetics of asthmatic disorders.
9. Inhaled glucocorticoids and or leukotriene receptor blockade is the presently accepted therapy for asthma. What are leukotrienes? How are they generated? What are the roles of phospholipase A_2 and phospholipase C in leukotriene production?
10. Explain why chemokine receptor antagonists are under investigation as possible therapeutic agents for the treatment of asthma.

RECOMMENDED APPROACH

Implications/Analysis of Family History

Given the fact that both husband and wife are chronic asthmatics, their offspring would be at high risk for developing asthma. Although there is a major genetic component to the underlying cause of asthma, the inherited pattern cannot be classed as autosomal, X-linked, or recessive.

Recent studies using positional cloning have attempted to address the issue of genetic associations. Positional cloning is a technique that attempts to identify polymorphic genes located close to known positions (markers) on chromosomes. The assumption is that the allelic forms of polymorphic genes, relevant for developing allergies, will be common to atopic individuals. Various criteria have been used to identify atopic individuals, including levels of IgE antibodies, a diagnosis of asthma, atopic dermatitis, and so on. On the basis of these studies, common allelic forms of polymorphic genes have been identified because of their link to known gene clusters (markers) on chromosome 2 (close to the interleukin [IL]-1 cluster), chromosome 5 (cytokine gene cluster), chromosome 6 (major histocompatibility complex genes), chromosome 11 (FcεR1-β, receptor for IgE), chromosome 12 (near the interferon gamma [IFNγ] gene cluster), and chromosome 13 (cysteinyl leukotriene 2 receptor), as well as several other chromosomes. Nevertheless there are still hundreds of genes encoded within the clusters of interest. Several cytokines encoded within the cytokine gene cluster on chromosome 5 have been implicated in allergic responses (e.g., IL-4, IL-5, IL-13, granulocyte-macrophage colony-stimulating factor).

Implications/Analysis of Clinical History

A common clinical presentation in infants and children is wheezing, coughing, and shortness of breath as a result of airway obstruction. About 50% of children who are genetically predisposed to asthma have at least one wheezing illness before entering primary school. Many, however, will have one wheezing episode before the age of 1 year. Most of these wheezing incidents are triggered by a viral infection of the respiratory tract. It is important to rule out other causes of wheezing, which include cystic fibrosis, anatomic anomalies, and so on. In adults, the clinical presentation is similar to that described for infants/children, but nonasthmatic causes of wheezing need to be ruled out. In adults this includes emphysema, chronic bronchitis, upper airway obstruction, and so on.

Implications/Analysis of Laboratory Investigations

The initial assessment is the pulmonary function test to determine the baseline level of airflow obstruction. Although more sophisticated equipment and techniques are available in some laboratories, simple spirometry is available in most laboratories. This test is used to obtain two measures (1) FEV_1, which is the volume of air that is forcefully exhaled in 1 second, and (2) FVC (forced vital capacity), which is the maximal volume of air that can be forcefully exhaled. The ratio of FEV_1/FVC is expressed as a percentage.

Individuals are retested 10 minutes after inhalation of a bronchodilator (e.g., albuterol) to determine reversibility of the FEV_1, a basic characteristic of asthma. An improvement in FEV_1 of 12% is considered significant. Because asthma has both an inflammatory and a bronchospastic component, a bronchodilator will not necessarily result in an increase in the FEV_1 if the airways are only inflamed. Results of these tests can be used to assess response to pharmacologic intervention. Individuals suspected of having exercise-induced asthma can be tested in a similar manner, repeating spirometry after exercise on a treadmill or other exercise unit.

Additional Laboratory Tests

Airway hyperresponsiveness may be assessed to confirm a diagnosis of asthma when the FEV_1 is not reversible and physical findings and clinical histories are insufficient to make a diagnosis. In this approach, a provocation challenge (e.g., with methacholine in aerosol form) is done. Spirometry results before and after the provocation challenges are compared. Asthmatics respond to provocation challenge with a 20% fall in FEV_1 at a lower concentration of methacholine. In other words, they are hyperreactive to methacholine. This is a more sensitive test than reversibility using a bronchodilator.

DIAGNOSIS

On the basis of the tests performed, a diagnosis of asthma may be made.

THERAPY

Long-term asthma control has traditionally been achieved with inhaled glucocorticoids. In recent years, however, therapeutic interventions have focused on blocking leukotriene receptor binding sites. For many patients, optimal therapy requires a combination of both inhaled corticosteroids and leukotriene receptor blockade. Leukotrienes are the end products of a biochemical cascade triggered by the action of 5-lipoxygenase on arachidonic acid. Leukotrienes (LTC4, LTD4, and LTE4) play an important role in the pathophysiology of asthma in that they mediate bronchoconstriction, chemotaxis of inflammatory cells, mucus production, and mucosal edema.

Arachidonic Acid: Precursor of Leukotrienes

Arachidonic acid is released from the No. 2 position of membrane-bound glycerophospholipids (e.g., phosphatidylinositol) by the action of phospholipase A_2 (PL-A_2). Arachidonic acid may also be released from the No. 2 position of 1-2 diacylglycerol (DAG) by DAG lipase. DAG is generated after the hydrolysis of phosphatidylinositol bisphosphate by phospholipase C (PL-C). Activation of PL-A_2 and PL-C occurs after the ligand interaction with a plasma membrane receptor on cells. A variety of different receptor/ligand interactions can trigger these signaling cascades, and these, in turn, may vary with the cell type (e.g., neutrophils). (Prostaglandins are produced after the action of cyclooxygenase 1 on arachidonic acid.) Cells do not synthesize the arachidonic (fatty) acid and so it,

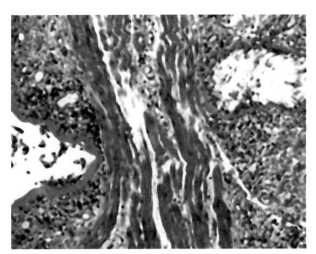

FIGURE 19–1 Lung tissue from asthmatic patient. The bronchi show hyaline thickening of the basement membrane with hypertrophy of underlying smooth muscle. Note the inflammatory infiltrate (eosinophils) and epithelial cells and eosinophilic mucinous material in the bronchial lumen. (Hematoxylin & eosin, ×200.)

or its precursor linoleic acid, must be derived from the diet.

ETIOLOGY: ASTHMA

Asthma is a multifactorial disease with a marked inflammatory component and bronchial smooth muscle spasm, both of which can lead to airway obstruction. Inflammatory cells and mucus accumulate in the airway (Fig. 19–1). In susceptible individuals this inflammation causes recurrent episodes of wheezing, dyspnea, and cough, particularly at night and in the early morning. Airway obstruction is generally reversible with appropriate pharmacologic therapy. However, in some cases there is evidence for only partial reversibility, suggesting that structural remodeling of the airway may develop in the long term.

Environmental Factors

In the western world there has been a general increase in the incidence of allergic diseases in association with improved public health. There is speculation that allergic diseases are a consequence of the absence of the habitual bacterial and parasitic infections with which we co-evolved. This is supported by epidemiologic data indicating that rural lifestyles tend to be protective for allergic diseases and that in nonfarming households the presence of a dog is protective.

Interestingly, the gene encoding CD14 is located within the chromosome 5 cytokine cluster. CD14 forms part of the receptor for lipopolysaccharide (LPS), a bacterial cell wall component and major stimuli of nonspecific inflammation. The segregation of CD14 with the cytokine cluster on chromosome 5 suggests that these act in concert. For example, CD14 triggers an inflammatory response that is then down-regulated by cytokines (e.g., IL-10) expressed in that cluster.

Asthma and Gene Polymorphism

Polymorphism within the gene encoding the receptor for the Fc region of IgE (FcεR1-β) is linked with high levels of IgE in some Australian aborigines parasitized with helminths. Engagement of FcεR1-β provides the major trigger for production of allergic mediators by mast cells. Interestingly, linkage of a particular FcεR1-β allele at this gene locus to atopy (high IgE levels) is seen only when the gene was inherited from the mother. If that allele is inherited from the father, that particular allelic form of FcεR1-β does not result in high levels of IgE.

This may reflect a maternal-fetal interaction through the placenta and/or breast milk (which explains early-onset irritable airways during the period of passive immunoglobulin acquisition from the mother). For later-onset disease, genomic imprinting may be in operation, where genes from one parent are preferentially expressed in comparison to genes from the other parent, as a result of the inactivation of either the maternal or paternal allele of a particular locus. This imprinting has also been observed where there is evolutionary conflict between maternal and paternal genes, such as in genes controlling fetal growth.

Role of Th2 Cytokines in Asthma

Recent data have documented unequivocally the important role of IL-13, as well as IL-4, in allergy and asthma. Both cytokines not only share significant structural homology but also share IL-4Rα as a receptor component. Although abundant data implicate IL-4 in Th2 development and isotype switching to IgE, it is clear that IL-4–independent (IL-13–dependent) pathways exist. T cells, eosinophils, mast cells, and NK cells have all been shown to secrete IL-13 *in vitro.*

More recently it has been shown that IL-13 mediates a nonoverlapping (with IL-4) role in mucus overproduction and eosinophilia seen in the bronchial airways of asthmatics. (IL-13 also plays a role in intestinal worm expulsion.)

Not surprisingly, more recent studies are focusing on the role of polymorphisms in the IL-4Rα chain as contributory factors to the genetics of asthmatic disorders. One polymorphism identified so far maps within the ITIM (immunoreceptor tyrosine-base inhibition motif) of this receptor molecule. In general, ITIMs are linked to inhibitory signaling cascades.

Role of Chemokines in Asthma

Any discussion of the immunogenetics of allergy/asthma must include consideration of chemokine biology. Chemokines and their receptors (seven-transmembrane G protein–coupled receptors) are essential for leukocyte trafficking from the circulation to inflamed tissues. (Chemokines are small secreted proteins that bind to receptors on cells, with the resulting effect being the movement of that cell toward the highest concentration of that chemokine.)

There is high promiscuity in this family, with many ligands binding different receptors and vice versa. Recently it has been shown that Th1 and Th2 cells express different chemokine receptors (CXCR3, CCR5 on Th1; CCR3, CCR4, and CCR8 on Th2). Thus, there is speculation that antagonists of these receptors (on Th2 cells) might be fruitful for treatment of allergic disorders. In asthma, recruitment of eosinophils to the airway might be targeted by blockade of chemokines implicated in this attraction (RANTES [CCL5] or eotaxin [CCL11]).

A 38-year-old female, MM, is seen in your office complaining of malaise for the past several months, a chronic cough, and pain in the left flank with hematuria (red blood cells in the urine). There is no medical history of note. There is no recent travel; she is afebrile, a nonsmoker, and not on any medication (either over-the-counter or prescribed). There is a family history of kidney stones, but her diet is not particularly rich in proteins, oxalates, or dairy products.

You order a routine chest radiograph and blood work/urinalysis. The report from the laboratory shows increased serum/urinary calcium concentrations and urinary red blood cells, and bilateral hilar lymphadenopathy (enlargement of the lymph nodes where the blood vessels and nerves enter the lung) is evident on the radiograph. Otherwise the blood work is normal, including serum/urinary urate levels. Urate elevation is a common cause of stone formation with genetically linked altered purine metabolism.

QUESTIONS FOR GROUP DISCUSSION

1. Hematuria and pain in the left flank, combined with the family history, is suggestive of renal colic. Explain why this does not account for all of this patient's symptoms.
2. What diseases might affect both the lungs and kidney, as well as contributing to this patient's feeling unwell? Review Case 17.
3. The laboratory studies showed normal serum/urinary urate levels. Explain why this would rule out kidney stones as an explanation for this patient's symptoms described in question 1. Why might drug-induced allergies cause a similar presentation?
4. The laboratory report also indicated that this patient had an increase in serum calcium concentration. Discuss some of the causes of this finding.
5. Explain how you would rule out (a) lytic bone disease (e.g., myeloma with osteolytic lesions) and (b) parathyroid adenoma (tumor of the parathyroid gland).
6. The chest radiograph indicated bilateral adenopathy (enlargement of glandular tissue, particularly of the lymph glands). Given the results of the chest radiograph, it is likely that infection with *Mycobacterium tuberculosis* would be high on the list of probabilities. What test could you administer to your patient to indicate whether this patient had been exposed to this infectious agent? What antigen would you use as a positive control? Explain why a positive control would be necessary.
7. Having ruled out tuberculosis as a consideration to explain this patient's symptoms, a computed tomographic (CT) scan was performed for more definition of the lungs. Results suggest granulo-matous lesions in the peripheral lung fields with confirmation of hilar adenopathy, which is suggestive of sarcoidosis. What would you expect a biopsy of the lung tissue to show?
8. Compare/contrast the granulomas in tuberculosis with those in sarcoidosis.
9. Patients with sarcoidosis have elevated levels of angiotensin-converting enzyme (ACE). Although a positive result supports a diagnosis of sarcoidosis, it is not confirmatory. Explain.
10. Describe the Kviem test. Discuss the limitations of the test and provide a rationale for the fact that it is not approved by the U.S. Food and Drug Administration (FDA).

RECOMMENDED APPROACH

Implications/Analysis of Family History

A familial history of kidney stones in a female directs us away from any X-linked disorders.

Implications/Analysis of Clinical History

The hematuria, combined with MM's family history, is suggestive of renal colic (intense pain in the lower back on one side as a result of passing a small stone down the ureter). But, if this is the problem, what is causing the kidney stone formation? Of note is the fact that both the lungs and kidneys are affected. We have already encountered two autoimmune diseases, Goodpasture's syndrome (see Case 17) and systemic lupus erythematosus (see Case 18), that cause a similar type of presentation owing to immune complex deposition in these tissues. Some drug-induced allergies can also manifest like this.

Implications/Analysis of Laboratory Investigation

We need to consider the implications of the increased serum/urinary calcium concentrations. MM's blood work indicated hypercalcemia, which is significant because kidney stones may develop in the presence of high serum calcium or urate. In this case, the serum urate value was normal. There are multiple causes of elevated serum calcium, including high doses of dietary supplements, altered bone metabolism (increased osteolysis [bone breakdown] vs. osteoblastogenesis [bone formation]), altered renal excretion, and parathyroid gland problems (this gland produces parathyroid hormone [PTH], which with vitamin D is an essential regulator of calcium/bone metabolism). None of these, however, clearly links the radiographic findings with calcium metabolism changes. Nevertheless you need to ensure that this patient does not have a lytic bone disease that could be causing this problem (e.g., myeloma with osteolytic lesions). A skeletal survey and/or bone scan will answer this.

Additional Laboratory Tests

Tests to investigate the possibility of a parathyroid adenoma (tumor of the parathyroid gland) were negative, but the levels of parathyroid hormone were elevated, suggesting that this may be contributing to (or the cause of) the increased calcium levels. A CT scan performed for more definition of the lung lesions revealed granulomatous-like lesions in the peripheral lung fields and confirmed the hilar lymphadenopathy.

Mantoux Test

Granulomatous-like lesions are present in the lungs of patients with tuberculosis; however, the classic presentation is a bilateral posterior apical lesion. Still, given the chronic cough and malaise, a Mantoux test, with an appropriate positive control, should be administered to rule out tuberculosis. In the Mantoux test tuberculin protein (purified protein derivative) isolated from cultures of *Mycobacterium tuberculosis* is injected intradermally and the effect examined 48 hours later. In this case, both the Mantoux test and the positive control were negative, and so one cannot definitively rule out tuberculosis. Anergic skin testing,

along with the bilateral hilar adenopathy, are consistent with sarcoidosis, a multisystemic disease of unknown etiology. It is thought that the low ratio of circulating CD4+ T cells to CD8+ suppressor and cytotoxic T cells explains this nonresponsiveness. Additionally, it is thought that the low CD4+ T helper cell count is the result of these cells migrating to the granulomas.

Biopsy

Fiberoptic bronchoscopy with transbronchial lung biopsy revealed noncaseating granulomas, consistent with sarcoidosis. In caseating granulomas the degraded tissue is converted to a dry cheesy mass, whereas in noncaseating granulomas this change does not occur. Although noncaseating granulomas are present in conditions other than sarcoidosis, the granulomas in tuberculosis are caseating, which would also rule out tuberculosis.

Angiotensin-Converting Enzyme

Diagnosis of sarcoidosis is mainly one of "exclusion" in that there is no test that functions as a "gold standard." To support this presumptive diagnosis, the serum level of ACE should be determined. In its active form, ACE plays a role in the regulation of blood pressure by stimulating the production of a hormone (aldosterone) and by inducing vasoconstriction, both of which lead to an increase in blood pressure. MM's serum indicated an elevated level of ACE, which is consistent with sarcoidosis but is not diagnostic in that patients with miliary tuberculosis will have elevated levels of ACE as will patients with inflammatory reactions occurring after inhalation of metal dust (e.g., beryllium dust), mold, and so on.

Pulmonary Function Tests

A spirometer is used to measure how rapidly a person can blow air out of the lungs following deep inhalation. Another lung test measures how much air the lung can hold (lung volume). (See Case 19.) Both of these were lower than normal when MM was tested, which is consistent with a diagnosis of sarcoidosis.

Kviem Test

This is a skin test, similar to the Mantoux test, in that it involves the subcutaneous injection of a substance and examination 48 hours later. In the Kviem test, which was developed in the late 1930s, a spleen homogenate from a person with sarcoidosis is injected intradermally into the person suspected of having sarcoidosis. Although a positive result can be seen after 48 hours, the area is not sampled for 4 to 6 weeks to allow time for granuloma formation. Formation of a noncaseating granuloma supports a diagnosis of sarcoidosis. A positive result is obtained in about 80% of all patients with active sarcoidosis (50% nonactive disease) but less than 1% of the normal population. This test is not FDA approved, nor has it been standardized.

DIAGNOSIS

Although there is no definitive test for sarcoidosis, the number of test results consistent with this disease strongly suggests that this is the correct diagnosis.

THERAPY

Not all patients with sarcoidosis require corticosteroid therapy. In some patients the disease follows a benign course. When required, long-term treatment with corticosteroids (to arrest granulomatous inflammation) is suggested. Other immunosuppressive therapies include cyclosporine and methotrexate. Electrocardiograms should be performed on all patients with sarcoidosis to ensure that there is no nonspecific granulomatous involvement of cardiac tissue and no evidence of cardiac ischemia (secondary to impaired lung function). In rare cases renal involvement can also occur. (See also amyloidosis, a condition characterized by the deposition of amyloid in tissues or organs.)

ETIOLOGY: SARCOIDOSIS

Sarcoidosis is a multisystemic disease of unknown etiology that may affect any organ in the body. However, most patients have some degree of lung involvement. The highest incidence of the disease occurs in young African American males. Sarcoidosis is a type IV hypersensitivity reaction, precipitated by chronic Th1

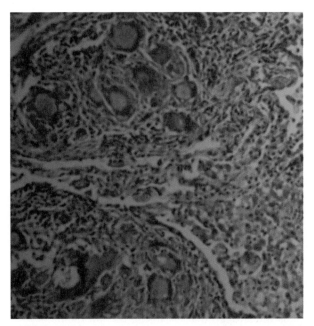

FIGURE 20–1 Sarcoid granulomas in the lung. The center of the lesion contains endothelioid cells, some of which fuse to form giant cells but (unlike the lesions of *M. tuberculosis*) without caseation and a peripheral ring of leukocytes. (Hematoxylin & eosin, ×200.)

sensitization/activation in response to ill-defined antigens, leading (as in tuberculosis) to chronic granuloma formation. A granuloma consists of an aggregate of cells arranged in almost concentric layers focused about macrophage-derived epithelioid cells (so named because histologically they resemble epithelial cells). Giant cells resulting from the fusion of macrophages may be present. Lymphocytes surround this region (Fig. 20–1). Older granulomas develop a circle of fibroblasts that define the outer region along with fibrous connective tissue.

Macrophages and epithelioid cells in these granulomas often produce an excess of ACE, an enzyme normally produced locally within the renal architecture that regulates filtration pressures and calcium absorption in the glomerulus. In those patients with active disease, the levels of ACE increase and can be used to monitor response to medication and disease progression. Granulomas may also produce 1,25-dihydroxyvitamin D, a hormone that increases intestinal absorption of calcium and increases the likelihood of kidney stone formation.

Ten-year-old Jimmy is brought to your office by his mother the day after he returned from summer camp, with diffuse blisters over his arms and legs. He has never had these before, and there is no family history of autoimmune disorders. He is not febrile and has taken no medications. Other than these blisters, which are associated with moderately itchy skin, he does not feel ill. How do you determine the underlying cause of the problem and how do you treat it?

QUESTIONS FOR GROUP DISCUSSION

1. List some autoimmune disorders that would present in this manner.
2. Given the absence of a family history of blistering disease, travel history becomes very significant. This child has been at "summer camp." Contact with the leaves of some plants can result in blistering in the sensitized individual. Name one common plant to which contact sensitivity is common. What is the antigen that is causing this problem?
3. Explain why this would need to be a re-exposure and not the result of an initial contact.
4. The summer camp history strongly suggests this is the result of re-exposure to urushiol, a small molecule present in the leaves of the poison ivy plant. Urushiol functions as a hapten following binding to a carrier protein. Define the terms *hapten* and *carrier protein*.
5. Describe the etiology of a type IV hypersensitivity reaction. Include in your description each of the following terms: dendritic cells, naive CD4+ T cells, memory CD4+ T cells, cytokines, macrophages, inflammatory mediators.

RECOMMENDED APPROACH

Implications/Analysis of Family History

There is nothing presented in this case that would indicate that family history is of significance.

Implications/Analysis of Clinical History

Epidermolysis bullosa is a term that refers to a group of disorders characterized by blister formation after mechanical trauma. Unless the condition is very mild, symptoms would have occurred as an infant. As well, one would have expected a family history of blistering disease. Another consideration is pemphigus foliaceus

(a benign form of pemphigus), an autoimmune disorder that is characterized by blisters; however, the most common age at onset is 60 years. In both of these disorders one would expect some family history of blistering. Drug-induced pemphigus would present in a similar fashion, but this patient has not taken any medication recently.

The importance of the clinical history needs to be stressed. Drug-induced hypersensitivity reactions and some infectious diseases can present in this fashion. Drugs can cause an autoimmune injury (antigens expressed at the border between the dermis and epidermis). These drug-induced reactions can be so severe that "skin sloughing" can occur, and patients need to be treated in a fashion analogous to a burn victim. There are also inherited autoimmune diseases that can look like this (e.g., bullous pemphigoid—a disease caused by autoantibodies against the epidermis). A variety of infections result in blistering before blister breakage and healing (e.g., chickenpox, molluscum contagiosum).

None of these really fits this clinical presentation in general because the clinical history is suggestive of something recent, causing an acute change.

Implications/Analysis of Laboratory Investigation

Laboratory investigations were not necessary to determine therapy.

DIAGNOSIS

The fact that these blisters appeared after summer camp suggests that this is a classic presentation of a contact sensitivity reaction (see Etiology).

THERAPY

The appropriate therapy here is simply topical corticosteroid creams, which generally produce complete resolution in days. Note that avoidance of poison ivy is crucial because subsequent exposure is likely to produce an even more dramatic reaction (immune memory!).

ETIOLOGY: TYPE IV HYPERSENSITIVITY REACTION

This is clearly a contact sensitivity type IV hypersensitivity reaction. These reactions are caused by T cell–mediated immune reactions, where a sensitization phase generates primed T cells specific for a plant hapten (urushiol) present in poison ivy leaves. Because urushiol is a hapten, an immune response occurs only if the hapten binds to cell surface proteins on the epidermis. When the proteins are released from the epidermis, Langerhans cells (dendritic cells of the epidermis) endocytose the protein-hapten complex, process it, and migrate to the nearest draining lymph node, where fragments are displayed on the cell surface complexed with class II major histocompatibility complex proteins. CD4+ T cells that recognize these complexes (and receive appropriate costimulatory signals) are activated. Some of these activated CD4+ T cells become memory cells and circulate in immunosurveillance.

Subsequent exposure to urushiol leads to the activation of the memory T cells and cytokine release at the site of re-exposure. These cytokines alter endothelial permeability and, in addition, can often directly stimulate other cell types (e.g., macrophages) to produce inflammatory mediators that result in pustular lesions.

FURTHER READING

Agostini C: Tailoring immunosuppressive therapy in interstitial lung diseases. Sarcoidosis Vasc Diffuse Lung Dis 21:3, 2004.

Berentsen S, et al: Favourable response to therapy with the anti-CD20 monoclonal antibody rituximab in primary chronic cold agglutinin disease. Br J Haematol 115:79, 2001.

Borza DB, Neilson EG, Hudson BG: Pathogenesis of Goodpasture's syndrome: A molecular perspective. Semin Nephrol 23:522, 2003.

Braem PP, et al: Diagnosis of cardiac sarcoidosis and follow up of 24 consecutive patients. Rev Med Interne 25:357, 2004.

Brantley TA: Diagnosing hemolytic disease of the newborn. Clin Lab Sci 15:140, 2002.

Brashington RD, et al: Immunologic rheumatic disorders. J Allergy Clin Immunol 111:S593, 2003.

Chang AB, et al: Effect of inspiratory flow on methacholine challenge in children. J Asthma 41:349, 2004.

Chaves CJ: Stroke in patients with systemic lupus erythematosus and antiphospholipid antibody syndrome. Curr Treat Options Cardiovasc Med 6:223, 2004.

Coker RK: Diagnosing and managing sarcoidosis. Practitioner 248:246, 2004.

Crawford GH, McGovern TW: Poison ivy. N Engl J Med 347:1723, 2002.

Cunard R, Kelly CJ: Immune-mediated renal disease. J Allergy Clin Immunol 111:S637, 2003.

David M, et al: Induction of the IL-13 receptor alpha2-chain by IL-4 and IL-13 in human keratinocytes: Involvement of STAT6, ERK and p38 MAPK pathways. Oncogene 20:6660, 2001.

Engeman TM, et al: Inhibition of functional T cell priming and contact hypersensitivity responses by treatment with antisecondary lymphoid chemokine antibody during hapten sensitization. J Immunol 164:5207, 2000.

Erlich JH, Sevastos J, Pussell BA: Goodpasture's disease: Antiglomerular basement membrane disease. Nephrology 9:49, 2004.

Etienne A, et al: Severe hemolytic anemia due to cold agglutinin complicating untreated chronic hepatitis C: Efficacy and safety of anti-CD20 (rituximab) treatment. Am J Hematol 75:243, 2004.

Evans RS, et al: Chronic hemolytic anemia due to cold agglutinins: II. The role of C′ in red cell destruction. J Clin Invest 47:691, 1968.

Fogg MK, Pawlowski NA: Anaphylaxis. Pediatr Case Rev 3:75, 2003.

Goodall J: Oral corticosteroids for poison ivy dermatitis. Can Med Assoc J 166:300, 2002.

Greenough A: Rhesus disease: Postnatal management and outcome. Eur J Pediatr 158:689, 1999.

Hoshi K, et al: Successful treatment of fulminant pulmonary hemorrhage associated with systemic lupus erythematosus. Clin Rheumatol 23:252, 2004.

Hudson BG, et al: Alport's syndrome, Goodpasture's syndrome, and type IV collagen. N Engl J Med 348:2543, 2003.

Janson S, Weiss K: A national survey of asthma knowledge and practices among specialists and primary care physicians. J Asthma 41:343, 2004.

Kitamura T, et al: Severe hemolytic anemia related to production of cold agglutinins following living donor liver transplantation: A case report. Transplant Proc 35:399, 2003.

Lamanske RF, et al: Asthma. J Allergy Clin Immunol 111:S502, 2003.

Nelson HS: β-Adrenergic bronchodilators. N Engl J Med 333:499, 1995.

Oddy WH, et al: Ratio of omega-6 to omega-3 fatty acids and childhood asthma. J Asthma 41:319, 2004.

Ovaly E: Late anaemia in Rh haemolytic disease. Arch Dis Child Fetal Neonatal Ed 88:F444, 2003.

Park MC, Park YB, Lee SK: Elevated interleukin-18 levels correlated with disease activity in systemic lupus erythematosus. Clin Rheumatol 23:225, 2004.

Parkinson G: Images in clinical medicine: The many faces of poison ivy. N Engl J Med 347:35, 2002.

Prince JE, Kheradmand F, Corry DB: Immunologic lung disease. J Allergy Clin Immunol 111:S613, 2003.

Ramos-Casals M, et al: Sarcoidosis of Sjögren syndrome? Clues to defining mimicry or coexistence in 59 cases. Medicine (Baltimore) 83:85, 2004.

Reich JM: Adverse long-term effect of corticosteroid therapy in recent onset sarcoidosis. Sarcoidosis Vasc Diffuse Lung Dis 20:227, 2003.

Riha RL, Allen RK: Cryptococcosis and sarcoidosis: Strange bedfellows: A report of five cases. Sarcoidosis Vasc Diffuse Lung Dis 21:71, 2004.

Sampson HA: Utility of food specific IgE concentrations in predicting symptomatic food allergy. J Allergy Clin Immunol 107:891, 2001.

Sampson HA: Food allergy. J Allergy Clin Immunol 111:S540, 2003.

Shah MK, Hugghins SY: Characteristics and outcomes of patients with Goodpasture's syndrome. South Med J 95:141, 2002.

Steinke JW, Borish L, Rosenwasser LJ: Genetics of hypersensitivity. J Allergy Clin Immunol 111:S495, 2003.

Van Kamp IL, et al: The severity of immune fetal hydrops is predictive of fetal outcome after intrauterine treatment. Am J Obstet Gynecol 185:668, 2001.

Violi F, Loffredo L, Ferro D: Premature coronary disease in systemic lupus. N Engl J Med 350:1571, 2004.

Wensing M, et al: Patients with anaphylaxis to pea can have peanut allergy caused by cross reactive IgE to vicilin (Ara h 1). J Allergy Clin Immunol 111:420, 2003.

SECTION III

Autoimmunity

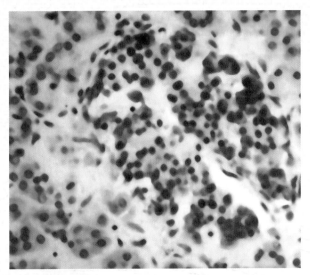

One of the most important characteristics of the mature immune system is its capacity for self:non-self discrimination. Failure to appreciate self (and thus to react against it) results in "*horror autoxicus*," or autoimmune disease. As biologic design specialists, we could all come up with mechanisms to avert autoimmunity—few would reach to the levels of sophistication, with a plethora of "back-up" systems in place, which nature has designed, ranging from "*deletion*" (specifically avoiding development of reactivity to self components), to "*ignorance/anergy*" (having recognition systems in place, but making sure they are not activated), to "*suppression*" (generating another system that serves to regulate anti-self reactive cells). As an acknowledgment of how well this system works, we point out how difficult it has been for us to duplicate this specific tolerance system for our own use (as, for instance, in transplantation biology—covered in a subsequent section).

Interestingly, while the autoimmune diseases can be classified in terms of organ-specific versus more generalized disorders, it will become apparent that a classification in terms of the immunopathology that underlies their existence (antibody-based or cellular-based) is reminiscent of our earlier section on hypersensitivity disorders. As in the field of clinical immunology in general, there have been some major breakthroughs in understanding in the past few years. Accordingly, while the reader can find, as expected, cases in systemic lupus erythematosus (Cases 22, 31), diabetes (Case 24) and rheumatoid arthritis (Case 23), which are arguably the "bread and butter" of autoimmunity, the case of APS (Case 26) is an excellent example of how newer molecular biology tools have significantly helped us understand the multiple immune manifestations of a single mutation.

Induction of self tolerance occurs during the maturational stages of lymphocytes in primary lymphoid organs. However, additional mechanisms exist in the periphery by which tolerance can be maintained. Loss of self tolerance leads to autoimmunity.

INDUCTION OF SELF TOLERANCE

T cells and B cells, effector cells in the immune system, are antigen specific. This specificity is the result of gene rearrangements within the DNA region coding for their antigen-specific receptors. Because gene rearrangements are random, some rearrangements will lead to the expression of receptors that recognize "self." Clones that recognize "self" are autoreactive. Deletion, or inactivation, of these self-reactive clones is believed to occur in the thymus and bone marrow during T cell and B cell development (see Cases 1 and 2). This process leads to tolerance induction of self antigens.

Some self-reactive clones, however, have been identified in the periphery, suggesting that tolerance to self antigens must also be acquired by some peripheral mechanism. These peripheral mechanisms for tolerance induction include suppression by T cells; lack of T cell help for B cell activation; absence of appropriate major histocompatibility complex (MHC) molecules for antigen presentation; and absence of co-stimulatory molecules. In some cases there is evidence that sequestration of self antigens leads to tolerance (because these antigens are not accessible to the immune system (e.g., lens crystallin in the eye). Immune responses to a self antigen leading to autoimmune disease indicate a loss of self tolerance.

LOSS OF SELF TOLERANCE

Loss of self tolerance has been postulated to occur via a number of mechanisms that include those that are (1) antigen related, (2) superantigen related, (3) genetic, and (4) hormone related.

Antigen-Related Mechanisms

Antigen-related mechanisms include the release of previously sequestered antigen; altered antigen presentation by nonprofessional antigen-presenting cells (e.g., after novel expression of MHC proteins); and so-called molecular mimicry after infection. In this case it is postulated that the host tissues share a common antigenic epitope with that of the virus or bacteria. However, loss of self tolerance may occur even if the foreign antigen displays only similar, not identical, antigens to those present on host tissues. In this situation, loss of self tolerance is due to cross reactivity. One example is the known cross-reactivity between human leukocyte antigen (HLA)-B27 epitopes and antigens of *Klebsiella pneumoniae* (a potential inciting agent for spondylarthritis). Ninety percent of individuals with the autoimmune disease "ankylosing spondylitis" have the HLA-B27 allele, whereas only 7% of the normal population has this allele.

Superantigen-Related Mechanisms

Loss of self tolerance may also be induced by superantigens. Superantigens can polyclonally activate subsets of lymphocytes. Because the mode of superantigen recognition by the T cell receptor differs from that of nominal antigen, it is possible that this polyclonal stimulation activates previously anergized, autoreactive lymphocytes and thus leads to the clonal expansion of self-reactive cells.

Genetic Defects

A number of genetic defects can lead to autoimmunity, including defects in the normal regulation of lymphocyte development/activation (e.g., Fas/FasL [CD95/CD95L]) defects leading to hyperproliferation (loss of apoptotic stimuli). It is possible, however, that the genes that contribute to the development of disease are those in linkage disequilibrium with the HLA allele, rather than the gene coding for the HLA allele itself.

Hormone Related

There are clearly some hormonal influences of importance in the development of autoimmune disorders. Many autoimmune diseases are more common in females than in males. However, the specific role of female hormones on the development of disease is unknown.

PATHOLOGIC PROCESSES ASSOCIATED WITH AUTOIMMUNE DISORDERS

Pathology Resulting from Direct Effect of Immunoglobulin

The presence of autoreactive antibodies can lead to different pathologic processes. One example is in the hemolytic anemias. "Warm hemolytic anemia" occurs when immunoglobulins bind to the cell surface (e.g., anti-Rh immunoglobulin binds to red blood cells), leading to phagocytosis/lysis. The direct Coombs' test is used to detect cell-bound immunoglobulin. In cold agglutinin disease, which is often seen after *Mycoplasma* infection, anti-glycophorin/anti-Ii antibodies bind to red blood cells to form immune complexes that activate complement and polymorphonuclear cells. This disease is referred to as "cold" agglutinin because the immunoglobulins dissociate from the target cell at 37°C (see Case 15). Often hemolytic anemias are drug induced (the drug is a hapten on the cell surface).

In Goodpasture's disease, anti–basement membrane immunoglobulins are generated and this leads to lung/renal pathology. Often anti-receptor immunoglobulins bind to the cell surface and cause pathology not from opsonization and complement activation leading to cell lysis but by increasing/decreasing cell bioactivity. Myasthenia gravis is caused by anti-acetylcholine receptor antibodies that block impulses across the neuromuscular junction. In Graves' disease, the generation of anti–thyroid-stimulating hormone receptor antibodies leads to hyperthyroidism (Fig. III–1). Acanthosis nigricans is associated with anti–insulin receptor antibodies.

Pathology Resulting from Immune Complex Formation

Systemic lupus erythematosus (SLE) is the classic example of an immune complex disorder. These patients have high levels of anti-dsDNA antibody, along with dsDNA, itself, in the serum (related to ultraviolet [UV] light and/or drug-induced cell death, for instance). Immune complexes formed in the serum are trapped in the basement membrane of glomeruli, of skin/endothelium, and in synovia of joints. Subsequent complement activation with release of chemical mediators and attraction and activation of phagocytes

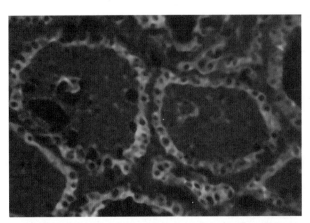

FIGURE III–1 Antithyroglobulin and antimicrosomal antibody staining of normal thyroid tissue. After binding of serum (from patients with Hashimoto's thyroiditis) containing human antibodies to thyroglobulin/microsomal antigens, the slide is stained with FITC/antihuman IgG and viewed under fluorescent microscopy. Microsomal antibodies stain the cytoplasm of epithelial cells lining the thyroid follicle; antithyroid antibodies stain thyroglobulin in the lumen of the follicle. (Indirect immunofluorescence, ×400.)

(and release of their enzymes, e.g., neutral proteases) causes pathology. In some cases dsDNA itself binds direct to basement membranes and traps immunoglobulins there (e.g., in the kidney).

Pathology Due to T Cells or T Cell Products

Activated T cells (recognizing autoantigens) produce a delayed-type hypersensitivity (DTH) reaction with Th1-type cytokine production (e.g., interferon gamma [IFNγ], interleukin [IL]-2, tumor necrosis factor [TNF]) and inflammatory infiltrates. An excellent example is Hashimoto's thyroiditis, in which T cells/monocytes are seen throughout the infiltrated gland. Antimicrosomal immunoglobulins are also produced, but this occurs *after* the release of antigens following gland destruction. These antibodies are *not* the cause of the disease. Multiple sclerosis is another autoimmune disease likely of T cell etiology. Oligoclonal, not polyclonal, immunoglobulin bands are seen in the cerebrospinal fluid (CSF), indicating an immunoglobulin response to limited sets of antigens. Histopathology confirms that the infiltrate in lesions is delayed-type hypersensitivity like and so it is not immunoglobulin (plasma cell) mediated. In an experimental model (allergic encephalomyelitis), which is induced by myelin basic protein, a limited set of T cells responds to antigens. This is an example of restricted Vβ usage (variable region of the T cell receptor beta chain).

SPECTRUM OF AUTOIMMUNE DISORDERS

Autoimmune disorders may be organ specific, non–organ specific, or a mixture of organ specific with systemic symptoms.

Organ Specific

Organ-specific autoimmune disorders include Hashimoto's thyroiditis, Goodpasture's disease, and Addison's disease (the adrenal glands).

Non–Organ Specific

The classic autoimmune disorder in this category is SLE, in which the spectrum of disease is very similar to graft versus host disease (GvHD) (see Transplantation Immunology, Section V). This is likely due to hyperstimulation of multiple components of the immune system, with hyper-Ig, and chronic production of nonspecific inflammatory/growth-promoting cytokines.

Mixture: Organ Specific with Systemic Symptoms

The classic autoimmune disorders in this category are rheumatoid arthritis and scleroderma. In rheumatoid arthritis joint involvement is common (immune complex mediated and possibly T cell mediated) along with lung/cardiac/skin and central nervous system (CNS) pathology. Scleroderma primarily manifests in the skin/ectodermal tissues but can cause multiorgan pathology as a result (e.g., affecting the gastrointestinal tract, skin, heart, or lung).

SPECIFIC AUTOIMMUNE DISORDERS

Systemic Lupus Erythematosus

SLE is a chronic inflammatory disorder, occurring predominantly in females (10:1). There is some MHC association with HLA-DR2/DR3. SLE is a multisystem disease associated with polyclonal B cell activation, antinuclear antibodies, and putative defects in B cells (regulation) and/or T cells (regulation). The etiology is unknown.

Rheumatoid Arthritis

Rheumatoid arthritis is another chronic inflammatory disease with female preponderance (3:1) and association with HLA-DR1/DR4. Generally, this disease affects joints. However, there is systemic involvement. The so-called rheumatoid factors are IgM (or IgG/IgA) antibodies specific for the Fc region of IgG. These antibodies may be important for immune complex formation and subsequent complement activation. Rheumatoid factors are *not* essential for disease. The etiology of rheumatoid arthritis is unknown, but the disease has been reported to follow infection with Epstein-Barr virus (human herpesvirus 4) or human T cell lymphotropic virus (HTLV-1).

Insulin-Dependent Diabetes Mellitus

Insulin-dependent diabetes mellitus (IDDM) is an endocrine disorder leading to a deficiency of insulin. There is some evidence for linkage with HLA-DR3/DR4. Autoantibodies to pancreatic islet cells and to insulin have been described. Prior infections with coxsackievirus/cytomegalovirus/mumps or rubella have been reported in patients with IDDM. An early sign of impending IDDM may be development of antibody to glutamic acid decarboxylase (GAD). Trials are underway to treat these individuals (immunosuppress) before development of IDDM.

Pernicious Anemia

Pernicious anemia is a disorder that manifests in defective red blood cell maturation due to malabsorption of vitamin B_{12}. In this disorder autoantibodies are produced to gastric parietal cell antigens, including autoantibodies to intrinsic factor. Normally, intrinsic factor is required for transport of vitamin B_{12} into the body. In pernicious anemia, binding of vitamin B_{12} to intrinsic factor is blocked by antibody, leading to a megaloblastic anemia.

AUTOANTIBODIES IN DISEASE STATES

Autoimmune disorders are particularly difficult to treat because the antigen is always present such that autoantibodies bind to these antigens to form immune complexes. When the antigen is soluble, immune complexes that form and circulate become lodged in small vessels where they trigger complement activation, neutrophil recruitment, and activation, such that pathology ensues (type III hypersensitivity reaction, e.g., SLE). Removal of antibodies would provide short-term relief and allow healing of damaged tissue.

When the antigen is a cell surface molecule, immune complexes form on the cell surface such that a type II hypersensitivity reaction is initiated. Pathology ensues as complement and neutrophils are recruited to the site (e.g., Goodpasture's syndrome, autoimmune hemolytic anemia). Because the antigen cannot be eliminated, this immune assault is ongoing. Removal of antibodies would provide short-term relief and allow healing of damaged tissue.

Hyperviscosity syndromes are syndromes in which the concentration of antibodies in circulation is very high, particularly if IgM antibody titer is very high. As a result, patients are at increased risk from hypoxemia (due to sluggish blood flow) and thrombotic events (stroke). Removal of antibodies would provide temporary relief.

Removal of Antibodies

One of the ways to gain temporary reprieve is to remove the antibodies from circulation. This can be achieved using plasmapheresis. In this procedure blood is separated into plasma and cells and the plasma is replaced with fresh frozen plasma and albumin. The antibodies are present in the plasma fraction and so they are removed from circulation.

Removal of Cells: Leukapheresis

In leukaphoresis, circulating leukocytes are collected by a continuous-flow cell separator. This is used rarely. Conditions for use include cryopreservation of stem cells before therapy, management of leukemia, and post-bone marrow transplantation.

IMMUNOTHERAPY FOR AUTOIMMUNE DISORDERS

The spectrum of therapies for autoimmune diseases includes (1) nonspecific immunosuppression, (2) specific immunosuppression, and (3) cytokine modulation.

Nonspecific Immunosuppression

In nonspecific immunosuppression the suppression is rather general and not limited to antigen specific B cells and T cells. It may, however, affect entire subsets of T cells (or B cells).

Anti-inflammatory Agents

Nonsteroidal anti-inflammatory drugs (NSAIDs), prednisone, methotrexate, and azathioprine (Imuran) are general nonspecific anti-inflammatory agents. One of the mechanisms by which the NSAIDs mediate their effects is through inhibition of products of the arachidonic acid pathway (e.g., prostaglandins, leukotrienes).

T Cell (But Non-Antigen)–Specific Agents

T cell–specific agents include cyclosporine, antibodies to CD3, antibodies to the IL-2 receptor (IL-2R), and antibodies to the T cell receptor-β (TCRβ) chain variable segments. These T cell–specific agents inhibit primarily the CD4+ T cell population such that IL-2, the T cell growth factor, is not transcribed, secreted, or bound by its receptor. In each case, the goal is to prevent the amplification of the response by inhibiting the proliferation and clonal expansion of those T cells that would secrete more IL-2, IFNγ, and TNF because these cytokines perpetuate the response.

Antigen-Specific Immunosuppression

Anti-TCR Antibodies

Anti-TCR antibodies recognizing unique sequence in the variable region (anti-idiotypic antibodies) have proven successful in experimental allergic encephalitis, an animal model for multiple sclerosis. Anti-idiotypic antibodies target only the clone of T cells binding the relevant autoantigens, and immunity to other pathogens is unaffected. Although intriguing because of their exquisite specificity, these may not be routinely useful clinically (each patient will likely have a unique idiotype). Evidence for limited expansion of the *same* TCR-bearing T cells would imply a useful role for anti-Vβ TCR antibodies (antibodies that target the variable region of the TCRβ chain).

Anti-MHC Antibodies or Peptide Antagonists

Anti–class II MHC antibodies prevent CD4+ T cell activation because the antibody binds to the peptide/class II MHC complex, blocking its binding to the TCR. Although this inhibits the recognition of all antigenic peptides that bind to a particular class II MHC allele, most individuals express other allelic forms of class II MHC, owing to the codominant expression of the MHC proteins.

Peptide antagonists are synthetic molecules, differing from the putative autoantigen only at those amino acids that confer a signaling function after engagement of the TCR. Binding of the antagonist functionally neutralizes autoantigen specific TCRs, without activating the T cells. This approach successfully treats experimental allergic encephalitis. Clinically, some information on the putative autoantigen is a prerequisite to synthesize potentially inhibitory ligands.

Cytokine Modulation

Pathology associated with multiple sclerosis and Hashimoto's thyroiditis, to name but two diseases, often results from unregulated production of type 1 cytokines (IL-2, IFNγ, and TNF). Under normal circumstances, naive CD4+ T cells differentiate to both Th1 and Th2 cells with one response predominating. When pathology is attributable to type 1 cytokines, there is a rationale for administration of type 2 cytokines (e.g., IL-4, IL-10, TGFβ, and IL-13) because these cytokines dampen further Th1 develop-ment. In experimental conditions this has not been as effective as would have been expected with the exception of the use of IL-4 in mice suffering from IDDM (NOD mice).

Anticytokine Antibodies

Monoclonal antibodies to cytokines themselves may be effective in some autoimmune diseases. TNF is found at elevated levels in inflamed joints where it causes activation of inflammatory cells within the joint and upregulates expression of a number of so-called adhesion molecules and their counter receptors (e.g., ICAM/LFA-1), which play a role in regulating migration of inflammatory cells to the joint synovium. Ongoing clinical trials are examining the use of antibodies to TNF to "shut down" the stimulation of inflammatory cells within the rheumatoid joint by released TNF. Human trials, with rheumatoid arthritis patients, have met with some success.

Clinical trials in which patients with multiple sclerosis are orally fed brain extract are in progress and have met with some success. Note that current (experimental) data suggest that the mechanism of regulation involved after oral feeding of antigen is quite complex, with local (mucosal) increased expression of monocyte chemotactic protein (MCP-1), decreased expression of IL-12, and thus dampening of type-1 cytokine production. These data in turn suggest that later trials might also include manipulation of chemokine production. This therapy requires some knowledge of the relevant antigen.

Dawn, a 15-year-old African American girl, was debating whether she should go on the spring ski trip that she had planned for so long. She had noticed stiffness in both her hips (and hands) each morning and wondered if that would affect her skiing. However, since the stiffness abated during the day, she thought that she would go, even if it meant only skiing in the afternoons. She enjoyed the trip, particularly since the weather was so warm and sunny, but she was concerned when she noticed a rash on her face. The rash persisted after she returned and so she went to see her family physician, who recognized the rash as being a classic presentation of systemic lupus erythematosus (SLE), and so he referred her to a local rheumatologist.

On questioning, the rheumatologist learned that there was no history of arthritic-type diseases in the family, although a distant cousin had recently been diagnosed with an inflammatory bowel disorder. A urine sample was found to be normal, indicating that glomerulonephritis was not a problem. A complete blood cell count was performed, along with an assay for antinuclear antibodies (ANA). The white blood cell count indicated a mild lymphopenia and neutropenia, reduced red blood cell count, and a severe drop in platelet count (see Appendix for reference values). The ANA antibody titer was significantly high (normal range: 1:40 to 1:120 depending on the laboratory). How would you proceed?

QUESTIONS FOR GROUP DISCUSSION

1. Dawn's physician recognized the rash across her face as a classic presentation of SLE. What is the underlying cause of this rash? Explain the underlying cause of the arthritis. (*Hint:* laboratory investigation revealed that Dawn had a high ANA titer.)

2. Dawn has a significant ANA titer. Define *antibody titer*. Explain why a negative result in this test would rule out SLE but a positive result would not confirm this diagnosis.

3. What follow-up antibody titer tests could you request to further investigate the presumptive diagnosis of SLE? Explain the principles underlying an indirect immunofluorescence antibody (IFA) test.

4. Explain why you would want to measure the levels of complement proteins C3 and C4. Explain what is meant by the expression "Levels of C3 and C4 are concordant with disease activity in patients with SLE."

5. Dawn's blood work indicated that she was anemic. Consequently, the physician requested the indirect and the direct Coombs' tests. Explain the principles underlying these tests and the rationale for requesting these tests in this patient.

6. Dawn's urine sample was normal, indicating that glomerulonephritis was not a problem. Explain why patients with high antibody titers often present with glomerulonephritis.

7. Explain why UV light exacerbates SLE.

8. Review B cell activation after encounter with antigen. Why would autoimmune B cells never be activated if T cell tolerance is intact?

9. Explain why a biopsy of the lymph nodes in a patient with active SLE would reveal hyperplasia in the cortex.

10. Explain why there are so many different autoantibodies of different specificities produced in SLE.

RECOMMENDED APPROACH

Implications/Analysis of Family History

The absence of a strong genetic link would not negate the presumptive diagnosis of SLE because susceptibility to SLE is multifactorial. The combined effect of hormones, genes, and environment determine disease prevalence, with females having a greater risk of disease, as does being African American. Dawn is an African American female and, as such, is in the highest risk group.

Implications/Analysis of Clinical History

A red butterfly rash on cheeks after sun exposure in a teenage female is a classic presentation of SLE and has been shown to lead to early testing and diagnosis. The rash results from blood leaking out of damaged blood vessels (immune complex–mediated inflammation) into the skin. However, recent studies have shown that when the initial presentation is arthritis (joint inflammation) and/or arthralgia (joint pain), diagnosis is often delayed, despite the fact that these are the most common initial symptoms (60% of patients studied).

Implications/Analysis of Laboratory Tests

Blood Cell Counts

Dawn's white blood cell count indicated a mild lymphopenia and neutropenia, which is very common in SLE patients and most likely results from autoantibodies to white cells. Low platelet count (thrombocytopenia), also common in SLE patients, can result in bleeding that manifests as bruises and/or rash. Dawn's red blood cell count was low, indicating anemia, and thus direct and indirect Coombs' tests were ordered to determine whether the anemia was due to the presence of autoantibodies that target proteins on the red blood cells. (See Additional Laboratory Tests.)

ANA Assay

Dawn had a significant ANA titer. ANA are autoantibodies that are specific for proteins and nucleic acids in the nucleus (e.g., histones, dsDNA, ssDNA). In the ANA assay, a patient's serum is serially diluted and then layered on nuclear components of human epithelioid cells (HEp-2). If ANA antibodies are present they will bind to the nuclear components of the HEp-2 cells. The presence of ANA antibodies is detected using a fluorescent-labeled immunoglobulin (antihuman) antibody that targets the Fc region of a particular antibody isotype (e.g., Fcγ, Fcμ, or Fcα). This is an indirect immunofluorescence assay (IFA). (Some laboratories may use rat liver or kidney cells instead of HEp-2 cells.)

Antibody titer is defined as the serum dilution beyond which autoantibodies cannot be detected. A positive ANA titer greater than the reference range, in that particular laboratory, is indicative of disease when accompanied by clinical symptoms. Although a negative result rules out a diagnosis of SLE, a positive result is only suggestive because other inflammatory conditions can also have ANA autoantibodies.

Additional Laboratory Tests

A variety of other tests were performed (anti-DNA, antiphospholipid, C3 and C4, direct and indirect Coombs' test) to examine evidence for abnormalities characteristic of SLE.

Antiphospholipid Antibodies

Antiphospholipid antibodies are a heterogeneous group of autoantibodies that can cause thrombotic events, leading to deep vein thrombosis or strokes.

Anti–Red Blood Cell Antibodies

In patients with anemia, the direct and indirect Coombs' tests are used to establish whether there is evidence of autoimmune hemolytic anemia, which can occur in SLE when autoantibodies against erythrocytes are present. In Dawn's case, both the direct and indirect Coombs' tests were negative (see Case 15), indicating that this was not the cause of the anemia.

Anti-DNA test

To support a positive ANA result, the patient's serum is screened for anti-dsDNA using an enzyme-linked immunosorbent assay (ELISA) and, if positive, a titer is determined using the IFA technique (see ANA assay earlier). A negative anti-dsDNA antibody test result does not eliminate SLE as a possible diagnosis, because not all SLE patients have anti-DNA antibodies (moderate sensitivity, high specificity test). However, significant titers of both anti-ANA and anti-dsDNA antibodies, as in Dawn's case, make a diagnosis of SLE very likely.

Complement C3 and C4

Dawn's serum C3 level was significantly reduced (normal: see Appendix). In general, the serum level of C3 and C4 complement proteins in SLE patients is decreased because immune complexes bind to and activate the classical pathway of complement. Complement activation triggers an enzymatic cascade in which C3 and C4 are cleaved and biologically active fragments are produced. Often the depletion in these proteins is proportional to the severity of the disease (i.e., number of immune complexes). In such cases the level of C3 and C4 is said to be "concordant" with disease activity, and thus can be used to monitor disease and its response to therapy. Successful immunosuppressive therapy is reflected in a rise in the serum level of C3 and C4. Nephelometry of either C3 or C4 (see Case 11) is sufficient to monitor disease in such patients.

DIAGNOSIS

Dawn was diagnosed with systemic lupus erythematosus.

THERAPY

Dawn should obviously avoid sunlight in the future (see later). Topical corticosteroids and hydroxychloroquine (Plaquenil), an antimalarial drug that has a beneficial effect for SLE for unknown reasons, have both been shown to be effective in treating the rash; however, the hydroxychloroquine has also been shown to be effective in controlling the arthritis. Depending on the severity of the arthritis, NSAIDs or mild doses of corticosteroids may be required, and in more severe cases high doses of corticosteroids will be necessary.

Dawn will have to be monitored carefully because immune complex deposition in the glomerulus is the trigger for inflammation and glomerulonephritis (Fig. 22–1). Proteins or red blood cells in the urine would signal this type of inflammation and so Dawn's

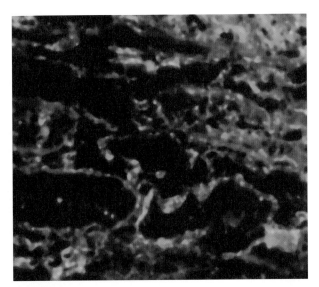

FIGURE 22–1 IgG deposited along tubal basement membrane in kidney of patient with SLE. (×100.)

immunosuppressive therapy would need to be increased and accompanied by periodic administration of cyclophosphamide intravenously.

ETIOLOGY: SYSTEMIC LUPUS ERYTHEMATOSUS

Systemic lupus erythematosus is a multisystemic disease involving increased size of lymph nodes as well as the production of several autoantibodies, immune complex formation, and deposition with consequential clinical manifestations. Sunlight (UV light) exacerbates the disease because UV light results in the crosslinking of DNA in cells. The release of DNA in an immunogenic form (UV linked) can lead to autoimmunization. As we shall see later, other autoimmune reactions may have different triggers for tolerance breakdown.

Polyclonal B Cell Activation

It is common in SLE to see evidence for polyclonal B cell activation with increased levels of serum immunoglobulin. Presumably, the increased lymph nodes are reflective of this B cell hyperplasia. Should you be concerned about this (e.g., premalignant or malignant lesions), a biopsy of an easily accessible lymph node could be ordered. Most likely this would reveal follicular hyperplasia in the cortex and increased numbers of plasma cells in the medulla.

There are often a plethora of autoantibodies of different specificities produced in SLE. In part, this is because the antigen(s) implicated in initiation of the disease are complex ones, such as the whole (or part thereof) of a nucleosome or a ribonucleoprotein particle (RNP), which contains several different molecular entities. Patients can produce autoantibodies against each of the different epitopes represented, with each epitope stimulating antibody production by a specific and unique B cell. Following this, in principle, any of these antibodies may form an immune complex with the whole nucleosome (or RNP).

Breakdown in Tolerance

Potentially autoreactive B cells probably exist normally in the circulation of all individuals, but it must be noted that we normally do not activate these B cell clones. Autoimmunity in general, and SLE in particular, represent a breakdown in normal "self tolerance" mechanisms. Exactly why this occurs remains unclear. For SLE, it seems that tolerance breakdown may result from a failure in normal immunoregulatory populations of T cells.

If T cell tolerance is intact, autoimmune B cells are never activated because the appropriate "help" for B cell differentiation to produce autoantibodies does not occur by virtue of T cell–induced regulation. An alternative hypothesis suggests that immune tolerance is broken by virtue of a generalized vigorous inflammation (e.g., UV light exposure). In this scenario, inflammation results in provision of a bystander milieu (of cytokines and other mediators) conducive to polyclonal B cell activation and a resulting differentiation of, at least some, B cells producing autoantibodies. Once these, in turn, produce cellular damage the reaction can become self perpetuating.

Jurgat is a 45-year-old woman of Indian descent with severe erosive deforming rheumatoid arthritis (RA) that began at the age of 22. She has had ongoing joint problems and more recently has experienced early signs of renal failure and some chest discomfort. She has tried without benefit all conventional anti-inflammatory therapies, including NSAIDs and chronic prednisone therapy (which left her with severe osteoporosis), as well as methotrexate and even cyclosporine. She became a good candidate for more experimental approaches but she has already experienced failure in a trial using antibody to human intercellular adhesion molecule (ICAM). What was the rationale for use of this agent? What is the potential pathophysiology behind her disease manifestations?

QUESTIONS FOR GROUP DISCUSSION

1. RA is a chronic inflammatory condition. Use a schematic to illustrate a typical inflammatory response. Include the following in your schematic:
   (a) tissue damage
   (b) activation of the intrinsic coagulation pathway
   (c) activation of prekallikrein, leading to the generation of C5a and bradykinin
   (d) C5a-mediated degranulation of mast cells leading to histamine release
   (e) histamine-mediated expression of P-selectin on the endothelium
   (f) bradykinin- and histamine-mediated increase in vascular permeability
   (g) activation of tissue macrophages leading to the release of interleukin (IL)-1, tumor necrosis factor (TNF), IL-6, and chemokines
   (h) effect of IL-1 and TNF on vascular endothelium including increase in ICAM-1, vascular cell adhesion molecule-1 (VCAM-1) and E-selectin, as well as chemokine secretion
   (i) effect of IL-1 and TNF on leukocytes (increase in integrin [e.g., LFA-1] expression
   (j) firm adhesion
   (k) secretion of matrix metalloproteinases by tissue macrophages, activated endothelium, and activated leukocytes
   (l) diapedesis (including PECAM-1/PECAM-1 interaction)
   (m) chemotaxis to site of inflammation
   (n) role of IL-6 in release of C-reactive protein (heat shock protein) from hepatocytes
2. Explain why C-reactive protein is a measure of inflammation.
3. The above steps (listed in question 1) represent an acute inflammatory response. In chronic inflammation, B cells and T cells also play a role. Explain how B cells and T cells would exacerbate the inflammatory process.

4. This patient has failed to improve during a trial using anti-ICAM antibodies. What is the rationale for this therapeutic approach?
5. Explain the rationale for using anti-TNF neutralizing agents for therapy.
6. Discuss the advantages and disadvantages (if any) for each of the following anti-TNF neutralizing agents: (a) murine antibodies, (b) chimeric antibodies, (c) humanized antibodies, and (d) fusion proteins.
7. Review the role of TNF in bacterial infections (see Case 12).
8. Discuss the innate and adaptive host defense mechanisms against *Mycobacterium tuberculosis*.
9. Explain why the Mantoux test should be administered to Jurgat before initiating therapy with a TNF-neutralizing agent.
10. Discuss the evidence that supports the fact that RA has a genetic component.

RECOMMENDED APPROACH

Implications/Analysis of Family History

Although we are not provided with any family history, RA does have a genetic component. A major genetic risk factor for RA is HLA-DR4, with about 70% of patients with RA expressing this HLA allele (control 28%). Studies with monozygotic twins also support a genetic component for RA (~17% concordance). This indicates that environmental factors also play a role in the genesis of RA.

Implications/Analysis of Clinical History

The course of RA varies from patient to patient. In Jurgat's case, disease progression has been very aggressive. The ineffectiveness of therapies to control the inflammatory processes reflects the fact that the underlying cause of RA remains unknown.

Implications/Analysis of Laboratory Tests

Although we are not provided with information regarding rheumatoid factor (autoantibodies), 66% of patients with RA have rheumatoid factor, an antibody that targets the Fc portion of IgG (control population 5%). Furthermore, patients with high titers of these autoantibodies have a more severe disease. Generally, tests for rheumatoid factor detect IgM isotype, but IgG and IgA isotypes may also be present. Rheumatoid factor is present in several infectious diseases (e.g., malaria, syphilis, leprosy) and other autoimmune disorders (e.g., systemic lupus erythematosus). Another test with prognostic significance is the C-reactive protein test, which is an indicator of inflammation. There are, however, no specific tests to confirm a diagnosis of RA.

Additional Laboratory Tests

In cases of severe erosive deforming arthritis, radiography to assess the bone erosion and cartilage destruction would be of value, particularly to monitor the efficacy of new therapies.

DIAGNOSIS

Jurgat has severe rheumatoid arthritis that requires a novel therapy.

THERAPY

Antibodies to Block Cells from Entering Synovial Tissues

One of the key features of inflammation is the recruitment of circulating leukocytes to the site of inflammation. The migration of cells from the blood vessels is dependent on the expression of adhesive molecules that sequentially induce rolling and firm adhesion on the vascular endothelium, followed by diapedesis as cells squeeze between endothelial cells. The expression of adhesive molecules depends primarily on the presence of the inflammatory cytokines, TNFα and IL-1, which are secreted by activated tissue macrophages.

Adhesive molecules that are expressed on the activated endothelium and induce rolling are referred to as selectins (P-selectin, E-selectin), and their counter molecules (carbohydrates) are present on circulating leukocytes. In contrast, the integrins (heterodimer proteins) are expressed on circulating leukocytes and their counter molecules are expressed on the activated endothelium.

TNFα and IL-1 alter both the expression (upregulate) and affinity (increase) of the integrins on leukocytes and upregulate their counter molecules on the activated endothelium (see question #1 and Case 8). Transmigration of cells into tissues requires the homo-interaction of PECAM-1, which is constitutively expressed on both leukocytes and endothelium. Activated endothelium and leukocytes also secrete enzymes (metalloproteinases) that degrade the basement membrane and permit diapedesis into the tissue.

Thus, one novel approach to treating nonspecific inflammatory diseases such as RA would be to prevent integrin/counter molecule interaction. In early clinical trials murine antibodies to block these interactions were administered, but the effectiveness of these antibodies was dramatically reduced when patients developed human anti-mouse antibodies (HAMA) responses. More recently, a human antibody (Fab fragment MOR 101, MorphoSys) that targets ICAM-1 has been developed using recombinant technology. Because LFA-1:ICAM-1 interactions are probably more important for migration at sites of inflammation than for normal recirculation, antibodies to these have been among the first under consideration. Data to date suggest these may prove of value, although this patient failed to benefit.

TNFα Neutralizing Agents

Another novel approach to use would involve agents that block the action of cytokines believed to be important in the pathophysiology of disease. IL-1 and TNFα were two of the cytokines believed to be most suited for targeting, based on experimental studies and clinical observation. Reagents designed to block inflammation caused by TNFα were shown to be effective. One of these reagents is a human anti-TNF monoclonal antibody (adalimumab). The other is a fusion protein consisting of the extracellular TNF-binding portion of the TNF receptor that has been linked to the Fc portion of human IgG1 (Enbrel/Etanercept). Both of these reagents bind TNF so that it is not available for binding to its cognate receptor on endothelial (and other) cells.

There is a major proviso worthy of note for patients using TNF-neutralizing reagents. TNFα is important in signaling intracellular destruction of chronic pathogens (e.g., *Mycobacterium* species). Patients receiving this therapy have often had a recrudescence of tuberculosis. It would be wise to question this patient about any past history of tuberculosis and, if positive, to monitor her closely while she receives this therapy.

Anti-Interleukin Antibodies

Interestingly, a natural antagonist of IL-1 exists (IL-1ra) so in addition to anti–IL-1 antibodies this molecule has also been tried clinically. Neither of these reagents has proved to be of great benefit clinically.

ETIOLOGY: RHEUMATOID ARTHRITIS

RA is an autoimmune disease, associated initially with inflammation and tissue destruction in the joints. Inflammation is associated with the presence of a number of immune cells (T cells/B cells) in the joint fluid along with a variety of inflammatory cytokines. These cytokines are intimately involved in many facets of the disease process, not the least of which includes the recruitment of the lymphoid cells to the inflamed joint and activation of bystander cells (monocytes/macrophages), with subsequent release of other inflammatory mediators (e.g., neutral elastases) that can further destroy tissue architecture.

Immune Complexes in RA

Note that some of Jurgat's complaints may represent inflammation caused by immune complex deposition. Thus, often patients with RA have circulating rheumatoid factor in their serum, an antibody to serum

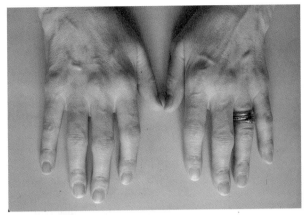

FIGURE 23–1 Early stages of rheumatoid arthritis. Hand shows swelling of proximal interphalangeal joints and effusions in metacarpophalangeal joints. (From Hochberg M, et al: Practical Rheumatology, 3rd ed. St. Louis, Mosby, 2004.)

immunoglobulin itself. This, in turn, can lead to immune complex deposition in various tissues (serosal lining of lungs and heart) and joints with subsequent inflammation (Fig. 23–1). Both T and B cells sensitized to autoantigens (likely collagen of the connective tissue) can also stimulate inflammatory responses.

Migration of Lymphocytes into Tissues

Normal lymphocyte recirculation through lymphoid/nonlymphoid tissues occurs in a nonrandom fashion, under the control of the expression of a number of receptors/counter receptors expressed on the lymphocyte/target tissue respectively. During the development of an inflammatory response the expression of a number of adhesion molecules also changes quite dramatically, as described earlier. Newer therapies are focused on inhibiting/blocking molecules that facilitate entry of circulating leukocytes to the site of inflammation.

CASE

24

MM, a 3-year-old white monozygotic twin boy was brought to the emergency department by his mother after suffering from a viral-like illness for nearly 3 weeks. Previously, she had taken MM to the family physician, but he had reassured her that the symptoms would resolve with acetaminophen (Tylenol). At the present time her son is not eating well; his urine output has been diminished for over 24 hours; he is quite listless with sunken eyes, and he is feverish.

This boy is obviously quite sick. All routine blood work is ordered, as is a chest radiograph and urinalysis. An intravenous line is obtained and fluid resuscitation is begun. The laboratory director calls approximately 1 hour later with urgent results. MM's blood glucose concentration is elevated, and his potassium concentration is low. Urinalysis was positive for glucose. Intravenous administration of insulin and potassium chloride is immediately initiated. Hyperglycemia in a young white child is highly suggestive of type 1A diabetes mellitus (type 1 DM). What would you expect the family history to reveal? Which Class II human leukocyte (HLA/major histocompatibility complex [MHC]) genes confer susceptibility to type 1 DM? What autoantibodies would you measure?

QUESTIONS FOR GROUP DISCUSSION

1. This patient's clinical history and presentation looks like the typical picture of type 1 immune-mediated diabetes (type 1 DM), an autoimmune disorder resulting from a breakdown in tolerance. What tissue does the immune system target? What is the role of these cells in the normal state?
2. Discuss the evidence that supports a genetic basis for this autoimmune disorder.
3. Discuss the putative environmental factors that have been investigated as triggers for type 1 DM.
4. What are the metabolic complications in type 1 DM? Explain the significance of a decrease in potassium levels and the presence of glucose in the urine. How does the presence of glucose in urine contribute to dehydration?
5. What autoantibodies are detected in the serum of patients in the early stage of the disease, long before clinical symptoms appear? How can this be used to benefit the patient?
6. What is the mainstay of treatment for type 1 DM? Why did patients (in the past) develop anti-insulin antibodies? Why is this not a problem today?
7. Explain why there has been a move toward more frequent injection of short-acting insulin in some individuals.
8. What is the significance of the fact that immunization with hsp60 peptide was associated with a shift from Th1 to Th2 cells specific for this peptide?
9. Explain why CD4+, CD25+ T cells have come under scrutiny in autoimmune disorders.

10. Explain the significance of identifying a patient with type 1A DM who has already been diagnosed with X-linked agammaglobulinemia (see Case 3).

RECOMMENDED APPROACH

Implications/Analysis of Family History

Although we have not been given any family history, disease susceptibility for type 1 DM depends on the degree of genetic similarity that an individual has with the proband. For example, MM's monozygotic twin, whose genetic makeup is identical to MM, has a 50% risk of also developing type 1 DM. The remaining risk is thought to be due to environmental factors (see Implications/Analysis of Clinical History).

More than 20 different genes have been identified that contribute to type 1 DM disease susceptibility, but the highest predisposing risks are associated with the inheritance of particular groups of class II MHC antigens. Individuals at highest risk for developing type 1 DM are those whose haplotype includes HLA-DR3, DQ2 and HLA-DR4, DQ8. Risk is somewhat lower, but still substantial, for individuals who express HLA-DR3, DQ2 or HLA-DR4, DQ8 (i.e., not both). Close to half of the patients with type 1 DM express all four of these HLA genes. Interestingly, some patterns of HLA-DR/DQ linkage patterns are protective. Given MM's age when the disease manifested, one would predict that MM (and his twin) would express the HLA genes that have the highest predisposing risk.

Individuals with type 1 DM and their relatives are at increased risk for a number of autoimmune disorders, including celiac disease, Addison's disease, pernicious anemia, and autoimmune thyroid dysfunction. About 14% of children with type 1 DM (without celiac disease) have IgA anti-tissue transglutaminase (tTG) autoantibodies. These tTG autoantibodies are also present in about 7% of nondiabetic first-degree relatives (without celiac disease). We would expect, therefore, that a family history would reveal autoimmune disorders in immediate or related family members.

Implications/Analysis of Clinical History

In the last 24 hours, MM's urine output has been diminished, an indication that dehydration might be a problem. Severe dehydration can lead to hypovolemic shock, and so an intravenous line was inserted and fluid resuscitation begun.

MM has been suffering from a viral-like infection for the past 3 weeks. Type 1 DM is often described in the aftermath of an (inciting?) infectious disease (e.g., coxsackie virus and cytomegalovirus).

Viruses, bovine milk, and toxins are only a few of putative environmental factors that have been investigated as triggers for type 1 DM in susceptible patients. Bovine milk has been included in this list because (in some studies, but not others) a comparison of the incidence of type 1 DM in countries with high/low rates of breast feeding showed that early introduction of bovine milk in an infant's diet could lead to induction of cross-reactive T cells/antibodies that might have pathogenic potential. Congenital rubella, in susceptible individuals, has also been included in the list of environmental factors that increase the likelihood of becoming diabetic.

Knowing whether MM has been breast fed, has had congenital rubella, or has had other viral infections would not affect the course of treatment or disease outcome, but for completeness this information should be included in the patient's file.

Implications/Analysis of Laboratory Investigation

The blood glucose concentration is elevated, and so dehydration is of concern. As mentioned, fluid resuscitation and insulin therapy have already been initiated. Potassium levels are decreased, suggesting severe diabetic ketoacidosis (see Etiology), and so potassium

chloride was administered. The initial presentation of ketoacidosis is usually accompanied by a normal or elevated plasma potassium level. This is because insulin deficiency leads to the movement of potassium ions from inside cells to the extracellular fluid. Urinalysis was positive for glucose, a classic indicator of diabetes mellitus.

One would expect that the chest radiograph would be normal, as would the white blood cell count and differential; however, the lymphocyte count would be at the high end of normal. The total serum immunoglobulin level would be increased because MM would have significant titers of autoimmune antibodies.

Enzyme-linked immunosorbent assays (ELISAs) for autoantibodies for islet antigens (glutamic acid decarboxylase [GAD], protein tyrosine phosphatase IA-2) and insulin should be requested. Anti-insulin and anti-GAD autoantibodies are often the first to develop, long before clinical symptoms. These autoantibodies serve as markers for disease. Autoantibodies are indicative of type 1A DM, rather than type 1B DM, which presents in a similar manner but patients do not have autoantibodies or any immune involvement.

Additional Laboratory Tests

An enzymatic approach is used to diagnose and monitor one of the ketone bodies (β-hydroxybutyric acid). However, patients can monitor their ketone levels using a urine dipstick assay.

DIAGNOSIS

MM's diagnosis was type 1A diabetes mellitus, with diabetic ketoacidosis.

THERAPY

Exogenous insulin, for life, is considered the mainstay of treatment for type 1 DM. Because many of the long-term complications of diabetes (cardiac/coronary atherosclerosis, blindness, neuropathy, gastroparesis) are believed to reflect the chronic effect of poor glucose control (oscillations between high/low blood glucose levels), there has been a move toward tighter control (more frequent injection of short-acting insulin, mimicking the natural response) in those individuals deemed suited to this treatment.

In the past, most patients, irrespective of the source of insulin, developed anti-insulin antibodies. With the human insulin and insulin analogs, development of anti-insulin antibodies is not common.

More recently, interest has been spurred into assessing whether vigorous immunosuppression before or at the first signs of diagnosis of type 1 DM can thwart the evolution of the full-blown disorder, and salvage at least some β cell function from autoimmune attack (see later). In part, at least, these studies were precipitated by the growing realization that there was clearly a genetic linkage with immune susceptibility genes. As well, the presence of serum antibodies to GAD seemed to presage the development of diabetes and so could serve as a marker for early therapy. Pilot studies using cyclosporine, a T cell immunosuppressant, have been tried, although with few revolutionary positive results.

ETIOLOGY: TYPE 1A DIABETES MELLITUS

Type 1 DM is an autoimmune disorder that occurs in genetically susceptible individuals when exposed to, as yet hypothesized, environmental factors. In type 1 DM, the immune system targets the β cells of the pancreatic islets, which results in their destruction and a loss of insulin synthesis and secretion. Irrespective of the environmental factor(s), the issue remains one of a breakdown in tolerance.

Metabolic Complications

In the nondisease state, insulin is synthesized and stored within cytosolic granules of β cells of the pancreatic islets (Fig. 24–1) and released into circulation when there is a rise in blood glucose concentration. Insulin increases the rate at which glucose is transported into cells, where it plays a role in several anabolic processes. In type 1 DM, glucose generated from simple or complex dietary carbohydrates is unable to enter cells and so the cells are, in effect, starving. Under these conditions, fatty acids are oxidized in the liver and one of the products (acetyl CoA) is converted to ketone bodies, which can serve as a metabolic fuel. However, elevated levels of ketone bodies in the blood lead to a condition known as ketosis.

Because the majority of ketone bodies are "acids" their high concentration in the circulation triggers buffering systems, which results in the excretion of

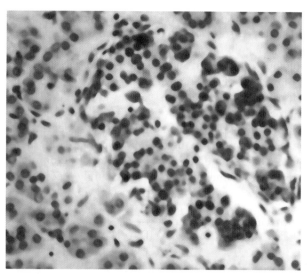

FIGURE 24–1 Normal pancreas. Pancreas stained with immunoperoxidase for glucagon (*red staining*) to show alpha cells in islets of Langerhans (~30% of islets are alpha cells). (Immunoperoxidase staining for glucagons, ×400.)

excess hydrogen ions into the urine. This is accompanied by the loss of water and other ions, including potassium, resulting in dehydration. The high concentration of glucose in the blood leads to urinary excretion of glucose, which is accompanied by a loss of water, owing to the osmotic effect of glucose, further contributing to the dehydration. This results in excessive thirst and decrease in blood volume that is characteristic of uncontrolled type 1 DM.

Breakdown in Tolerance: Stimulation of TLR4

Much of the progress in our understanding of type 1 DM has come from studies with rodents that have served as models for human studies. One pilot study with a heat shock protein (hsp) peptide addressed the relevance of toll-like receptors (TLR) recognition in the immunopathogenesis of type 1 DM. Hsps play an important role, functioning as chaperones for newly synthesized or aberrantly folded proteins. From an evolutionary point of view, hsps are highly conserved in all organisms ranging from bacteria to humans. Hsp60, one of the most studied hsps, has also been shown to activate macrophages and dendritic cells (antigen-presenting cells) after binding to TLR4 on these cells. Peripheral blood cells of both type 1 DM patients and a diabetes-susceptible nonobese diabetic (NOD) strain of mice have a greater number of T cell clones that are specific for hsp60 than do normal populations. In one study, immunization of NOD mice with an hsp60 (amino acids 437 to 460) peptide, prior to the development of overt symptoms of diabetes, led to protection from diabetes. This immunization was associated with a shift from Th1 to Th2 cells specific for the hsp60 peptide. This is consistent with other studies that showed that infusion of Th2 cytokines, particularly IL-4, could ameliorate disease.

Breakdown in Tolerance: Role of Treg Cells

Gut-derived gamma/delta T cells are implicated in regulation of type 1 DM. In animals in which this population of cells was deliberately abolished, diabetes was much easier to induce by deliberate feeding of proinsulin as an autoantigen. Moreover, in these mice, early immunoregulation by gamma/delta TCR+ cells seemed later to evolve to Treg cells, expressing both CD4+ and CD25+.

The CD4+, CD25+ Treg cells have come under intense scrutiny over the past several years as being of major importance in natural immunoregulation, with loss of their function underlying many autoimmune problems (e.g., rheumatoid arthritis, multiple sclerosis, and autoimmune gastritis).

In an interesting model of autoimmune diabetes using a susceptible NOD strain of mouse, induction of such Treg cells by immunization with an insulin peptide (B9-23) was indeed found to protect these mice against diabetes, a protection that could be transferred to other mice by T cells. Similar treatment in pilot studies in humans has been reported to arrest β cell destruction, with preservation of insulin levels at the pretreatment values, along with induction of CD4+, CD25+ Treg.

Role of Autoantibodies

The role of antibodies in the initiation of disease is controversial, although, once generated, they can certainly contribute to the pathogenesis. It is difficult to rationalize a role for antibody in the initiation of disease given reports of type 1 DM in a patient with X-linked agammaglobulinemia (see Case 3). Not surprising, this patient did not have autoantibodies, which are the diagnostic marker of type 1A DM. Rather, involvement of the immune system was shown to be the *in vitro* proliferation of T cells to islet-specific autoantigens. Additionally, the patient's class II MHC haplotype was consistent with that for the highest risk susceptibility (see earlier).

Late-Onset Diabetes

Late-onset (adult) diabetes is often caused by other autoimmune conditions (including anti-insulin receptor antibody and general refractoriness of triggering at the cell surface insulin, receptor, etc). Endogenous insulin is still produced but not in adequate quantities. In such cases, stimulation of existing beta cells with oral antidiabetic medications (e.g., glyburide) to secrete insulin leads to a lowering of blood glucose levels.

CASE

25

Anna is a 27-year-old woman who has been in your practice for many years. She is a teacher, a mother of two young boys, and a nonsmoker and has had no significant ailments of which you are aware. She now presents with generalized fatigue for several months that is significantly impacting on her home life and work. Your immediate concern is that Anna is anemic, which can occur as a result of a poor diet. On questioning, however, Anna is emphatic that she eats a balanced diet and is not a vegetarian. Strict vegetarians can become anemic from a diet-related deficiency of vitamin B_{12} (cobalamin).

Routine physical examination is unremarkable, and chest radiograph is normal. Her blood work shows thrombocytopenia, leukopenia, and anemia (see Appendix for reference values). A peripheral blood smear reveals macrocytic anemia (large red blood cells) and hypersegmented polymorphonuclear neutrophils (PMNs). (Hypersegmented neutrophils have five or more lobes, whereas normal ones have three or four.) Anna is not aware of anyone else in her immediate family who has ever had this sort of problem, although her only siblings are two brothers. What are your thoughts so far?

QUESTIONS FOR GROUP DISCUSSION

1. This patient has had general fatigue for several months and you are concerned that she might be anemic. What is the most common cause of anemia? How would you treat this? What would you recommend for patients who do not absorb iron well?
2. List some of the conditions that you should rule out as causes of anemia due to occult loss of blood.
3. Anna's blood smear revealed macrocytic red blood cells and hypersegmented polymorphonuclear neutrophils. This is consistent with megaloblastic anemia. What is the most common cause of megaloblastic anemia?
4. Review the steps of vitamin B_{12} intestinal absorption. Include in your discussion each of the following: parietal cells, intrinsic factor, vitamin B_{12}, and cubilin.
5. Anna's serum level of vitamin B_{12} is below normal. She is not a vegetarian so it is unlikely that this is a dietary deficiency. How would you test for impaired absorption of this vitamin? Explain the general principle underlying this test and the general procedure.
6. A positive Shilling test indicates only that the absorption of vitamin B_{12} is abnormal. To determine the etiology of the disorder, what autoantibodies would you measure?
7. Discuss the factors that could cause impaired absorption of this vitamin.
8. Explain why measures of homocysteine and methylmalonic acid are not used regularly to test for vitamin B_{12} deficiency.

9. Compare and contrast Imerslund-Grasbeck syndrome and pernicious anemia.
10. Explain how deficiencies in vitamin B_{12} (or folate) can result in anemia.

RECOMMENDED APPROACH

Implications/Analysis of Family History

There is no strong evidence for a genetic component of Anna's clinical presentation, although we are only provided with information regarding the immediate family.

Implications/Analysis of Clinical History

Anna is a nonsmoker, has had no significant ailments, but has been experiencing fatigue for several months, suggesting that she might be anemic. Otherwise, the clinical history is unremarkable.

Implications/Analysis of Laboratory Investigation

Anna's blood work is consistent with megaloblastic anemia. Although there are a number of conditions that can lead to megaloblastic anemia, one of the most common is a deficiency in vitamin B_{12} or folic acid. Because Anna is not a strict vegetarian, a diet-related deficiency of vitamin B_{12} is unlikely. Many patients with a deficiency of vitamin B_{12} have normal serum levels of folate because these levels fluctuate with diet. An appropriate next step would be to test for serum levels of vitamin B_{12}.

Additional Laboratory Tests

Anna's serum vitamin B_{12} levels were low. In the absence of dietary deficiency, impaired absorption of vitamin B_{12} is the most common cause of low serum levels.

Intrinsic Factor and Vitamin B_{12} Absorption

Impaired absorption is generally due to a deficiency of intrinsic factor, the molecule to which dietary vitamin B_{12} must bind before it can be transported across the intestinal wall. Intrinsic factor is produced by gastric parietal cells and so any clinical condition that destroys these cells will lead to a deficiency in intrinsic factor (see Etiology). In some autoimmune disorders, normal levels of intrinsic factor are produced but it is unavailable for binding vitamin B_{12} because anti–intrinsic factor autoantibodies compete with vitamin B_{12} for the intrinsic factor. Therefore, this effectively reduces the amount of vitamin B_{12} that can be transported.

The Shilling Test

Although in some clinical laboratories the Shilling test has been replaced by other tests (see Etiology), this test is still performed in some centers to determine whether orally administered vitamin B_{12} is being transported across the intestinal membrane. In essence, this test determines whether sufficient intrinsic factor is available to transport vitamin B_{12} across the intestine.

In this test, the patient is given an *oral* dose of radiolabeled vitamin B_{12}, which is then measured in urine that has been collected over the following 24 hours. To ensure that radiolabeled vitamin B_{12} does not bind to sites in the body (causing a false low measure), unlabeled vitamin B_{12} is injected intramuscularly. Anna's Shilling test result was shown to be grossly abnormal.

To confirm that the low serum levels of vitamin B_{12} are due to a deficiency of intrinsic factor, the test is repeated with the exception that intrinsic factor is given along with the oral administration of vitamin B_{12}. On the basis of this test, it was concluded that Anna did have a deficiency of intrinsic factor and was diagnosed as having pernicious anemia.

Testing for Autoantibodies

Although you begin treatment immediately (see Therapy section), you also continue to investigate the ultimate etiology of this disorder and request screening for serum autoantibodies to parietal cells and intrinsic factor. The results are made available to you 3 weeks later. Your patient is producing autoantibodies both to gastric parietal cell antigens and to intrinsic factor.

DIAGNOSIS

Megaloblastic anemia resulting from a deficiency of vitamin B_{12} absorption is also referred to as pernicious anemia. Anna was diagnosed with pernicious anemia.

THERAPY

Accordingly, you elect to treat this problem with injectable vitamin B_{12} (every 2 to 3 weeks), which resolves the problem within 3 months. Contrary to conventional medical practice, a number of studies with patients diagnosed with malabsorption of vitamin B_{12} and megaloblastic anemia have concluded that oral administration of very high doses of vitamin B_{12} is as effective as intramuscular injections of vitamin B_{12}. The rationale for this approach is that about 1% of vitamin B_{12} is absorbed in the absence of intrinsic factor.

ETIOLOGY: PERNICIOUS ANEMIA

Deficiencies in vitamin B_{12} and/or folic acid cause megaloblastic anemia, a general term for anemias characterized by enlargement of proliferating cells, particularly red blood cell precursors. Cell enlargement is the result of delayed mitosis despite continuing DNA synthesis and normal synthesis of cytoplasmic proteins and RNA. As a result, megaloblasts accumulate in the bone marrow so few red blood cells are released into the circulation, resulting in anemia. Contributing to the anemia is the fact that the enlarged red blood cells undergo increased hemolysis.

Genetic Component

There is no strong evidence of a genetic component to pernicious anemia, although there are scattered reports that individuals inheriting HLA-A2, HLA-A3, HLA-B7, or HLA-DR5 are predisposed to disease. Some genetic component may yet be identified in that concordance has been reported in sets of monozygotic twins. Since these studies were reported in the 1960s, the monozygotic twins may, in fact, have had a congenital intrinsic factor deficiency, which would manifest as malabsorption and vitamin B_{12} deficiency.

Source and Absorption of Vitamin B_{12}

Our bodies do not synthesize either folate or vitamin B_{12}, and so both must be obtained from our diets. Commensal bacteria, however, can synthesize this vitamin B_{12}, and so we get this vitamin from this source as well. Vitamin B_{12} is absorbed after complexation with intrinsic factor, a protein synthesized by gastric parietal cells. There are two immunologic reasons for a decrease in the availability of intrinsic factor: the first is the production of anti-intrinsic factor autoantibodies, and the other is the autoimmune destruction of parietal cells such that the amount of intrinsic factor secreted is severely decreased.

Vitamin B_{12}–Intrinsic Factor Receptor, Cubilin

Intestinal absorption of B_{12} occurs only when vitamin B_{12} and intrinsic factor form a complex that binds to the cognate receptor, cubilin, present on the intestine and kidney epithelium. This receptor is encoded on chromosome 10.

New Strategies in Laboratory Testing

Elevations in total homocysteine are considered a good indication of vitamin B_{12} deficiency. In fact, increased levels of homocysteine can be detected before symptoms occur. One downside to using this measure as an indicator of vitamin B_{12} deficiency is that other deficiencies and causes can also lead to an increase in homocysteine.

Elevations in methylmalonic acid are also good indicators of vitamin B_{12} deficiency and are more specific than measures of homocysteine, but other causes for elevation in methylmalonic acid have also been reported. Furthermore, assays are expensive and not available in most laboratories.

Imerslund-Grasbeck Syndrome: a Megaloblastic Anemia

Defects in the intrinsic factor/vitamin B_{12} receptor (cubilin) can also lead to a megaloblastic anemia that has been named Imerslund-Grasbeck syndrome. Defects in the synthesis of this receptor or mutations that affect binding of the intrinsic factor/vitamin B_{12} complex lead to Imerslund-Grasbeck syndrome, which is also characterized by a deficiency of serum vitamin B_{12} levels. In a recent report, the functional intrinsic factor/vitamin B_{12} receptor was shown to be a complex, consisting of two subunits, cubilin and amnionless, referred to as "cubam." Whether mutations in amnionless will also prevent absorption of vitamin B_{12} is the focus of ongoing studies.

Folic Acid Deficiencies

Folic acid deficiencies occur primarily in individuals who have had inadequate diets, as may be the case in drug addicts and alcoholics. However, impaired absorption of folate may also occur.

Iron Deficiency Anemia

In contrast, iron deficiency anemia (generally diet related) is not uncommon (microcytic anemia) and is easily treated with iron replacement. In this type of anemia, you should make sure the patient is not losing blood in an occult manner (gastrointestinal tract tumor or chronic gastritis/ulcer; heavy menses). Occasionally, patients do not absorb iron well, and you may have to resort to more readily absorbed oral formulations, or even injectable iron.

Brad, a 25-year-old man, was referred to your endocrinology service by his family physician with apparently multiple autoimmune-type manifestations. He first came to his family physician's attention several years earlier with weight gain, listlessness, general fatigue, and coarsening of the skin. After multiple attempts to establish a diagnosis his physician finally arrived at the conclusion (seemingly confirmed by thyroid function tests) that he was hypothyroid. There was no antecedent viral illness that anyone could remember, and no other family members were affected. These problems seemed to resolve with conventional thyroid replacement therapy with levothyroxine. About 2 years later fatigue recurred despite evidence for normal thyroid replacement. Blood work at this time was suggestive of adrenocortical involvement, and indeed a diagnosis of Addison's disease was pursued. Measurement of serum and urinary adrenocortical hormones supported this hypothesis too, and again he was treated effectively with replacement mineralcorticoid, fludrocortisone (Fluorcortef/Florinef). Once again there was no evidence of any precipitating event to this disorder (drugs/infection) and no family members were affected. Finally, just 3 weeks ago he presented with an oral *Candida albicans* infection, which has been inordinately resistant to topical antifungal agents, and his physician is at a total loss. He is essentially unsure whether Brad is just "unlucky" or whether all of these events are tied together and are independent manifestations of some disorder he has not heard of. The answer is in fact likely to be the latter.

CASE

26

QUESTIONS FOR GROUP DISCUSSION

1. Autoimmune polyendocrinopathy syndrome (APS-1) has been mapped to a unique gene, AIRE (**A**uto**I**mmune **RE**gulator), on chromosome 21. What is the role of the protein that it encodes?
2. What is the criteria for a diagnosis of APS-I? Of APS-II? What technique is used to confirm a mutation in the AIRE gene?
3. Review the role of the thymus in tolerance induction (see Case 2 and the discussion on positive and negative selection).
4. Explain the significance of the fact that an equivalent gene in the mouse has been shown to be expressed in the thymus at sites where negative selection occurs (see Case 2).
5. What is the significance of the fact that a number of organ-specific antigens are actually now known to be expressed in the thymus (e.g., insulin, myelin/oligodendrocyte glycoprotein (MOG), proteolipid protein (PLP), and glutamic acid decarboxylase)?
6. Knockout mice for the AIRE gene equivalent do not express the AIRE equivalent protein. Explain the significance of the fact that they have multiple organ-specific immune syndromes (e.g., orchitis, retinitis), and have antibody titers to multiple organ-specific antibodies.

7. The knockout mice (question 4) have no obvious immune cell abnormalities when compared with wild-type mice. However, there is a subtle increase in thymic epithelial cells in the medulla, as determined using CD80 (B7-1) and CR-1 (antibody specific to thymic epithelial cells). What is the role of CD80 in T cell activation?
8. The knockout mice (question 4) also had an increased number of activated cells in the periphery as determined using CD44 (high) and CD62L (low). CD44 is a glycoprotein that binds to hyaluronan. CD62L is also known as L-selectin, an adhesive molecule that binds to carbohydrates on the endothelium to induce cell rolling. What is the significance of an increase in activated T cells in the periphery in these knockout mice?
9. In further studies with the knockout mice (question 4), thymuses were removed and treated to remove mature T cells. Then these thymuses were transferred into athymic mice (nu/nu); the mice all have the AIRE phenotype described in question 4. On the basis of these studies, hypothesize a role for the AIRE gene in tolerance induction.
10. Why could negative selection of T cells specific for organ-specific genes not occur in the absence of promiscuous transcription of those genes in the medulla?

113

RECOMMENDED APPROACH

Implications/Analysis of Family History

No other affected family members were identified. This does not rule out a genetic disorder in that diseases that have an autosomal recessive inheritance are quite rare. In this type of inheritance disease manifestation occurs only when the individual inherits two defective copies of the gene.

Implications/Analysis of Clinical History

There was no antecedent viral illness that anyone could remember, nor was there any evidence of any precipitating event to this disorder (drugs/infection). The weight gain, listlessness, general fatigue, and coarsening of the skin are symptoms that present in a patient whose thyroid is underactive. The presentation of Addison's disease in a patient who is receiving therapy for hypothyroidism should have steered the physician into considering disorders that affect multiple endocrine systems, in particular autoimmune polyendocrine syndrome (APS).

APS is classified as either APS-I or APS-II. The APS-I classification applies to those syndromes that include Addison's disease, autoimmune thyroid dysfunction, and chronic mucocutaneous candidiasis. The APS-II classification differs from the APS-I in that these patients present with type 1A diabetes instead of mucocutaneous candidiasis (along with Addison's disease and autoimmune thyroid dysfunction). The fact that Brad had recently presented with a *Candida albicans* infection that was inordinately resistant to topical antifungal agents, in addition to the other endocrine disorders, strongly suggests that Brad has APS-I.

Implications/Analysis of Laboratory Investigation

The laboratory investigations over the past few years had confirmed a diagnosis of hypothyroidism, Addison's disease, and now *Candida albicans* infection.

Additional Laboratory Tests

Patients with APS have mutations in the AIRE (AutoImmune REgulator) gene, which maps to human chromosome 21 (see Etiology). Polymerase chain reaction (PCR) and sequencing are used to confirm a mutation in the AIRE gene.

DIAGNOSIS

Brad was diagnosed with the autoimmune polyendocrinopathy syndrome, type I, which is a rare autoimmune disease with autosomal recessive inheritance. Patients with APS-I present with hypothyroidism, Addison's disease, and candidiasis.

THERAPY

Continue with levothyroxine and fludrocortisone. Treat infections as they arise.

ETIOLOGY: AUTOIMMUNE POLYENDOCRINOPATHY SYNDROME

APS-I has been mapped to a unique gene, AIRE, which maps to human chromosome 21. More than 42 different mutations in the AIRE gene have been described. The AIRE gene encodes a transcription factor for many genes. Immunologic tissues, particularly the thymus, show high expression of AIRE. The high expression of the AIRE gene in the thymus, combined with the widespread autoimmune disorders that develop in mice in which this gene has been knocked out, has led to the proposal that the normal AIRE gene encodes a protein that plays a significant role in tolerance induction during T cell development.

In particular, it has been proposed that the AIRE gene product enhances the ectopic expression of peripheral tissue proteins within the thymus (medullary epithelial cells), the site of negative selection during central tolerance induction. It follows, therefore, that self tolerance to peripheral tissue antigens would not occur in the absence of a functional AIRE gene because promiscuous transcription of these peripheral proteins would either not occur or they would be expressed at only low levels in the thymus. The diseases represented in APS-I are presumably those (multiple ones) whose proteins escaped tolerance induction by virtue of low level (or absence of) thymic (medulla) expression. In the absence of this expression, autoreactive T cells are not deleted and tolerance induction does not occur, which leads to multiple autoimmune disorders.

A number of known organ-specific antigens are now known to be ectopically expressed in the presence of a normal AIRE protein (e.g., myelin/oligodendrocyte glycoprotein [MOG], proteolipid protein [PLP], insulin, and glutamic acid decarboxylase), particularly in the medulla, where negative selection occurs.

Murine Studies

An equivalent gene has been discovered in the mouse (~80% homology at protein level). The mouse gene encodes a protein, some 540 amino acids, made up of 14 exons. It is expressed in the thymus, in the medullary epithelium, in dendritic cells, and in essentially all sites of negative selection.

Knockout Mice

A homologous deletion mutant for the mouse gene (knocking out exon 2, which introduces a frameshift and early termination, with no detectable protein) leads to multiple organ-specific immune syndromes (e.g., orchitis, retinitis) in association with development of multiple organ-specific antibodies, much like APS.

Comparison of Knockout Mice with Wild-Type Mice

The knockout mouse has no other obvious abnormalities. It has equivalent numbers to wild-type mice of CD4+/CD8+, αβTCR+, γδTCR+, CD69+ cells, and the same number and function of B cells; its polymorphonuclear cells are equivalent to those of wild-type mice, as are the splenic dendritic cells and antigen-presenting cells. Mixed lymphocyte responses (MLRs) are equivalent, and there is the same cytokine profile after concanavalin A stimulation. There is a subtle increase in thymic epithelial cells in the medulla, marked by CD80 (B7-1) and CR-1, and an increased number of activated T cells in the periphery (CD44hi, CD62Llo [L-selectin]).

Role of the Thymus in the AIRE Phenotype

In an attempt to understand the human disorder, thymuses were removed from the knockout mice, depleted of all mature lymphocytes with 2-deoxyguanosine *in vitro* (thus eliminating the possibility of transferring known immunoregulatory CD4+CD25+ Treg), and transplanted to nu/nu (athymic) mice. At 8 weeks, all mice have the AIRE phenotype. When detailed molecular biology comparisons were performed by gene chip expression in the thymic medullary epithelium of wild-type and knockout mice, some 200 to 1000 genes were found to be affected.

Survival of Autoreactive T Cells

A number of organ-specific tissue-antigen encoding genes are downregulated in knockout mice (e.g., insulin but not glutamic acid decarboxylase). Thus, one possible explanation for these data hypothesizes that AIRE protein enhances organ-specific antigen expression in thymus. Failure to express those organ-specific antigens (in the thymic medulla during development of the T cell repertoire) results in failure to delete autoreactive T cells, tolerance induction does not occur, and this results in multiple autoimmune diseases.

Arnold, a 28-year-old man, recently returned from a camping trip in Massachusetts and has noticed several large, itchy, erythematous (red) patches (that seem to "move around") on his arms. He remembers being bitten by some "bugs" while camping, but otherwise there is no significant medical history of note and no drug history. You recall reading about Lyme disease while you were at medical school and order a serum test for antibodies to *Borrelia burgdorferi*. The test comes back positive, confirming your suspicions (and the recognition of a classic "erythema migrans" picture).

You treat Arnold with a 28-day course of doxycycline with complete resolution of the symptoms. Several months later, Arnold reappears in your office with severe arthritic symptoms of several weeks' duration, predominantly in the large joints (knees). He has been taking over-the-counter anti-inflammatory medication with no relief. An aunt suffers from rheumatoid arthritis, and he is concerned that he is developing the same disease.

You are concerned instead that this represents a persistent manifestation of the Lyme disease. In fact, titers to *B. burgdorferi* are even higher than when you first saw him. Despite further rounds of antibiotic therapy there is no obvious resolution of the arthritic picture, and indeed over the next 3 years his disease is marked by frequent exacerbations. What are some current thoughts regarding this picture? What is known about the pathophysiology?

QUESTIONS FOR GROUP DISCUSSION

1. Review the mode of infection with *Borrelia burgdorferi*.
2. Describe the tests used to diagnose infection with *B. burgdorferi*. What is the confirmation test in North America?
3. Review the inflammatory process (see Case 23). What evidence is there that *B. burgdorferi* synovitis is the result of antigen-driven activation?
4. Spirochete survival has been used to explain persistent synovitis. Discuss.
5. Discuss how molecular mimicry could lead to an autoimmune basis for persistent synovitis.
6. Explain *dominant antigenic epitope* and how this could account for the fact that resident Lyme disease is rare in Europe.
7. Discuss various forms of therapy and the rationale for each.

RECOMMENDED APPROACH

Implications/Analysis of Family History

A major genetic risk factor for therapy failure in patients with Lyme disease is HLA-DR4. Interestingly, Arnold's aunt has rheumatoid arthritis, which is

not linked to Lyme disease, but about 70% of patients with RA express the HLA-DR4 allele (control, 28%).

Implications/Analysis of Clinical History

There is no significant history of note and no drug history. Arnold's "bug" bites were, in fact, tick bites. Ticks are arthropods that belong to the same class as mites. Life stages of ticks include egg, larvae, nymph, and adult. The larvae, nymph, and adult tick obtain their blood meal from mammals and humans. During the blood meal, nymph and adult ticks that are infected with *B. burgdorferi* (in saliva) transmit these bacteria to the host. Because the nymph form is so tiny, it can attach to the host unnoticed and feed for days.

Sixty to 80 percent of patients infected with *B. burgdorferi* initially develop a red spot that expands to form the characteristic ring shape with an outer red shape with a clear center, often described as "bull's-eye" in appearance. Doxycycline is the treatment of choice for men and nonpregnant women and appeared to be effective for Arnold. However, the later presentation of arthritis and the fact that there was no obvious resolution of the arthritic picture suggests that bacterial persistence is not likely the cause of the arthritis. Patients who fail therapy continue to have reactivity to *B. burgdorferi* outer surface lipoprotein A

(OspA), suggesting that this antigen cross reacts with a host protein.

Implications/Analysis of Laboratory Investigation

Laboratory testing plays an important role in diagnosis. Serum tests for antibodies to *B. burgdorferi* include enzyme immunoassay (EIA) and indirect immunofluorescence test. Depending on the laboratory, diagnosis is confirmed with a Western blot. Arnold's EIA results came back positive. In fact, the EIA antibody titers to *B. burgdorferi* were even higher than they were at the initial diagnosis.

Additional Laboratory Tests

A polymerase chain reaction (PCR) test might be considered; however, given the many rounds of antibiotics it is unlikely that *B. burgdorferi* persists in serum. Furthermore, in most patients resistant to drug therapy, PCR technology has generally failed to detect spirochetes.

DIAGNOSIS

Arnold is diagnosed with persistent synovitis, which is seen in about 10% of individuals with so-called antibiotic-resistant Lyme disease.

THERAPY

Patients who do not respond to antibiotic therapy are treated with anti-inflammatory drugs or synovectomy (removal of joint tissue that is inflamed).

ETIOLOGY: LYME DISEASE

Immunologic Response

B. burgdorferi stimulates both innate immune responses (via toll-like receptors), causing release of inflammatory cytokines and other mediators from neutrophils and macrophages, as well as adaptive immune responses. In general, it is thought that Th1-type immunity is engaged as part of the protective immune response.

The final synovial pathology in both rheumatoid arthritis and Lyme arthritis is quite similar. Synovial inflammation and hypertrophy are noted, as are vascular proliferation, mononuclear cell infiltration, and increased expression of adhesion molecules. Multiple nodular aggregates of T cells and B cells with follicular dendritic cells and even germinal center B cells are consistent with ongoing antigen-driven activation, as expected from an autoimmune process. Inflammatory cells express mRNAs for proinflammatory cytokines and a few anti-inflammatory cytokines (e.g., IL-10). Abundant matrix metalloproteinases (MMPs) predominate in the joint fluid (e.g., MMP8), which probably contribute to joint erosion. This picture has led to the idea that understanding the cause of this infectious arthritis may hold key information to the study and understanding of RA.

Persistent Synovitis

The persistent synovitis seen in about 10% of individuals, often in the absence of evidence for persistent infection (so-called antibiotic treatment resistant Lyme disease) has been explained as potentially representing one, or a combination of, the following.

Spirochete Survival?

One hypothesis suggests the spirochetes are protected from host immunity by virtue of modulation of outer surface (immunogenic) epitopes, or following coating by host proteins. Consequently, they are not targeted by B cells, macrophages, or complement. However, in general, even sensitive PCR technology has failed to detect spirochetes in most patients. A "rescue" position for this hypothesis is that there is some long-term retention of spirochete antigens (without viable organisms), which leads to continued stimulation of an arthritogenic response.

Another hypothesis put forth is that the spirochetes survive in a niche (e.g., the cytosol of synoviocytes) where they are not accessible to B cells, phagocytes, or complement. Antigens present in the cytosol are generally processed by the proteasome and displayed on the cell surface of the infected cell where they are recognized by cytotoxic T cells. In this scenario, synoviocytes would be destroyed and *B. burgdorferi* released from the infected cell. To comment on the fate of the bacteria released from these cells would be mere speculation.

Molecular Mimicry?

More interesting is the hypothesis of *Borrelia*-induced autoimmunity, following epitope mimicry. In this model, antigenic determinants on *B. burgdorferi* are similar or identical to a series of amino acids in a host protein (e.g., OspA and LFA-1). Therefore, B cell and T cell activation in response to OspA would generate immune cells and antibodies that would target LFA-1.

Dominant Antigenic Epitope?

The dominant epitope in the *B. burgdorferi* protein, OspA, in the North American form of disease is distinct in sequence from that of the European variant, where treatment-resistant disease is rare. T cells from a susceptible North American population show a higher frequency of responses to this epitope than a North American population with simple Lyme disease. Finally, there is some (albeit weak) evidence that this T cell epitope in OspA shows some relatedness with a sequence in the LFA-1 molecule.

Loss of Tolerance: Autoimmunity?

General inflammation, associated with large-scale tumor necrosis factor-α/interleukin-1β release after *B. burgdorferi* infection, triggers autoimmunity in a bystander fashion (e.g., perhaps potentiated by loss of regulatory T cells). This general mechanism may hold true for several autoimmune-type disorders but has yet to be shown unequivocally for any one particular disorder.

Fred, a 40-year-old man, is well known to the local shelters, including the one you supervise, because he has lived on the streets for several years. He is a known alcoholic and has had tuberculosis in the past, for which he was successfully treated under careful supervision. You have noticed that he has been moving more slowly over the past few days and inquire whether he is feeling like himself. He admits to some general fatigue, particularly in the legs, which just "don't seem to want to carry him around anymore like they used to." The following morning, the fellow who sleeps in the cot next to Fred indicates to you that Fred cannot seem to get out of bed. You confirm this problem, and you call the emergency medical service (EMS) to transport him to the hospital. To your surprise, when you get to the hospital to visit him, the receptionist tells you that he is seriously ill, is in the intensive care unit, and has been intubated because he was no longer able to breathe for himself.

You arrive at the intensive care unit to find Fred in the condition reported. The attending physician describes Fred's condition as one of ascending paralysis, typical of Guillain-Barré syndrome. He asks if Fred has recently suffered from a diarrheal illness (which he did, you recall, about 4 weeks ago), as well as about Fred's alcohol history and other medical disorders. A stool culture was ordered to test for enteric bacteria.

The physician ordered a blood test for creatinine kinase (an enzyme released from destroyed muscle), a stool sample, and assays to detect antibodies that target the gangliosides GM_1 and GQ_{1b}. These are distributed throughout peripheral nervous system myelin.

QUESTIONS FOR GROUP DISCUSSION

1. This patient is an alcoholic. Despite this, alcoholic myopathy is low on your list of considerations. Explain. How would you rule out myopathy as a cause of Fred's problem?
2. What factors, other than alcoholic myopathy, have been shown to cause altered neurotransmission with resulting paralysis?
3. Why would botulism toxin not be a consideration as the cause of Fred's clinical presentation?
4. Fred's condition is one of ascending paralysis, typical of Guillain-Barré syndrome. In this syndrome the myelin sheath of nerves is destroyed such that the nerve conduction is altered. Explain how this would lead to loss of muscle mass with time.
5. Antecedent infection with *Campylobacter jejuni* or cytomegalovirus may lead to Guillain-Barré syndrome and production of autoantibodies to gangliosides present in myelin, GM_1 and GM_2, respectively. Explain how an infection can lead to the production of autoantibodies.
6. What is the most common source of *C. jejuni* infection? What are the symptoms?
7. Describe possible mechanisms for destruction of myelin sheath after production of anti-GM_1 or anti-GM_2 autoantibodies.
8. Explain why Fred's cerebrospinal fluid (CSF) analysis would show an elevated level of protein.
9. Explain why muscle paralysis is life threatening.
10. Describe the two recommended therapies for Guillain-Barré syndrome.

RECOMMENDED APPROACH

Implications/Analysis of Family History

We are not provided with any family history; however, congenital disorders are clearly unlikely again given the historical context in which this disease is presenting. We are told that the symptoms are typical of Guillain-Barré syndrome, which is an autoimmune disorder that is directed at myelin sheaths, resulting in progressive demyelination and altered nerve conduction, which leads to altered neuromuscular contraction. Familial cases of Guillain-Barré syndrome are almost nonexistent, as are data to support a linkage with any particular HLA haplotype.

Implications/Analysis of Clinical History

Alcoholism and Drug Reactions

Alcoholism itself causes muscle wasting, particularly of the proximal muscle girdles (hip/shoulder muscles). However, the tempo of this disorder is too severe for an alcoholic myopathy. Some drug-induced inflammatory disorders (causing myositis) would potentially present in this fashion, but again the tempo is severe.

Metal or Toxin Poisoning

Lead poisoning (with altered neuromuscular transmission) is possible, as are toxins, but neither you nor the attending physician has been given any history suggestive of toxin ingestion. Botulism toxin, which presents in a similar manner, causes descending, not ascending, paralysis. A variant of Guillain-Barré syndrome (Fischer variant) also causes descending paralysis and is difficult to distinguish from botulism toxin.

Campylobacter jejuni Infection

Of significance is the fact that Fred has had gastroenteritis during the past month. Some infectious agents, particularly *C. jejuni*, are known to precede development of Guillain-Barré syndrome. Stool samples of patients infected with *C. jejuni* may contain viable bacteria for 2 to 4 weeks after cessation of diarrhea. Studies have shown that the lipo-oligosaccharide fraction of *C. jejuni's* outer capsular structure is similar to gangliosides. Furthermore, anti-ganglioside antibodies from patients with Guillain-Barré syndrome do cross react with the *C. jejuni* lipo-oligosaccharide fraction.

C. jejuni is the most common bacterial cause of diarrhea in the United States, with 1% of the population infected annually. Contaminated poultry is the cause in more than 60% of cases. Symptoms (fever, diarrhea, abdominal pain) usually resolve in 1 week, with few (<0.02%) cases having more severe sequelae.

Other Infectious Agents

Other infectious agents that are associated with Guillain-Barré syndrome include Epstein-Barr virus, *Mycoplasma pneumoniae*, and cytomegalovirus, but severe axonal degeneration in Guillain-Barré syndrome is associated with *C. jejuni* infections more often than with other infectious agents. About 66% of patients with Guillain-Barré syndrome report antecedent illness with one of these infectious agents. Recent immunization may also precede Guillain-Barré syndrome (e.g., swine influenza vaccine).

Implications/Analysis of Laboratory Investigation

Stool cultures confirmed *C. jejuni* infection. Assays to detect autoantibodies indicated that anti-GM_1 antibodies were present; however, autoantibodies to GQ_{1b} were not detected. High titers of anti-ganglioside autoantibodies (GM_1) may occur in patients when Guillain-Barré syndrome is preceded by *C. jejuni* infection. Autoantibodies to ganglioside GQ_{1b} are associated with the Fischer variant of Guillain-Barré syndrome. Autoantibodies to ganglioside GM_2 may be present when cytomegalovirus is the antecedent infectious agent.

To rule out myopathy as a cause of Fred's problem, a blood sample was tested for creatinine kinase enzyme, which is released from destroyed muscle. Fred's creatinine kinase enzyme level was normal (see Appendix for reference value).

CSF analysis was requested to test for the presence of protein and white blood cells, a nonspecific test for inflammatory processes of the central nervous system. Nerve conduction studies were also requested to determine whether myelin was being destroyed.

Additional Laboratory Tests

CSF analysis indicated an elevated CSF protein level, again suggestive of inflammation, without an increase in leukocytes (pleocytosis). Nerve conduction studies were confirmatory, showing a slowing of conduction velocities, indicating loss of myelin. This is not surprising given that anti-myelin had been detected in Fred's serum.

DIAGNOSIS

Fred was diagnosed with Guillain-Barré syndrome.

THERAPY

The key problem (at least initially) is overcoming the wasting that is causing difficulty with respiratory muscles. Plasma exchange therapy (plasmapheresis) and high doses of intravenous immunoglobulin (IVIG) have been tried with some success. The choice of therapy seems to vary from area to area.

Plasmapheresis

Plasmapheresis is a technique in which autoantibodies (and other proteins) are mechanically removed from the patient. Basically, in this approach, the plasma is separated from the blood cells in a cell separator. The cells are returned to the patient, and intravenous fluid (or antibody-free donated plasma) is used to replace the plasma (the plasma containing antibodies is discarded). Treatment of this problem using this therapy, thus depends on plasmapheresis until such time as production of anti-myelin antibodies decays to levels inadequate to cause symptoms.

Intravenous Immunoglobulin

IVIG is pooled human plasma that consists primarily of IgG antibodies of different specificities, collected from thousands of healthy individuals. The mechanism by which this therapy works is unclear, but it has been proposed that the high concentration of IgG antibodies downregulates B cells by binding to inhibitory Fcγ receptors on these cells.

ETIOLOGY: GUILLAIN-BARRÉ DISEASE

Guillain-Barré disease is an autoimmune disorder in which the myelin sheath of peripheral nerves is attacked by the immune system. It is now believed these attacks represent a classic example of antigen mimicry, where antigens at the surface of infectious agents (e.g., *C. jejuni*) result in production of antibodies that react with, and form, immune complexes that activate complement and destroy the myelin sheath of nerves, preventing nerve conduction. Muscle biopsy shows that, at least initially, the muscle tissue is absolutely normal, although nerves show demyelination. With time, loss of muscle mass occurs from wasting (absence of nerve impulses).

Most individuals recover completely from this disorder (in 3 to 6 months), although a small unfortunate population (<5%) is left with some residual infirmity. In the most severe cases this can even necessitate a life-long tracheostomy with ongoing ventilatory assistance.

C A S E
29

PD is a 38-year-old woman whom you see in follow-up for investigation of abnormal results of liver function tests and vague chronic fatigue. During an otherwise uneventful pregnancy, 2 years earlier, some transient moderate increase (twofold to threefold) in liver enzymes was noted, with simultaneous complaints of abdominal cramps and bloating.

At that time, stool cultures for *Clostridium difficile* toxin were positive and her symptoms resolved after treatment with metronidazole. She is currently experiencing diarrhea of 2 weeks' duration, with fatty foul-smelling stools and frequent abdominal cramps, but on questioning she admits that these symptoms have been essentially intermittent for 10 years or more. However, she does casually mention that when she is on a lactose-free diet the abdominal cramps are less frequent and less severe.

On questioning she is emphatic that there is no family history of inflammatory bowel disorders, that she is not a drug user and that she does not drink alcoholic beverages, has taken no medications, has not been exposed to hepatoxins (as far as she knows), and has not traveled. Blood work revealed a moderate elevation (twofold) in liver enzymes and a deficiency in production of clotting factors synthesized exclusively by the liver. Stool culture was normal, and B cell and T cell numbers and function were normal, as were serum immunoglobulin titers. An enzyme-linked immunosorbent assay (ELISA) for human immunodeficiency virus (HIV) was negative.

QUESTIONS FOR GROUP DISCUSSION

1. Our investigation should begin by considering the possible causes for diarrhea and increase in liver enzymes. Explain why each of the following is not a likely explanation.
   (a) *Clostridium difficile* infection
   (b) Intestinal malignancy
   (c) Cystic fibrosis
   (d) Primary biliary cirrhosis
   (e) Amyloidosis
2. Given the chronic nature of the disorder, evidence for malabsorption, and the relapsing/remitting nature of the disease, an intestinal biopsy was performed. What did this biopsy reveal?
3. Based on the clinical history and the intestinal biopsy, PD was diagnosed with celiac sprue. What causes this disease?
4. Explain how you would confirm a diagnosis of celiac sprue (gluten-sensitive enteropathy).
5. What factor differentiates celiac sprue from other diseases that mimic it (parasitic infections and/or chronic duodenitis)?
6. What recommendations would you give to this patient?

RECOMMENDED APPROACH

Implications/Analysis of Family History

No family history of inflammatory bowel disorders was noted.

Implications/Analysis of Clinical History

The initial discovery of elevated liver function tests in the context of pregnancy was certainly potentially indicative of a pregnancy-related liver disease, including intrahepatic cholestasis, acute fatty liver, and disorders associated with preeclampsia and eclampsia. However, we are told the pregnancy itself was uneventful, and these pregnancy-related changes generally resolve after birth.

Infections

We are told that a previous infection with *C. difficile* has been eradicated; moreover, *C. difficile* infection is not associated with liver abnormalities. Infections would be a consideration for the diarrhea and altered liver function tests, particularly in immunocompromised individuals, but T cell and B cell numbers and function were normal. Tuberculosis, amebiasis, and schistosomiasis could all fit this picture (of gastrointestinal complaints and liver abnormalities), but the chronic course, lack of travel history, and negative stool cultures reduce their likelihood. Bacterial overgrowth in the upper intestine is a plausible consideration.

Disorders That Present Similarly

Intestinal malignancy could present this way, although again the lengthy history suggests this is an unlikely explanation. Cystic fibrosis would certainly fit this picture, although such a late presentation would be extraordinary. Primary biliary cirrhosis, an idiopathic disease generally affecting females of this age group, is a rare autoimmune-type disorder that fits this picture; in a male, sclerosing cholangitis is a disorder also associated with idiopathic inflammation of the bile ducts. A liver biopsy should be ordered to rule out this option (see Additional Laboratory Tests).

Chronic amyloidosis, another rare multisystemic immunologic disorder associated with overproduction and deposition (with induction of nonspecific inflammatory processes) of various proteins (e.g., serum amyloid protein) could also explain the picture. Biopsy would rule this out (also test for elevated serum amyloid protein).

Implications/Analysis of Laboratory Investigation

Blood work should include elimination of HIV infection and simple tests to exclude generalized immunodeficiency (e.g., T cell and B cell numbers/function; serum immunoglobulin). Given the chronic nature of the process, the evidence for malabsorption symptoms, and the relapsing/remitting nature of the disease, an intestinal biopsy is warranted (see Additional Laboratory Tests).

Additional Laboratory Tests

Liver and intestinal biopsies were performed. Liver biopsy was essentially normal. The intestinal biopsy reveals flattening of the crypts, villous atrophy, a lymphoplasmacytic infiltration of the mucosal wall, and increased intraepithelial lymphocytes (see Diagnosis).

Further confirmation of the diagnosis can be sought with tests for antigliadin antibodies. In addition, antiendomysial antibodies are increased in titer; these recognize a tissue transglutaminase that has gliadin as its preferred substrate.

DIAGNOSIS

The best diagnosis after the intestinal biopsy results and clinical history is celiac sprue, or gluten-sensitive enteropathy.

THERAPY

Eliminate gluten from the diet.

ETIOLOGY: CELIAC DISEASE

Celiac sprue, or gluten-sensitive enteropathy, is caused by immunologic reaction to wheat gliadin and similar proteins in the diet. The disease has an incidence of some 1:500 in Western Europeans. The importance of increased intraepithelial lymphocytes in this disorder has been stressed as a factor differentiating celiac sprue from other diseases that mimic it, including the altered histopathology and absorption that occurs in association with some parasitic infections and/or chronic duodenitis. These intraepithelial lymphocytes are, in general, cytotoxic T cells that decrease in number when gluten is withdrawn from the diet, rapidly recurring (within hours) with reintroduction of gluten in the diet. The relief of symptoms with elimination of gluten from the diet is also diagnostic.

Sam is a 44-year-old, previously healthy man who has been suffering from blurred vision and intermittent numbness in the left leg and right arm for 7 months. Over the past 4 weeks he has been incontinent of urine twice. His male companion is convinced he has a brain tumor or some other sinister disorder. All of his routine blood work is normal, as is his urinalysis, antinuclear antibody (ANA) titers, and complement C3 levels. His last HIV test (6 years ago) was negative, and he has lived with his current partner for more than 5 years. A repeat HIV test is negative.

QUESTIONS FOR GROUP DISCUSSION

1. Review the types of infection that cause chronic infection of the central nervous system (CNS) or encephalitis. What single piece of evidence would reduce the likelihood that Sam has an infection or a multifocal brain tumor?
2. Systemic lupus erythematosus (SLE) cerebritis might present in this manner. Review Case 18 and explain why this disorder might lead to cerebritis. How would you rule out SLE?
3. What disorders are associated with urine incontinence in males?
4. Multiple sclerosis (MS) is a waxing/waning disease that manifests at different sites, and so this disorder should be the focus of investigation. Explain how magnetic resonance imaging (MRI) and magnetic resonance spectroscopy could help in the diagnosis of MS. What would a biopsy show?
5. Oral feeding of antigen (bovine myelin) has been used as a therapeutic intervention in some clinical trials of patients with MS. Explain the rationale for this approach.
6. Explain why chemokine antagonists are being considered as therapeutic agents in MS. (*Hint:* review Case 23.)
7. Explain *tolerance induction* and how this might be achieved in patients with MS.
8. Discuss the pros/cons of targeting specific Vβ T cells as therapy for patients with MS.
9. What antibody isotype(s) is (are) found in the CSF of patients with MS? In the serum?
10. Review the steps of delayed-type hypersensitivity (DTH). Note, in particular, the role of interferon gamma (IFNγ). Explain why IFNγ would exacerbate MS.

RECOMMENDED APPROACH

Implications/Analysis of Family History

Although we are not provided with any family history, there is a genetic susceptibility for MS. However, risk for this autoimmune disorder involves more than gene inheritance. For example, living in a temperate zone (both north and south of the equator) has been shown to be a risk factor for MS. However, even within the same temperate climate the prevalence of MS is higher in whites.

Implications/Analysis of Clinical History

The altered vision and intermittent numbness in Sam's arm and leg are indicative of multiple, distinct sites in the nervous system and lead one to consider a multifocal brain tumor. However, the fact that the altered vision and changes in sensation are also occurring at different points in time suggests we are dealing with a waxing/waning disease entity, which is *not* characteristic of tumors but should make you think of other causes, especially immunologic ones.

Infection

Toxoplasmosis (and other chronic CNS infections [e.g., *Cryptococcus neoformans*]) could present as a multifocal disease. One might expect viral encephalopathies (e.g., herpes simplex virus, also referred to as human herpesvirus 1) to present more acutely than over months. Again, infection is unlikely to be intermittent. Immune complex deposition disease (lupus cerebritis) such as occurs in systemic lupus erythematosus (SLE), is a possibility because it is associated with intermittent inflammation in the CNS (see Case 31).

Urine Incontinence

The urine incontinence is puzzling in that Sam does not appear to have an infection and is not taking medications known to affect continence. In men, diabetic neuropathy, MS, and Parkinson's disease are known to be causes of incontinence. There is no evidence of diabetes or Parkinson's disease, but the symptoms of blurred vision and changes in sensation are consistent with a diagnosis of MS.

Implications/Analysis of Laboratory Investigation

His last HIV test (6 years ago) was negative, and a repeat test is negative, ruling out HIV-related neurologic disease. All of Sam's routine blood work is normal, as are his ANA titers and complement C3 levels, ruling out lupus cerebritis (see earlier). Having excluded SLE, viral infection, and diabetes, we are faced with the fact that there are multiple neurologic insults that manifest as a clinical symptom intermittently. The most plausible disease based on both exclusion and clinical presentation is MS.

Additional Laboratory Tests

There is no definitive diagnostic test for MS. A positive diagnosis requires that a number of criteria be fulfilled. MRI that reveals four distinct white matter lesions (or three if one is periventricular) is a criterion supporting an MS diagnosis. Results of Sam's MRI evaluation revealed multiple lesions with no ring enhancement after administration of a contrast agent (which is typical of "walled off" tumor/cryptococcal/ and *Toxoplasma* lesions). Magnetic resonance spectroscopy may be used to detect biochemical changes in the brain by following the levels of N-acetyl-aspartate (NAA), an amino acid found in neurons and axons. A reduction in NAA is indicative of axonal loss. This technique provides information regarding decreased activity in areas of the brain without lesions and so can be used to monitor the progression of MS. A biopsy revealed nonspecific inflammation with activated glial cells and lymphocyte infiltration.

DIAGNOSIS

Sam was diagnosed with multiple sclerosis.

THERAPY

At present, neither prednisone nor cyclophosphamide (potent anti-inflammatory agents) have proven to have the desired efficacy, and there is clearly a need for newer therapies, including investigational ones.

Oral Feeding of Antigen

One therapy that has incited great interest involves oral feeding of CNS antigens, which may be relevant to the disorder! Why would further antigen exposure be considered as a way of improving disease outcome, rather than making it worse? The rationale lies in the belief that pathology is secondary to Th1-driven cytokine production. If this is the case, "switching" T cell activation to Th2 cytokines might be beneficial. Transforming growth factor-β (TGFβ) and interleukin-10 (IL-10) are two cytokines that can alter this balance of Th cells from Th1 to Th2. The production of both these cytokines is increased (we do not know how) after oral immunization. Presumably, this has something to do with unique modes of antigen presentation in the gut. The expectation is that increased TGFβ and IL-10 will "switch off" cytokine production by Th1 cells, increase Th2 cytokine production, and thus lead to improvement of symptoms in MS. To date the results of clinical trials have not been very impressive.

One of the reasons for these disappointing results may lie in the fact that several studies have been published suggesting that Th2 cytokines also play a role in the pathogenesis of MS.

Chemokine Antagonists

Other notable changes occur within the CNS of MS patients, perhaps even before altered cytokine production. Included in the changes are altered production of certain chemokines, chemical messenger molecules that control a myriad of functions, including leukocyte migration, endothelial activation, cytokine production, and even lymphocyte activation. Thus, treatment with chemokine antagonists may prove beneficial.

Restoring Tolerance

In animal model systems, therapies aimed at restoring tolerance have shown some promise. The "targets" in this approach are T lymphocytes expressing T cell receptors specific for MS peptide and class II MHC proteins (i.e., class II MHC/MS peptide). This is accomplished by introducing altered MS peptides that will be presented to T cells in the groove of class II MHC proteins on antigen-presenting cells. The expectation is that the altered peptide will trigger signals that inhibit further T cell activation. Consequently, these T cells undergo apoptosis and result in nonresponsiveness to the class II MHC/MS peptide (i.e., tolerance).

Monoclonal Antibodies

In another approach, CD4+ T cells are targeted with monoclonal antibodies so that complement or phagocytes can destroy them. The specificity of the monoclonal antibodies is the particular Vβ segment present in the T cell receptors that recognize the class II MHC/MS complex (see Case 2). The downside to this approach is that many T cells specific for other peptide-MHC complexes also express that particular Vβ segment and so all of these T cells would also be destroyed.

A more pervasive deletion of immune cells can be accomplished by the deletion of leukocytes (which would include T cells) using a monoclonal antibody (alemtuzumab) specific for the leukocyte marker, CD52. The downside to this type of therapy is that all leukocytes are potential targets for elimination. A clinical trial using this monoclonal antibody is currently in progress in both the United States and Europe.

ETIOLOGY: MULTIPLE SCLEROSIS

MS is a chronic inflammatory disease of the CNS that results in scarring and demyelination (Fig. 30–1). There is evidence that a breakdown of tolerance to a variety of nerve-associated proteins/glycolipids plays a major role in the disease process. CD4+ T cells, secreting type 1 cytokines, have been the focus of investigations and novel therapies for MS. More recently, however, a role for type 2 cytokines (and CD8+ T cells) in the disease process has been proposed. Autoantibodies specific for myelin basic protein are generated in MS, but these are not thought to be the inciting agents of disease. They do, however, contribute to the

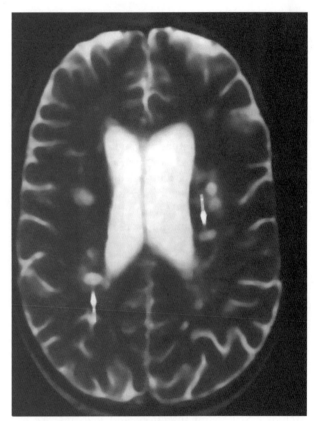

FIGURE 30–1 Multiple periventricular lesions seen in MR image of patient with late-stage multiple sclerosis.

pathogenesis of disease because their presence can activate phagocytes and complement processes.

Risk for Acquiring MS

From a genetic point of view, HLA-DR2 is a major risk factor for developing MS. Obviously, the contribution of genetic inheritance is best determined with monozygotic twins, which shows a concordance rate of 30%. Siblings and other relatives have an increased risk for disease, but this risk decreases as genetic similarity decreases. So, even though first-, second-, and third-degree relatives are all at risk, third-degree relatives would have the lowest risk (see earlier for risk associated with living in a temperate zone).

Immunoglobulin Profiles in CNS and Serum

CD4+ T cells recognize unique CNS antigens (e.g., myelin basic protein), and cytokine production from these T cells activates local inflammatory processes. Note that when cells in the immune system are activated by specific antigen, only T and B cells recognizing that particular antigen will proliferate. This results in so-called oligoclonal activation, not polyclonal activation.

In this case, the immunoglobulin profile in the CNS shows an oligoclonal pattern of IgG synthesized in the CNS. Various techniques are used to ascertain that these IgG antibodies are not serum antibodies that have crossed into the CNS. In contrast, all antibody isotypes are represented in serum. These antibody isotypes can be separated using immunoelectrophoresis; and because of the polyclonal nature of the antibodies in this disease, the pattern is smeared.

T Cell Receptor Specificity

In the T cell compartment, specific stimulation leads to recruitment of T cells expressing only some Vβ molecules in their antigen receptor. Again, Vβ analysis of T cells after specific stimulation will show oligoclonal expansion of the Vβ repertoire. Similarly, CNS T cells show limited Vβ patterns (oligoclonal activation).

Inciting Agent(s)

There often is evidence for both immunoglobulin and T cell reactivity to antigens that cross react with "measles-like" antigens, providing the basis for the belief that there may be a viral inciting agent as the cause of this disease. The geographic distribution of this virus might explain the preponderance of MS in those individuals born in the temperate zones.

Cytokine Production and a Delayed-Type Hypersensitivity Reaction

An inflammatory delayed-type hypersensitivity reaction (DTH) picture is characteristic of Th1 activation. Thus, in most circumstances you can expect to see evidence for IL-2, IFNγ, and tumor necrosis factor-α (TNFα) production. With effective treatment, production of these inflammatory-type cytokines decreases. The difficulty is in finding an effective treatment!

Interestingly, IFNγ was initially used as a therapy for MS, but it exacerbated the disease, despite the fact that it reduced symptoms in animal models. More puzzling is the fact that therapies that neutralize TNFα have induced inflammatory demyelination. Until recently, most studies supported a model in which disease process was due to the presence of type 1 cytokines and that the disease process could be ameliorated by enhancing the production of type 2 cytokines that downregulate type 1 cytokine production.

RR, a 17-year-old woman who was previously well, has been admitted to the hospital because of fever, rash, generalized fatigue, and acute pain in the left eye. In the last 2 months she has lost 12 kg in weight and reports an intermittent fever with fatigue of the same duration. She has had multiple sexual partners and a therapeutic abortion at 14 years of age. There has been no recent travel, and a tuberculosis skin test is negative (with positive control). She appears ill, has marked conjunctival infection, a tender sclera with palpation, and left retinal detachment with some peri-orbital swelling. Fundoscopic/ophthalmoscopic examination (of the optic disc, blood vessels, and retina) is otherwise normal. The remainder of the ears, nose, and throat examination is unremarkable, although she does have prominent nontender cervical nodes. There is also swelling of the inguinal nodes, a macular rash (small, flat spots) on the thigh, and a faint cardiac murmur in the upper chest.

An HIV (ELISA) and a syphilis (VDRL) test were ordered immediately, as was a urine and blood screen culture, and chest radiograph. HIV tests were negative, but a serologic test for syphilis was positive, although a hemagglutination test for *Treponema pallidum* was negative (i.e., a "false positive" syphilis test was seen). Urine showed 2+ (30 mg/dL) protein, some red blood cells, and some hyaline casts (generally reflecting inflammatory changes in the upper urinary tract, including the kidney). Blood screen indicated that she was moderately anemic (hemoglobin 80% of normal; see Appendix for reference value), with a lymphopenia (lymphocyte counts about 20% of normal) and low platelets. The chest radiograph was normal. A bone marrow aspirate with smear was performed. However, there was no evidence for lymphoma or leukemia, Hodgkin's disease, malignant histiocytosis (resident macrophages in connective tissue), or other immunolymphoproliferative disorders. Computed tomography (CT) showed swelling of the soft tissues around the left eye and evidence for cerebral atrophy. Blood cultures remained negative throughout hospitalization.

QUESTIONS FOR GROUP DISCUSSION

1. This clinical picture is consistent with multiple different disorders. So, the challenge is to exclude disorders by the judicious use of tests. Review the results of each of the following tests and the conclusions that could be drawn on the basis of these results.
   (a) Complete blood cell count
   (b) Urinalysis
   (c) Bone marrow aspirate and smear
   (d) Culture
   (e) Chest radiograph
   (f) Computed tomography (CT)
   (g) Antibody titer for HIV
   (h) Antibody titer for syphilis
2. The serologic test for syphilis (VDRL) was positive. Yet the confirmatory test (hemagglutination assay) was negative. Explain.
3. The CT scan showed evidence for cerebral atrophy. In addition, laboratory tests revealed lymphopenia and thrombocytopenia. These results coupled with the cardiac murmur, a macular rash, and a positive syphilis VDRL are consistent with an autoimmune disorder. Explain why you would consider or rule out each of the following:
   (a) Reiter's syndrome
   (b) Crohn's disease
   (c) sarcoidosis
   (d) Behçet's disease
   (e) rheumatoid arthritis
   (f) polyarteritis
   (g) Wegener's granulomatosis
   (h) systemic lupus erythematosus
4. What result would you expect if you were to test for each of the following?
   (a) antinuclear antibodies
   (b) anti-dsDNA antibodies
   (c) complement C3 or C4 levels
   (d) biopsy of the rash
5. What therapy would you recommend? Explain.

RECOMMENDED APPROACH

Implications/Analysis of Family History

No family history is provided. See Cases 18 and 22 for genetics of this disorder.

Implications/Analysis of Clinical History

This presentation is consistent with multiple disorders; and in attempting to exclude them, it is essential to be judicious in choice of tests. The picture seems to be one of an acute disorder, and our diagnostic decision tree should keep this in mind.

Implications/Analysis of Laboratory Investigation

Ruling Out Infection

Early testing ruled out the probability of acute or chronic infectious disorders as explanation for these symptoms in that the chest radiograph is normal, blood cultures are negative, as are the tests for HIV and syphilis. Although the VDRL assay, the screening test for syphilis, was positive, the confirmatory test was negative. The VDRL assay detects anticardiolipid antibodies. Because these antibodies may be present in patients with some viral, bacterial, and parasitic infections, and in some autoimmune disorders, there is a high incidence of false-positive findings. Therefore, a confirmatory test that detects antibodies specific for antigens expressed on *Treponema pallidum* (the causative agent of syphilis) is required. The confirmatory test was negative, indicating that RR did not have syphilis, but she does have anticardiolipin antibodies, and we must take this into consideration when determining a diagnosis.

Ruling Out Malignancy

The likelihood of a malignancy (lymphoma, leukemia, Hodgkin's disease, malignant histiocytosis, or other lymphoproliferative disorders) has lessened at this time in that the chest radiograph is normal and the white blood cell count is reduced (not elevated). As well, the bone marrow smear, which provides (1) a leukocyte estimate, (2) leukocyte differential, (3) the presence of abnormal cells (e.g., Reed-Sternberg cells

in Hodgkin's disease), (4) as well as erythrocyte, and (5) platelet morphology, was normal.

Anemia, Proteinuria, and Hyaline Casts

RR is moderately anemic, but a number of mechanisms can lead to anemia (e.g., trauma, autoantibodies, infections, iron deficiency, drug associated). Urinalysis revealed proteins, red blood cells, and hyaline casts. Hyaline casts consist of material shed from renal tubules but retain the shape of the tubule. Hyaline casts are made of gelled protein and are translucent.

The presence of protein, red blood cells, and hyaline casts in the urine is an indication that the kidneys are not functioning normally. Renal problems can develop as a result of immune complex deposition in the glomeruli. Because we have already ruled out an acute or chronic infection, as well as a malignancy, these could not be the source of antigen and so we should be focusing our attention to autoimmune disorders in which immune complexes contribute to the pathology. Circulating immune complexes could also trigger inflammatory reactions that result in swelling of soft tissues around the left eye and cerebral atrophy (as shown on CT).

Rheumatologic Disorders as Possibilities

Our focus has instead switched to the likelihood of a rheumatologic disorder as the primary diagnosis. The spondylarthropathies such as Reiter's syndrome or Crohn's disease are unlikely, given the lack of evidence for musculoskeletal symptoms (prominent in Reiter's disease, as is keratitis and iritis, not scleritis) or gastrointestinal symptoms (for Crohn's disease). Sarcoidosis might also explain the scleritis and renal involvement but is less likely in the absence of lung disease and arthritis. Behçet's disease, a chronic inflammatory disorder in which HLA-B51 is risk factor, is associated with ocular inflammation but generally presents as mucosal ulceration (absent in this patient). Rheumatoid arthritis is unlikely in the absence of any joint symptoms.

Vasculitis is an inflammation of the blood vessels that results from narrowing of the inflamed vessels and, hence, insufficient blood flow to the affected organ (Fig. 31–1). Therefore, manifestations or symptoms depend on the particular vessels involved. Polyarteritis nodosa, a multisystemic disease that often involves the skin, nerves, heart, gut, and kidneys

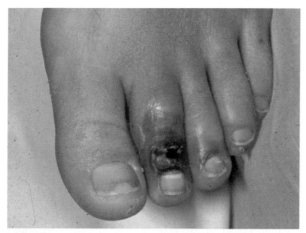

FIGURE 31–1 Necrotic digital ulceration in a patient with vasculitis (immune complex–mediated). (From Goldman L, Ausiello D: Cecil Textbook of Medicine, 22nd ed. Philadelphia, Saunders, 2004.)

might be considered except that most cases occur in 40- to 60-year-old patients. Dermatomyositis might be considered, bearing in mind the vague symptoms and the rash. Blood work to eliminate muscle inflammation essentially removes the latter from consideration.

Wegener's granulomatosis, a granulomatous vasculitis that can present with scleritis, rash, and renal involvement, is certainly a consideration. It affects both men and women of all ages. Typically, these patients produce high titers of anti-neutrophilic cytoplasmic antibodies (ANCA), and an ELISA could be ordered to rule out this possibility, but the false-positive syphilis test is not readily explained by vasculitis.

Immune Complex Disorder

High on the list of possibilities is systemic lupus erythematosus (SLE). Immune complex deposition in different tissues would explain the results of the urinalysis, CT, and false-positive VDRL assay. As well, lymphopenia, thrombocytopenia, cardiac signs (the murmur referred to earlier), and the rash are consistent with a diagnosis of SLE. The rash results from blood leaking out of damaged blood vessels during the inflammatory processes. The cerebral atrophy is striking in one so young, but it could represent lupus cerebritis, an inflammation of the brain. Therefore, tests to determine the ANA and anti-DNA titer, as well as a biopsy of the rash were ordered (see Additional Laboratory Tests).

Additional Laboratory Tests

A serologic test for ANA was performed (positive at a titer of 1:2000). Antibodies to double-stranded DNA were detected at high titer (1:640), and complement C3 and C4 were low, as were total serum complement levels (see Case 11). Biopsy of the rash showed features typical of leukocytoclastic (small vessel) vasculitis.

DIAGNOSIS

The laboratory results and clinical picture are suggestive of an actively aggressive picture of SLE, with severe ocular findings.

THERAPY

Appropriate aggressive treatment was instituted initially (with high-dose intravenous corticosteroids), given the immediate threat to the organ (the eye). Thereafter, maintenance therapy (oral corticosteroids) with monitoring of her serology and urine should begin. A cardiac ultrasound may be performed to get baseline estimate of cardiac performance and to ensure no pericardial fluid collection from serositis.

ETIOLOGY: SYSTEMIC LUPUS ERYTHEMATOSUS

Autoantibodies form soluble complexes with a number of autoantigens, and the resulting immune complexes deposit in small vessels in various tissues. These immune complexes serve as a target for neutrophil, macrophage, and complement activation, resulting in the production and release of inflammatory mediators that cause local damage.

The central nervous system inflammation can often cause very significant pathology. Seizures have been described in this scenario. Neuropsychiatric testing often reveals significant deficits (e.g., in memory, intellectual ability). These are generally not permanent if aggressive treatment of the underlying cause (i.e., SLE) is used. Presumably, the deficits reflect transient neurologic "stunning" from inflammatory processes.

FURTHER READING

Aminoff M, et al: Mutations in CUBN, encoding the intrinsic factor-vitamin B_{12} receptor, cubilin, causes hereditary megaloblastic anaemia 1. Nat Genet 21:309, 1999.

Andersen MS, et al: Projection of an immunological self shadow with the thymus by the AIRE protein. Science 298:1395, 2002.

Andres E, et al: Efficacy of short-term oral cobalamin therapy for the treatment of cobalamin deficiencies related to food-cobalamin malabsorption: A study of 30 patients. Clin Lab Haematol 25:161, 2003.

Ang CW, Jacobs BC, Laman JD: The Guillain-Barré syndrome: A true case of molecular mimicry. Trends Immunol 25:61, 2004.

Arbuckle MR, et al: Development of autoantibodies before clinical onset of systemic lupus erythematosus. N Engl J Med 349:1526, 2003.

Atkinson MA, Eisenbarth GS: Type 1 diabetes: New perspectives on disease pathogenesis and treatment. Lancet 358:221, 2001.

Au A, O'Day J: Review of severe vaso-occlusive retinopathy in systemic lupus erythematosus and the antiphospholipid syndrome: Associations, visual outcomes, complications and treatment. Clin Exp Ophthalmol 32:87, 2004.

Baudon JJ, et al: Diagnosing celiac disease: A comparison of human tissue transglutaminase antibodies with antigliadin and antiendomysium antibodies. Arch Pediatr Adolesc Med 158:584, 2004.

Bolaman Z, et al: Oral versus intramuscular cobalamin treatment in megaloblastic anemia: A single center, prospective, randomized, open-label study. Clin Ther 25:3124, 2003.

Brasington RD, et al: Immunologic rheumatic disorders. J Allergy Clin Immunol 111:S593, 2003.

Centers for Disease Control and Prevention: Lyme disease—United States, 2001-2002. JAMA 291:2810, 2004.

Cervera R, Asherson RA: Clinical and epidemiological aspects in the antiphospholipid syndrome. Immunobiology 207:5, 2003.

Ciccarelli O, Miller DH: Magnetic resonance imaging in multiple sclerosis. Practical Neurol 2:103, 2002.

Cohen SB, et al: Patient-versus physician-reported outcomes in rheumatoid arthritis patients treated with recombinant interleukin-1 receptor antagonist (anakinra) therapy. Rheumatology 43:704, 2004.

Cole P, Rabasseda X: The soluble tumor necrosis factor receptor etanercept: A new strategy for the treatment of autoimmune rheumatic disease. Drugs Today 40:281, 2004.

Csernok E: Anti-neutrophil cytoplasmic antibodies and pathogenesis of small vessel vasculitis. Autoimmun Rev 2:158, 2003.

Delarasse C, et al: Myelin/oligodendrocyte glycol-protein-deficient (MOG-deficient) mice reveal lack of immune tolerance to MOG in wild-type mice. J Clin Invest 112:544, 2003.

Devendra D, Eisenbarth GS: Immunologic endocrine disorders. J Allergy Clin Immunol 11:S624, 2003.

Devlin SM, Andrews CN, Beck PL: Celiac disease: CME update for family physicians. Can Fam Physician 50:719, 2004.

Eisenbarth GS, Gottlieb PA: Autoimmune polyendocrine syndromes. N Engl J Med 350:2068, 2004.

Ekerfelt C, et al: Lyme borreliosis in Sweden: Diagnostic performance of five commercial *Borrelia* serology kits using sera from well-defined patient groups. APMIS 112:74, 2004.

Fasano A, et al: Prevalence of celiac disease in at-risk and not-at-risk groups in the United States: A large multicenter study. Arch Intern Med 163:286, 2003.

Finkel HE, et al: Blindness in a vegan. N Engl J Med 343:585, 2000.

Fletcher DD, et al: Long-term outcome in patients with Guillain-Barré syndrome requiring mechanical ventilation. Neurology 54:2311, 2000.

Fyfe JC, et al: The functional cobalamin (vitamin B_{12})–intrinsic factor receptor is a novel complex of cubilin and amnionless. Blood 103:1573, 2004

Gill JM, et al: Diagnosis of systemic lupus erythematosus. Am Fam Physician 68:2179, 2003.

Gordon MM, et al: A genetic polymorphism in the coding region of the gastric intrinsic factor gene (GIF) is associated with congenital intrinsic factor deficiency. Hum Mutat 23:85, 2004.

Grimm D, et al: Outer-surface protein C of the Lyme disease spirochete: A protein induced in ticks for infection of mammals. Proc Natl Acad Sci U S A 101:3142, 2004.

Halonen M, et al: AIRE mutations and human leukocyte antigen genotypes as determinants of the autoimmune polyendocrinopathy-candidiasis-ectodermal dystrophy phenotype. J Clin Endocrinol Metab 87:2568, 2002.

Harrison MJ, Ravdin LD: Cognitive dysfunction in neuropsychiatric system lupus erythematosus. Clin Opin Rheumatol 14:510, 2002.

Hayes EB, Piesman J: How can we prevent Lyme disease? N Engl J Med 348:2424, 2003.

Homo-Delarche F, Drexhage HA: Immune cells, pancreas development, regeneration and type 1 diabetes. Trends Immunol 25:222, 2004.

Kang I, Park SH: Infectious complications in SLE after immunosuppressive therapies. Curr Opin Rheumatol 15:528, 2003.

Klein L, et al: Shaping of the autoreactive T-cell repertoire by a splice variant of self protein expressed in thymic epithelial cells. Nat Med 6:56, 2000.

Kroesen S, et al: Serious bacterial infections in patients with rheumatoid arthritis under TNF-α therapy. Rheumatology 42:617, 2003.

Lassmann H, Ransohoff RM: The CD4-Th1 model for multiple sclerosis: A crucial re-appraisal. Trends Immunol 25:275, 2004.

Londie M, Maiuri L: Gliadin as stimulator adaptive and innate immune responses in celiac disease. J Pediatr Gastroenterol Nutr 39:S729, 2004.

Martin S, et al: Development of type 1 diabetes despite severe hereditary B-cell deficiency. N Engl J Med 345:1036, 2001.

Muller WA: Leukocyte–endothelial-cell interactions in leukocyte transmigration and the inflammatory response. Trends Immunol 24:327, 2003.

Myhre AG, et al: Autoimmune adrenocortical failure in Norway autoantibodies and human leukocyte antigen Class II associations related to clinical features. J Clin Endocrinol Metab 87:618, 2002.

Nadelman RB, Wormser GP: Recognition and treatment of erythema migrans: Are we off target? Ann Intern Med 136:477, 2002.

Nyholm E, et al: Oral vitamin B_{12} can change our practice. Postgrad Med J 79:218, 2003.

Ochi K, et al: Changes in serum macrophage-related factors in patients with chronic inflammatory demyelinating polyneuropathy caused by intravenous immunoglobulin therapy. J Neurol Sci 208:43, 2003.

Oh R, Brown DL: Vitamin B_{12} deficiency. Am Fam Physician 67:979, 2003.

Ozbek S, et al: Delay in the diagnosis of SLE: The importance of arthritis/arthralgia as the initial symptom. Acta Med Okayama 57:187, 2003.

Pedotti R, et al: Multiple elements of the allergic arm of the immune response modulate autoimmune demyelination. Proc Natl Acad Sci U S A 100:1867, 2003.

Polman CH, Uitdehaag M: New and emerging treatment options for multiple sclerosis. Lancet Neurol 2:563, 2003.

Rossi T: Celiac disease. Adolesc Med Clin 15:91, 2004.

Seneviratne U: Guillain-Barré syndrome. Postgrad Med J 76:774, 2000.

Settles B, et al: Down regulation of cell adhesion molecules LFA-1 and ICAM-1 after in vitro treatment with anti-TNF-alpha agent thalidomide. Cell Mol Biol 47:1105, 2001.

Sollid LM, Gray GM: A role for bacteria in celiac disease? Am J Gastroenterol 99:905, 2004.

Steere AC, Coburn J, Glickstein L: The emergence of Lyme disease. J Clin Invest 113:1093, 2004.

Steere AC: Duration of antibiotic therapy for Lyme disease. Ann Intern Med 138:761, 2003.

Toh BH, van Driel IR, Gleeson PA: Pernicious anemia. N Engl J Med 337:1441, 1997.

Torrance GW, et al: Improvement in health utility among patients with rheumatoid arthritis treated with adalimumab (a human anti-TNF monoclonal antibody) plus methotrexate. Rheumatology 43:712, 2004.

Van Koningsveld R et al: Effect of methylprednisolone when added to standard treatment with intravenous immunoglobulin for Guillain-Barré syndrome: Randomized trial. Lancet 363:192, 2004.

Van Rhijn I, et al: Gamma/delta T cell non-responsiveness in *Campylobacter jejuni*–associated Guillain-Barré syndrome patients. Neurology 61:994, 2003.

Wanschiz J, et al: Distinct time pattern of complement activation and cytotoxic T cell response in Guillain-Barré syndrome. Brain 126:2034, 2003.

Ward PC: Modern approaches to the investigation of vitamin B_{12} deficiency. Clin Lab Med 22:435, 2002.

Watson JA, Clearman B, Mitros F: Effect of a gluten-free diet on gastrointestinal symptoms in celiac disease. Am J Clin Nutr 79:669, 2004.

White S, Rosen A: Apoptosis in systemic lupus erythematosus. Curr Opin Rheumatol 15:557, 2003.

Widhe M, et al: *Borrelia*-specific interferon-gamma and interleukin-4 secretion in cerebrospinal fluid and blood during Lyme borreliosis in humans: Association with clinical outcome. J Infect Dis 189:1881, 2004.

Williams AJK, et al: The high prevalence of autoantibodies to tissue transglutaminases in first degree relatives of patients with type 1 diabetes is not associated with islet autoimmunity. Diabetes Care 24:504, 2001.

Yang XF, et al: Essential role of OSpA/B in the life cycle of the Lyme disease spirochete. J Exp Med 199:641, 2004.

SECTION IV

Tumor Immunology

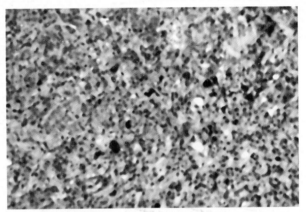

If we were to plot scientific enthusiasm for an important role for the immune system in response to autologous tumors as a function of time over the last 50 to 70 years, we would trace a sinusoidal curve. To a degree at least, this curve often reflects the introduction of newer technologies into the field. We are experiencing an upswing in enthusiasm at the current time, which owes much to an improved analysis of the evidence for tumor-unique (or at least tumor-associated) antigens, which could in principle be recognized by the host immune system (independent of normal tissue recognition), and to a major advance in our understanding of how to manipulate the important antigen presentation systems in the host (particularly the dendritic cell system). As a result, we have more definitive evidence that indeed tumor-bearing patients are making immune responses against their own tumor cells, and that there are now well-described techniques whereby we can intervene to augment that immunity, in the hope that a benefical effect on tumor growth can be realized.

Several of the cases presented in this section focus on these newer therapies in cancer immunology, including the use of cell-based therapies (renal carcinoma—Case 36) and autoimmunization with manipulated dendritic cells (Case 37). Case 35 (cervical carcinoma) represents a particularly innovative approach to cancer immunology and highlights contemporary studies behind clinical trials investigating vaccination against papilloma virus as a means to eradicate this particular disease in susceptible females.

Tumors are growths that may be benign or malignant. In general, encapsulated tumors whose cells are well differentiated and resemble normal tissues are considered benign. In contrast, malignant tumor cells are not encapsulated and possess the ability to invade adjacent tissues and metastasize to distant sites. Malignancies are categorized according to the tissue from which they derive. Thus, sarcomas, lymphomas, and leukemias are tumors of mesenchymal origin whereas carcinomas are tumors of epithelial origin (Fig. IV–1).

TUMOR ANTIGENS

Irrespective of the etiology of tumors, their eradication by the immune system requires recognition of some "foreign" molecule, a tumor antigen. Thus, we predict that (1) human tumor cells will have unique antigens; (2) those antigens can be recognized by the immune system; and (3) immunosuppression would thus *promote* tumor growth.

Tumor-Specific Antigens

Some tumor antigens arise after *de novo* expression of molecules as a result of activation of previously "silent" genes. This could occur as a result of altered transcriptional factor activity or inactivation of tumor suppressor genes (e.g., retinoblastoma gene product TP53). Alternatively, a mutation in a normal gene sequence could lead to the expression of mutant peptides. As example, point mutations in the ras protein have been observed during analysis of tumor cells, and it is conceivable that this mutated ras protein might serve as a tumor antigen. The cell membrane Ig (mIg) present on a B cell monoclonal tumor (chronic lymphocytic leukemia [CLL]) is an example of a tumor-specific antigen because the tumor cells all express a unique immunoglobulin molecule on their cell surface.

Proteins that are specific to a tumor are called "tumor-specific antigens"; if they induce immune responses leading to tumor rejection, they are referred to as tumor-specific transplantation antigens.

Tumor-Associated Antigens

In some cases, tumorigenesis is associated with the re-expression of a protein that had been expressed previously during the embryonic stages of differentiation, so-called oncofetal antigens. Examples are carcinoembryonic antigen (CEA) (found in colon, lung, breast, and stomach tumors); α-fetoprotein (AFP) (liver, testicular tumors); and melanocyte-associated epithelial antigens (MAGE) (melanoma). Note that antigens that signify the differentiation stage of the cell at which the block occurred in malignancy are termed *differentiation antigens*. Because these antigens are found in other cells, albeit in different quantities, and/or at different stages of development, they are called *tumor-associated antigens*. Tumor-associated antigens often aid in tumor diagnosis and prognosis.

Chemically Induced Tumors

In animal model systems using genetically identical mice, it has been found that chemically induced tumors do have quite unique antigens. Thus, two independent methylcholanthrene-induced tumors in mice

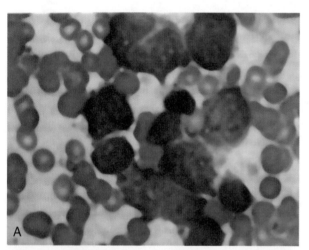
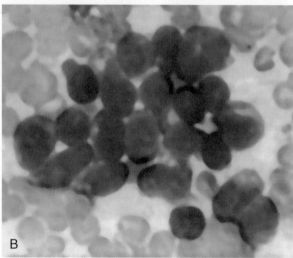

FIGURE IV–1   Blast cells in patients with leukemia. **A,** Acute myelogenous leukemia. **B,** Acute lymphocytic leukemia.

can be shown to possess different antigens, designated Tum1 or Tum2. When those tumors are excised and retransplanted in reciprocal fashion, mice with excised Tum1 are found to be immune to rechallenge with Tum1, but susceptible to Tum2, and vice versa.

Virally Induced Tumors

In contrast to these data, virally induced tumors have been found to express *common* tumor antigens. In this same experimental design, when two tumors (in different animals), TumA and TumB, were induced by the same virus (e.g., mouse sarcoma virus), following tumor resection, both mice resisted rechallenge with each of TumA and TumB.

In humans, Epstein-Barr virus (EBV; human herpesvirus 4) and human T lymphocyte virus-1 (HTLV-1) may be the etiologic agents for some tumors. Burkitt's lymphoma/nasopharyngeal sarcoma may be induced in susceptible individuals by EBV; some T cell leukemias are caused by HTLV-1 (e.g., Japan, Caribbean). However, a contrasting viewpoint suggests that the spontaneous tumors that we see clinically are a subset of the naturally occurring repertoire and are best characterized *by virtue of their poor (lack of) immunogenicity.*

TUMOR IMMUNOSURVEILLANCE

The role of immune surveillance as a means of thwarting the development of cancer is still disputed. Autopsies on young individuals dying of trauma during the Vietnam War revealed an incidence of metaplasia (thought to be indicative of early malignant transformation) far beyond the incidence of cancer in the population. Was this because the immune system eradicates most of these growths "silently"?

Individuals who are immunosuppressed have increased malignancies, but generally these are only lymphomas/skin cancers/Kaposi's sarcomas. Is this a direct effect of the immunosuppressive drugs/viruses? Why do we not see an increased incidence of all cancers? This may be able to be explained in part from what we know of the multiple genesis of tumors. Tumors induced after viral infections may be contingent on a previously compromised immune system. For example, infection with EBV leads to mononucleosis, a self-limiting disease in the general population; however, immunocompromised individuals who develop mononucleosis may subsequently develop a malignant lymphoma. Likewise, patients with AIDS

(already harboring chronic infection with one virus (human immunodeficiency virus [HIV]) are thought to develop Kaposi's sarcoma and other malignancies after exposure to secondary (viral) infections, in this case human herpes simplex virus-6 (HSV-6).

Arguments Against Immunosurveillance

A number of arguments have been raised against the concept of immunosurveillance as initially postulated by Thomas. Thus, there is no increased frequency of metastatic growth in the placenta during pregnancy (an immunoprivileged site). Bg/Bg mice (with marked natural killer [NK] defects) and Nu/Nu mice (athymic, lacking T cells) show no increased incidence of spontaneous malignancy (although they are more susceptible to virally induced tumors), despite the lack of NK cells or T cells, both of which have been implicated in antitumor immunity (see later). Finally, even a major population of immunosuppressed individuals (e.g., transplant patients) again do not show evidence for an overall increased incidence of (solid) malignancies, merely an increase in virally induced tumors (along with lymphomas and skin tumors).

EFFECTOR MECHANISMS FOR ELIMINATION OF TUMORS

Innate Immune Mechanisms

Macrophages

In vitro studies have shown that resting macrophages are ineffective in tumor destruction. Culturing macrophages with lipopolysaccharide or interferon gamma (IFNγ) induces their activation, and the subsequent secretion of cytokines, some at least of which are tumoricidal (e.g, tumor necrosis factor [TNF]). Although the mechanism of TNF cytotoxicity is debated, cell death is associated with (or mediated by) apoptosis. The *in vivo* role of macrophage in modulating tumorigenesis remains controversial, but tumors with massive macrophage infiltration are thought, in general, to have a better prognosis.

Natural Killer Cells

NK cells lyse tumors *in vitro* in a major histocompatibility complex (MHC)-unrestricted manner. Recognition of tumor antigen by the NK cell receptor is inhibited by the presence of MHC molecules, such that high MHC-expressing cells *are not killed* by NK cells (probably by CD8 cells instead [see later]). The receptor mediating this effect is the so-called killer-inhibitory receptor (KIR). Thus, NK cells may mediate surveillance against tumors that have down-regulated MHC (to avoid killing by CD8 cells). The efficacy of NK cell–mediated tumoricidal activity may be enhanced in the presence of cytokines derived from activated T cells. Included in the list of cytokines are interleukin (IL)-2, IL-12, and IFNγ.

Incubation of peripheral blood cells with high concentration of IL-2 leads to the generation of lymphokine-activated killer (LAK) cells. These LAK cells may be derived from NK cells, but after growth in IL-2 they show a marked enhancement in their ability to lyse tumor cells, relative to NK cells not exposed to high concentrations of IL-2. Note that NK cells may also participate in antibody-dependent cell-mediated cytotoxicity (ADCC), a form of killing in which tumor cells are destroyed by osmotic lysis, following recognition of the Fc region of an IgG/antigen bound to the tumor cell via Fab.

Acquired Immune Mechanisms

Antibodies: Enhancing Innate Immunity

Activated B cells differentiate to plasma cells secreting antibodies with a defined specificity. Antibodies may play a role in tumor cell destruction, as demonstrated by *in vitro* studies. However, the efficacy of antibodies depends on the presence of complement, phagocytes, or NK cells. Complement-mediated osmotic lysis of tumor cells, after activation by the classical complement pathway, has been observed for leukemic cells in culture. Similarly, phagocytic-mediated destruction of leukemias has been seen, where antibodies function as opsonins to enhance phagocytosis. In one mode of NK (and other) cell-mediated tumoricidal activity, destruction is mediated by ADCC. Antibodies bind to tumor antigens; the NK cell recognizes the Fc region of the IgG antibody, and a killing mechanism is activated. Whether these mechanisms play a role in preventing the development of spontaneous tumors remains to be elucidated. Antibodies may also mediate loss of adhesion receptors (antibody-induced downregulation), which can promote metastasis.

T Cells

Most studies of tumor destruction by T cells have focused on the role of CD8+ cytotoxic T cells (CTLs).

A tumoricidal role for CD8+ T cells *in vivo* is postulated because tumor-specific CD8+ T cells have been isolated from peripheral blood of cancer patients, as well as from excised tumor masses. Because differentiation of pre-CTLs to mature CTLs requires the presence of IL-2, it is likely that tumor-specific CD4+ T cells are also required for effective CTL-mediated antitumor immunity. Whether the preferential activation of Th2 cells, rather than Th1 cells, affects the course of tumorigenesis or tumor rejection is unknown. One might expect CD8-mediated tumor killing to be most relevant for virally induced tumors and perhaps to be a function of MHC expression. (*Note:* IFNγ could increase MHC expression and augment killing.)

EVIDENCE FOR EXISTENCE OF TUMOR IMMUNITY *IN VIVO?*

Studies with cancer patients have shown evidence for tumor-specific immunity in many patients, suggesting there is indeed often activation of the immune system in response to tumor antigens. However, the presence of detectable malignancy in these patients also indicates that immune responses have been inadequate.

Any of the following could be considered evidence for specific host immune reactivity to tumors: (1) presence of tumor-infiltrating lymphocytes (TIL); (2) existence of tumor-specific cytotoxic cells (CTLs); (3) evidence for local changes in cytokine production (e.g., increased IFNγ) suggestive of local antigen activation; (4) increased lymphocyte proliferation to tumor antigens *in vitro* (this may be difficult to measure if *in vivo* activation of cells has already occurred); and (5) evidence for restricted Vβ gene usage in expanded (T) cell populations.

HOW DO TUMORS EVADE IMMUNE SURVEILLANCE?

Many studies have tried to identify the mechanisms by which tumors evade immune-mediated destruction. A number of components of the immune system have been implicated in this process.

Tumor-Related Phenomena

1. *Sequestration:* The tumor may be in an immunologically privileged site (e.g., the anterior chamber of the eye), inaccessible to the immune system.

2. *Mutations of mutations:* Immune responses to foreign peptides are directed to discrete antigenic epitopes. Because there are few antigenic epitopes on most proteins, "mutations of mutations" might allow tumor cells to escape detection owing to a loss of antigenicity. Tumors could also escape detection by a process called "antigenic modulation." In this instance, an initial immune response to the tumor results in the formation of antigen/antibody complexes on the tumor cell surface, with a subsequent loss of antigen epitopes after endocytosis/shedding, allowing for tumor escape from immune recognition.
3. *Antigen masking:* Tumors may evade destruction by "antigen masking." This refers to a phenomenon by which tumor antigens are "hidden" from the immune system by complex carbohydrates on the cell surface.
4. *Antigen shedding:* The role of antibodies in tumor destruction *in vivo* remains elusive. Nevertheless it has been postulated that antibody complexed to soluble tumor antigen (shed from the tumor) might play a role in blocking tumor destruction. The exact mechanism(s) for this are not understood but may involve binding of immune complexes to antigen-specific receptors on the lymphocyte surface, without concomitant activation of those cells.
5. *Secretion of immunosuppressive molecules:* Tumors often produce molecules with potent, but nonspecific, immunosuppressive properties (e.g., prostaglandin E_2).

T Cell–Mediated Phenomena

1. *Decrease in MHC expression:* Tumor lysis by CTLs requires recognition of a tumor peptide by MHC class I. Cell transformation can lead to a decrease in expression of MHC, leading to tumor cell survival as a consequence of a deficiency in the expression of MHC molecules required for antigen presentation. Loss of MHC class I expression, however, would be expected to result in increased NK-mediated lysis of tumor cells (see earlier).
2. *Lack of type 1 cytokines:* The immune response could be also dampened if Th1 cells are not stimulated to release cytokines required for the differentiation of pre-CTLs to mature CTLs, or if inappropriate subsets of Th cells (e.g., Th2 cells?) are activated.
3. *Hole in the repertoire:* Tumors may escape immune detection if the T cell repertoire does not include

a TCR specific for the tumor antigen/MHC complex. This phenomenon is known as a "hole in the repertoire." A similar failure to recognize the tumor could result from an inability of a particular host MHC alleles to bind a potentially immunogenic tumor peptide for efficient antigen presentation, a phenomenon referred to as determinant selection.

Antigen-Presenting Cell–Related Phenomenon

Efficient antigen presentation for immune responses requires appropriate co-stimulatory molecules on the antigen-presenting cell. Absence of these (and/or their ligands on the host lymphocyte) often results in ineffective immunization.

ROLE OF ANTIBODIES IN DIAGNOSIS AND PROGNOSIS OF TUMORS

Tumor-specific antibodies are used in the diagnosis and prognosis of tumors, and to a lesser degree as therapy. For diagnosis and treatment of cancer, antibodies should ideally have a high level of sensitivity and specificity. For monitoring tumor recurrence, sensitivity is of more value.

Diagnosis

Diagnosis of tumors often uses immunologic tools. Included in these are (1) looking for products of the tumor (urinary Bence Jones proteins in myeloma); (2) detecting molecules (e.g., enzymes) known to be associated with a tumor; and (3) investigation of specific antitumor immune responses *in vitro* (enzyme-linked immunosorbent assay [ELISA]; proliferation; CTL, etc.). In general this approach will be unsuccessful if there are no tumor-specific transplantation antigens.

Prognosis

Because a diagnosis has generally already been made, use of reagents for monitoring tumor growth is restricted less by specificity considerations and more by sensitivity considerations. Accordingly, early recurrences in gastrointestinal malignancies are detected after CEA levels postoperatively, even though elevated CEA levels are seen in such a wide variety of (nonmalignant) conditions that this is not a useful diagnostic test. Similarly, in the case of choriocarcinoma, β-human chorionic gonadotropin (β-hCG) is such a sensitive and reliable test for recurrence that it is used (monitoring by ELISA) to guide treatment decisions regarding chemotherapy.

ROLE OF ANTIBODIES IN THERAPY

Based on the premise that tumors bear antigens that are tumor specific, it was believed that monoclonal antibodies would serve as "magic bullets" for the destruction of tumors. To make them more effective in the destruction of tumors, toxic, or radioactive, molecules were attached to the antibody so they would be internalized along with the antibody. The specificity of the antibody would ensure that only tumor cells would be destroyed.

Radiolabeled antibodies have been used with varying degrees of success to treat Hodgkin's patients when no other viable treatment exists; internalization is not required for destruction of tumors with radioisotopes. Nevertheless, monoclonal antibodies have not enjoyed great success as a tool for tumor treatment, although they are coming into more use in imaging studies (to detect micrometastases) and for purging tumor cells from bone marrow before re-infusion (e.g., autologous transplants in lymphoma). The use of anti-idiotypic monoclonal antibodies in the treatment of B cell CLL (the surface immunoglobulin idiotype represents the unique tumor-specific transplantation antigen in this case) is a special case, which, through cost/logistics, still limits universal applicability.

NOVEL AND NONSPECIFIC IMMUNOTHERAPIES FOR TUMORS

Nonspecific Immunostimulation

Advocates of the hypothesis that activation of the immune system is a requirement for elimination of tumors have proposed the use of various agents that can stimulate the immune response, particularly in patients with malignancies. Immune-enhancing molecules that are currently under consideration include levamisole, which was originally used in helminth infections and found to have immune-stimulating properties; bacille Calmette-Guérin (BCG), which is the attenuated form of *Mycobacterium bovis*, has also

been recognized for a number of years for its immunostimulating properties, as has *Corynebacterium parvum*. The mode of action is believed to be some modification of the local cytokine milieu and/or augmentation of innate immune mechanisms. More recently, attention has been paid to infusion of the cytokines themselves.

Introducing Cytokine Genes in Inactivated Tumor Cells

One strategy aimed at enhancing the immune response is the introduction of the IL-2 gene into inactivated tumor cells *ex vivo* and the reintroduction of these modified cells into the patient. Tumors may escape destruction if pre-CTLs do not differentiate into CTLs. Because IL-2 is required for differentiation, in addition to tumor recognition, introduction of the gene for IL-2 into the tumor would thus ensure that this cytokine was available after recognition of the tumor cell by the pre-CTL.

The introduction of cytokine genes, other than IL-2, into isolated/inactivated tumor cells for reintroduction into the patient is also being examined. Current trials include the introduction of the gene for IFNγ (an NK cell activator), and granulocyte-macrophage colony-stimulating factor (GM-CSF, a dendritic cell growth factor). Recognition of tumor cells by NK cells with the appropriate receptor would put the NK cell in the vicinity of the IFNγ-secreting tumor, where this cytokine would make the NK cells more potent killers. Note that IFNγ also upregulates the expression of MHC molecules on the tumor cell. Introduction of GM-CSF would enhance numbers of dendritic cells suitable for antigen presentation and induction of an immune response to the tumor.

Augmenting Antigen-Presenting Cells

More recently attention has focused on inserting genes for MHC or co-stimulatory molecules (e.g., B7-1 [CD80], B7-2 [CD86]), with or without cytokine genes, into tumor cells, so that they become "better" presenting cells for the tumor antigen. A modification of this approach is to "pulse" antigen-presenting cells (e.g., dendritic cells) *ex vivo* with a "soup" from tumor cells (in efforts to activate the antigen-presenting cells or allow surface expression of MHC class II/tumor peptide) and re-infuse this antigen-pulsed system into patients.

Re-infusion of Tumor-Infiltrating, or LAK, Cells

In this approach, the tumor is excised from the patient and T cells that have infiltrated the tumor are clonally expanded *in vitro* and are then re-infused into the patient, along with IL-2 (T cell growth factor); in some cases tumor-infiltrating cells are modified *in vitro* by insertion of the gene for IL-2 directly into the tumor-infiltrating cells before re-infusion.

A modified version of this strategy involves the insertion of the gene for tumor necrosis factor (TNF) in the tumor-infiltrating cell with infusion of the genetically modified cells into the patient. The rationale for this approach is that tumor-infiltrating cells will home to tumors and secrete TNF locally to kill the tumor. Both strategies have been applied in melanoma and renal cancer, with mixed success.

Specific Immunostimulation

Perhaps one of the promising immunospecific therapies that is evolving is the use of "transfer factor." Transfer factor consists of a peptide molecule complexed with oligonucleotides. Transfer factor is produced by T cells and can transfer a memory T cell phenotype to T cells that have not been in contact with the pathogen. Furthermore, transfer factor can augment a Th1 response by shifting the differentiation of Thp cell away from a Th2 phenotype. Diseases that are associated with a Th1 deficiency state could benefit from therapeutic intervention with transfer factor. These would include fungal infections, infection with *Mycobacterium tuberculosis*, cancer, and so on.

You are looking after a patient with B cell chronic lymphocytic leukemia (CLL). There are a number of conventional chemotherapeutic regimens available to treat this disease and a number of other investigational ones. Included among the investigational therapies is one involving infusion of antibodies made artificially (*ex vivo*) to the patient's own tumor cells. There is, in fact, a major accepted immunologic dogma behind this treatment and why it might be expected to work, although thus far in practice such therapy has not been as effective as we might have hoped.

QUESTIONS FOR GROUP DISCUSSION

1. In B cell CLL, membrane immunoglobulin (B cell antigen receptor) is considered a tumor-specific antigen. Explain.
2. There are two major types of CLL. Explain how these populations differ.
3. In what types of cells is ZAP-70 normally found? In general terms, what is its role?
4. How does CLL typically present clinically? How is it diagnosed?
5. Assuming that an antibody can be generated that is specific for the tumor-specific antigen (question 1), the immune complex that is formed on the cell surface could activate a number of immunologic processes to destroy these malignant cells. Explain how each of the following could be recruited to destroy the malignant B cells: (a) complement, (b) neutrophils, and (c) NK cells.
6. One would expect that the infusion of tumor-specific antibodies would lead to the effective killing and elimination of malignant cells. However, this approach has not been particularly effective. Explain why that might be the case (see Tumor Immunology, Section IV).
7. Describe the "Jerne idiotypic network theory." How would these networks produce the normal homeostasis in both T and B lymphocytes within the immune system?
8. Assuming that you could develop the appropriate anti-idiotypic antibody to target a particular population of T cells, what *in vitro* experiments could you perform that would provide information as to the potential efficacy of this approach?
9. The generation of antibodies specific for the idiotype on B cells would, in effect, represent the "magic bullet" therapy so long sought. The effectiveness of this therapy relies on the individual uniqueness (magic bullet) of the treatment. Yet, this is also its major limitation as a therapeutic approach in clinical practice. Explain.
10. Why would the use of T cell or B cell differentiation molecules as targets for antibodies tagged with toxins/radioactive material be more attractive for therapy than similarly labeled anti-idiotypic antibodies in clinical practice?

RECOMMENDED APPROACH

Implications/Analysis of Family History

B cell CLL is a monoclonal tumor, resulting from the proliferation and expansion of a single clone of B cells at a "frozen" point in time in their development. Studies of CLL and family history have shown an elevated risk of CLL for offspring and siblings of patients with CLL, as well as first- and second-degree relatives. However, no specific gene has been identified that is the cause of the disease *per se*. Recent literature reports have focused on the fact that patients with CLL can be divided into two major groups: those that have mutations in the variable region of the immunoglobulin heavy chain (VH) and those that do not have mutations in this gene. Patients with the mutated gene have a better prognosis than those without the mutation. It is now known that there are about 244 genes that are differently expressed in these two types of CLL. Of these 244 genes, ZAP-70 has been determined to be the best prognostic marker. ZAP-70, a tyrosine kinase, is a key signaling molecule in T cells and NK cells. It is not normally expressed in B cells. However, it is expressed in most patients with unmutated immunoglobulin VH gene, where it is recruited to the B cell receptor and enhances signaling.

Implications/Analysis of Clinical History

More than half the patients diagnosed with CLL are asymptomatic. For these patients diagnosis is made after a blood test for other reasons, including a yearly physical examination. Patients who are symptomatic will present with fatigue, weight loss, and generalized lymphadenopathy. The median age of CLL diagnosis is 64 years.

Implications/Analysis of Laboratory Investigation

An increased white blood cell count with more than 90% small lymphocytes (normal is about 30%) is suggestive of CLL. Bone marrow biopsy will generally show evidence for altered differentiation (myelodysplasia).

Additional Laboratory Tests

Immunotyping of cells using flow cytometry is also important in diagnosis. Panmarkers CD19 and CD20 will be present, as will CD5, CD43, and CD23. In this case, these cells were shown to be ZAP-70 negative, as determined by flow cytometry.

DIAGNOSIS

A diagnosis of B cell chronic lymphocytic leukemia was made. This patient was determined to have a mutated VH immunoglobulin gene and was negative for ZAP-70, suggesting a good prognosis.

STAGING AND PROGNOSIS

Two systems have been used classically to determine clinical staging and prognosis. The Rai system is based on the idea that nonfunctioning lymphocytes accumulate with time. There are four stages, with the first stage indicating increased numbers of lymphocytes in the bone marrow and in circulation. Stages II, III, and IV include enlarged spleen, anemia, and thrombocytopenia, respectively, along with the lymphocytosis referred to in stage I. The Binet system is similar but includes the number of enlarged lymphoid areas. Recent studies indicate that a better approach to predict progression of CLL is the detection of ZAP-70 in B cells, using flow cytometry for assessment.

THERAPY

There are a number of conventional chemotherapeutic regimens available to treat this disease and a number of other investigational ones (see later).

ETIOLOGY: CHRONIC LYMPHOCYTIC LEUKEMIA

CLL is a monoclonal tumor resulting from the proliferation and expansion of a single clone of B cells at a "frozen" point in time in their development. All tumor cells of the malignant clone are identical and express the same immunoglobulin molecule on their surface, and this immunoglobulin is unique to this B cell clone alone (an accepted principle of generation of diversity in the immune system). Thus the surface immunoglobulin on this cloned population is an example of a tumor-specific antigen.

Surface immunoglobulins are antigens expressed uniquely on a subpopulation of B cells. Therefore, if reagents (antibodies) could be made to it they would, in principle, be ideal targets in that only the tumor cells would be recognized.

Investigational Chemotherapeutic Regimens

Included among the investigational therapies is one involving infusion of antibodies made artificially (*ex vivo*) to the patient's own tumor cells. There is, in fact, a major accepted immunologic dogma behind this treatment, and why it might be expected to work, although thus far in practice such therapy has not been as effective as we would have hoped.

Mechanism of Tumor Destruction Using Monoclonal Antibody Therapy

As a result of such recognition, several, again conventional, immunologic reactions should occur:

1. Complement mediated lysis would be expected to destroy tumor cells (after activation of MAC, and osmotic lysis of cells). This has indeed been shown for some leukemic cells *in vitro*.
2. Increased phagocytosis of tumor cells by host cells with Fc (or C3) receptors should result in destruction by cells of the innate immune system.
3. Antibody-dependent cell-mediated cytotoxicity, after recognition by Fc or C3 receptor-bearing cells, even in the absence of phagocytosis, should suffice to activate either killing machinery, or growth-inhibitory machinery in the host cells, a mechanism referred to as ADCC. NK cells are believed to be particularly effective in this phenomenon.

Limitations to Antibody Therapy

Antigenic Modulation

As noted earlier, in general these mechanisms of tumor protection have not proven as effective in practice as in theory. One explanation for this has been that antibody-mediated downregulation of surface antigen (antigen modulation) occurs to render the tumor refractory to cell killing. The net observed result (outgrowth of populations of tumor cells with lower/absent surface immunoglobulin) could reflect a passive selection process (antibody merely allows for the selective "darwinian" outgrowth of [preexisting mutant] cells with little surface immunoglobulin), or an active process, resulting from engagement of surface immunoglobulin by the anti-immunoglobulin antibody and subsequent internalization of the complex with reduced re-expression in so-called tumor cell revertants. Whichever the mechanism, the loss of surface immunoglobulin makes these cells refractory to such treatment. It also unfortunately makes it less easy to monitor the presence of disease (decreased numbers of the surface immunoglobulin–marked tumor clone).

Individual Uniqueness

A major problem with consideration of this form of therapy in clinical practice is the very individual uniqueness of the treatment. What will work (be effective for) CLL with idiotype 1 will not work for CLL with idiotype 2. The cost and time frame of development of such tailored (to the individual) therapy is prohibitive.

Developmental Stage-Specific Differentiation Markers

This, in turn, has focused attention on the potential role of developing reagents directed against more common (e.g., developmental-specific) antigens. When B cells (and indeed) T cells, differentiate, they express unique stage-specific differentiation markers. There is some hope that reagents directed against these may be used alone, or after suitable tagging (with toxins/radioactive materials, etc.), to serve as diagnostic/immunotherapeutic tools.

Novel Genes

Finally, we have slowly come to realize that alterations in the normal patterns of differentiation that result in malignant transformation is itself often associated with overexpression of novel genes that can themselves serve as suitable targets for immunotherapeutic intervention. Kinase genes (e.g., ZAP-70), and other oncogenes, have proven to be just such molecules, and there is a growing interest in using both as target for either conventional pharmacotherapy and/or immunotherapy.

Jerne's Idiotypic Network Theory

As mentioned, the concept of producing antibody (or immunoreactive lymphocytes) to antigen-specific cell surface receptors on other immune cells forms the basis of a concept/theory of normal immunoregulation, the so-called Jerne's idiotypic network theory.

Jerne's idiotypic network theory suggests that normal immune regulation involves this mutual recognition of surface immunoglobulin, or T cell receptor, determinants by a network of interacting lymphocytes, producing the normal homeostasis in both B cells and T cells in the immune system. Jerne postulated that only by envisaging such a network could one imagine a realistic closed regulated immune system. Without it the system would be open ended. For each and every cell with a unique (idiotypic) surface immunoglobulin (or T cell receptor) Jerne postulated the existence of a (regulatory) cell with a counter-receptor (an anti-idiotypic receptor).

Anti-Idiotypic Antibodies to Target B Cells or T Cells

For the patient discussed, what we are essentially trying to do is develop this anti-idiotypic population, which would thus regulate expansion/development of the tumor clone expressing an anti-idiotypic surface immunoglobulin. Because Jerne's theory predicts idiotypy in T cells as well as in B cells, an alternative strategy might be to generate B cells whose surface immunoglobulin is specific for the idiotype of T cells that provide help for the tumorigenic B cell clone. An alternative approach is to produce B cells that are specific for the idiotype on the CLL cells.

Evidence for T Cell Immunity to CLL

Evidence for such immunization of T cells for anti-idiotypic regulation could be sought by exploring evidence for direct T cell immunity to CLL. Proliferation of T cells or production of cytokines

CD4 cells after stimulation with the surface immunoglobulin (antigen) specific for the T cell idiotype could provide such evidence. Evidence for antigen-restricted recognition by T cells *in vivo* implies the expansion of a (antigen-limited) T cell pool. In general, evidence for antigen immunization in a T cell pool is sought by asking whether there is evidence for limited Vβ T cell expansion after the immunization procedure.

Animal Studies

At least in animal studies there is some evidence that anti-idiotypic immunization of T cell immunity may be (more) effective (than induction of anti-idiotypic antibody). Why this is so is not clear, although this may reflect the engagement of unique T cell functions in a (presumed) regulatory T cell population. Note that there is (in Jerne's theory), however, no *a priori* difference (in initial function) between idiotype-bearing cells and anti-idiotype–bearing cells. Whichever is the "mirror" image depends on one's viewpoint!

A 22-year-old man is admitted to the intensive care unit (ICU) in severe respiratory distress. This unfortunate fellow was diagnosed with chronic myelogenous leukemia (CML) 6 months ago. His doctors advised both him and his family that a bone marrow transplant offered the only chance of cure. Extensive searching of relatives who were prepared to donate marrow failed to find a good match. However, searching the bone marrow transplant registry revealed one donor matched for all class I and II disparities. Transplant was performed 5 months earlier, after pretreatment with cyclophosphamide. He has had three episodes of graft-versus-host disease (GvHD), all of which resolved with pulses of anti-CD3 antibodies and corticosteroids. His current medications include cyclosporine, methotrexate, and prednisone. He has had hematuria for 10 days and watery diarrhea for 5. While in the ICU his respiratory distress worsens and there is an urgent intubation to allow for adequate oxygenation. All cultures are negative. At this stage you are not sure of what might be going on but are aware of a number of possibilities.

QUESTIONS FOR GROUP DISCUSSION

1. Explain why it is technically more difficult to closely match a solid organ compared with matching for bone marrow transplant.
2. Matching is generally done using restriction fragment length polymorphism (RFLP) or allele-specific polymerase chain reaction (PCR) to match for MHC antigens. Despite this, vigorous rejection may occur. Explain.
3. It is of interest that in the early years of clinical transplantation, concern was voiced that from our knowledge of how the T cell immune system developed one might predict that bone marrow transplant recipients might become immunologic cripples.
4. T cells expressing T cell receptors that can interact with self MHC (on thymic epithelium) with appropriate avidity are positively selected to leave the thymus. How do you reconcile the fact that in a bone marrow transplant, the antigen-presenting cells in the periphery would express donor MHC, yet the donor T cells have been educated on host thymic epithelial cells expressing host MHC (that is, how do T cells recognize these antigen complexes?)?
5. Patients who receive bone marrow transplants must receive immunosuppressive therapy to reduce the risk of HvGD and GvHD (host versus graft disease; graft versus host disease). To what type of infections are these patients particularly prone? How might these present?
6. GvHD itself presents often as a multisystemic disease with gastrointestinal, lung, genitourinary, and skin involvement. However, an alternative cause of these complaints could be that the patient has an infection (see question 5). Why is it important to rule out infection as the cause of these symptoms?
7. Why is it very important that you do not ignore GvHD as an unlikely cause of the symptoms while you investigate a possible viral infection? Discuss how you would proceed to "cover" both possibilities.
8. Within 2 days, the patient died of multiple organ failure. Blood culture showed gram-negative sepsis and disseminated cytomegalovirus (CMV) infection. CMV (human herpesvirus 6) has evolved strategies by which to hinder the immune response. Discuss these strategies.
9. With reference to question 8, one would expect that a decrease in class I MHC expression would hinder CD8+ T cells but a decrease in class I MHC should lead to NK cell activation. What cytokines are required to enhance NK cell cytotoxicity? What cell secretes these cytokines?
10. What cell population is the target of anti-CD3 therapy? Of cyclosporine therapy?

RECOMMENDED APPROACH

Implications/Analysis of Family History

CML is a clonal disorder of hematopoietic progenitor cells. Consequently, all cell types arising from that progenitor cell will be affected and increased in cell number. This would include granulocytes, monocytes, and platelets. Although the average age at which patients are diagnosed is 53, this disorder also occurs in young adults and children. White males are more likely to get CML than white women or African-American males. Hereditary factors are not known and may not play a role in disease susceptibility because an identical twin does not show greater susceptibility than a sibling when one twin has been diagnosed with CML.

Implications/Analysis of Clinical History

Nearly half of CML patients are asymptomatic, whereas others will present with fatigue, bleeding, abdominal fullness, and weight loss. Splenomegaly is the most common abnormality observed during the physical examination. Asymptomatic patients are often diagnosed after an abnormal blood test, which was requested for other reasons, including simply a physical checkup.

Implications/Analysis of Laboratory Investigations

In general, CML patients have an elevated white blood cell count (see Appendix for reference value) as well as an elevated platelet count (increase of ~ 40%), in the absence of infection or an inflammatory response.

Additional Laboratory Tests

When the clinical picture, physical diagnosis, and blood tests are suggestive of CML, cytogenetic tests are used to confirm the diagnosis. Diagnosis is typically based on the detection of the Philadelphia (Ph) chromosome, which is present in 90% of the patients. The Ph chromosome is a modified version of chromosome 22, secondary to a reciprocal translocation with chromosome 9. The net effect of this translocation is the creation of a unique fusion gene, termed BCR-ABL. The BCR gene (*N*-terminal) fuses with the ABL gene, which is the catalytic domain of the tyrosine kinase gene (ABL). This chimeric gene product is key to the development of CML in that it leads to uncontrolled proliferation of cells expressing this gene. These mutated cells predominate in the bone marrow and the circulation. The BCR-ABL transcripts are detected using reverse transcriptase polymerase chain reaction (RT-PCR).

DIAGNOSIS

Diagnosis of chronic myelogenous leukemia is generally made based on the detection of the Ph chromosome.

THERAPY

Treatment consists of high-dose chemotherapy that destroys proliferating cells, which includes both the leukemic cells and the normal hematopoietic cells. Such treatment necessitates allogeneic bone marrow transplantation. As mentioned earlier, the mean age of CML at diagnosis is 53 years, but bone marrow transplantation has a significant mortality risk for patients older than 40 years of age. In this case, the patient is only 22 years old and so this is the best option for him. Irrespective of the age of the patient, bone marrow transplants have a high risk of GvHD.

New Approaches to Treatment

Some patients can be treated and cured with allogeneic bone marrow transplants. For the elderly, GvHD obviates this as a treatment. Treatment of these patients has in recent years included interferon alpha (IFNα) as adjunctive therapy. IFNα is a cytokine that is known to have antiviral and antiproliferative effects. Not everyone can tolerate the side effects of this treatment. A promising new therapy is imatinib (Gleevec), an inhibitor of the BCR-ABL kinase.

ETIOLOGY: GRAFT VERSUS HOST DISEASE

GvHD is not uncommon after allogeneic bone marrow transplantation. This patient was closely matched for all MHC class I/II mismatches (technically easier to do for marrow transplants when time is on your side). In contrast, when a solid organ becomes available the ischemic time (for the potential graft) limits the time available to match carefully for all incompatibilities. Matching would generally be using RFLP and/or allele-specific PCR. However, note that even after careful complete matching for MHC incompatibilities, multiple minor histologic incompatibilities are likely to be present, and often immune responses to these can generate as vigorous a rejection response as that to MHC antigens.

MHC Restriction in Allogeneic Bone Marrow Transplantation

It is of interest that in the early years of clinical transplantation concern was voiced that, from our knowledge of how the T cell immune system developed, one might predict that bone marrow transplant recipients might become immunologic cripples. Thus, their T cells would become MHC restricted (in the host thymus) to MHC alleles (e.g., peptide/HLA-DR3) of host origin (expressed on drug-resistant and/or radioresistant persistent host epithelial cells) whereas antigen in the periphery would be presented to them in the context of donor MHC (e.g., peptide/HLA-DR4 on antigen-presenting cells developing from myeloid precursors in the marrow transplant). Some data in the animal literature supported this theoretical position. In practice, human transplants are performed in general across closely matched (MHC) alleles, and, perhaps for this reason, this problem has not, in general, been seen in practice.

Graft Versus Leukemia Effect

A potential benefit from bone marrow transplantation in cases of patients suffering from myeloid malignancies has been realized with the observation that lymphocytes differentiating in such transplanted individuals often develop a repertoire of cells capable of recognizing the tumor cells (graft versus leukemia T cells [GvL]), which are distinct from those recognizing host (graft versus host cells [GvH]) and could thus potentially be harnessed to assist clearance of the tumor. An early concern was that in fact the specificities of GvH T cells were not distinguishable from those of GvL. However, it has become increasingly apparent that the (multiple minor) histoincompatibility differences responsible for each reactivity are distinct, and thus therapies aimed at eliminating GvH do not necessarily eliminate the beneficial GvL effect.

Clinical Presentation: GvHD or Infection?

GvHD itself presents often as a multisystem disease with gastrointestinal, lung, genitourinary, and skin involvement. Treatment of GvHD would involve a pulse of increased immunosuppressive drugs. However, an alternative cause of the presenting complaints may itself be an infectious episode, secondary to the immunosuppression to which the patient has

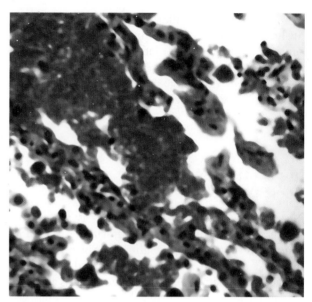

FIGURE 33–1 Lung tissue of bone marrow transplant patient with opportunistic infection by *Pneumocystis jiroveci*. Alveoli are filled with aggregates of *Pneumocystis* whereas alveolar septa are widened and infiltrated with mononuclear cells. (Schiff stain, ×400.)

been exposed already to allow engraftment (prevent rejection) of the bone marrow graft. This immunosuppression exposes the patient to multiple opportunistic infections (somewhat analogous to HIV infection or patients treated for autoimmune disorders), among which lung pathogens (CMV, *Pneumocystis*) would rank high on the list (Fig. 33–1). In addition, some of the immunosuppressive drugs used (methotrexate, in particular) can often induce hepatic and/or lung toxicity on their own accord.

Consequence of Misdiagnosis

It is important, before beginning a treatment plan, to at least have a working hypothesis concerning what you are treating and a backup plan should that hypothesis not be borne out by future events. If it is believed that the primary problem is infectious, more immunosuppression would obviously be to such a patient's detriment! Further administration of more toxic drugs would also not be useful if that is deemed to be the problem. However, if the problem really is GvHD and we do not treat it—that, too, could be fatal.

Therapy

A reasonable plan might be to treat the most likely pathogens (assuming infection), while at the same time trying to generate data (cultures of serum/urine/blood/cerebrospinal fluid) that would support that hypothesis and attempt to investigate further for signs of GvHD (biopsy of available tissue from affected organs [e.g., liver/bronchoscopy of the lung]) before beginning increased immunosuppressive therapy to treat that option.

Outcome

Within 2 days the patient became anuric (renal functioning ceased) and he required vasopressors to maintain his blood pressure. His lungs showed opacities throughout (on chest radiograph) that were read as evidence of acute respiratory distress syndrome by the radiologist. Taken together this multiple organ failure was thought likely to be due to terminal systemic sepsis. He died 12 hours later. Blood cultures showed gram-negative sepsis and disseminated CMV infection.

A patient of yours has just undergone surgery at your local hospital for cancer of the colon. You agreed to act as a surgical assistant for this operation. After completion of the surgery, the surgeon reminds you to draw a carcinoembryonic antigen (CEA) level. Why did the surgeon do this? What is this measurement? What is the significance of measuring this in this population?

QUESTIONS FOR GROUP DISCUSSION

1. What are the two most common colorectal cancers in which heredity plays a role? Explain why a mutation in a gene encoding proteins that play a role in DNA mismatch repair might make a person more susceptible to colon cancer.
2. Describe the clinical manifestations of colon cancer and the screening tests that are used for early detection.
3. What is the underlying assumption behind the concept of tumor immunology?
4. Explain the term *tumor-specific antigen* and give examples.
5. Explain the term *tumor-associated antigen* (oncofetal antigen). Give three examples.
6. Carcinoembryonic antigen (CEA) is an oncofetal antigen. What is its function? Given its function, what role might it play in embryogenesis? What role might it have in adults when it is re-expressed in malignant tissues?
7. Explain why CEA cannot be used as a specific marker for the detection of colon cancer.
8. Explain the term *magic bullet* as it refers to tumor therapy. Describe approaches that are used in attempts to achieve this.
9. Describe, in general terms, the assay for measuring CEA levels in a patient. Discuss why there is, to date, no well-described cell-mediated immune assay available for CEA detection. How might you approach this problem to develop an assay?
10. Regarding the patient in this case, if CEA has no value in the specific diagnosis of the tumor, of what value is it to measure CEA in this patient?

RECOMMENDED APPROACH

Implications/Analysis of Family History

Individuals with a family history of colorectal cancer or polyps in a parent or sibling (diagnosed before the

sixth decade) are at increased risk for colon and rectal cancer. Most cases of colorectal cancer occur sporadically; however, about 7% of cases are hereditary. The two most common colorectal cancers in which heredity plays a role include (1) hereditary nonpolyposis colorectal cancer (HNPCC) and (2) familial adenomatous polyposis (FAP). Patients with HNPCC have mutations in hMH1, hMSH2, hPMS1, or hPMS2 proteins, which play a role in the repair of DNA mismatches. Because DNA mismatches are not repaired, mutations occur more frequently. When these mutations are in growth-regulatory genes, cancer can arise. Individuals with FAP have hundreds/thousands of polyps at an early age, and, generally, some of these polyps will result in colorectal cancer.

Implications/Analysis of Clinical History

Common symptoms of colorectal cancer include (1) a change in bowel habits, irrespective of whether it is diarrhea or constipation; (2) blood in the stool; (3) stomach cramps; (4) decreased appetite; and (5) fatigue/weight loss.

Implications/Analysis of Laboratory Investigation

Colorectal cancer is often detected during screening procedures that include (1) digital rectal examination, (2) fecal occult blood test, and (3) either a colonoscopy, sigmoidoscopy, or barium enema.

Additional Laboratory Tests

A positive result from a fecal occult blood test should be followed by a complete blood cell count to check for anemia.

DIAGNOSIS

This patient was diagnosed with colon cancer. A staging system from O to IV is used to report the degree of spread through the colon/rectal wall and then through the body. Also, serum levels of CEA are determined after resection. This is done after resection because CEA levels have no diagnostic value (elevated levels are expressed in a number of malignant and nonmalignant conditions, including in heavy smokers and cirrhotics). CEA is a cell surface glycoprotein that occurs in high levels on colon epithelial cells during embryonic development, but expression is downregulated in adults. The sera of patients with colorectal cancer typically have elevated levels of the oncogenic tumor-associated antigen, CEA. Although there are a number of different tests that may be used to detect serum CEA, the enzyme-linked immunosorbent assay (ELISA) is used most often.

Why Measure CEA Expression?

To return to the patient of interest, one might now ask, if CEA has no value in the specific diagnosis of the tumor or as a therapeutic "tool" (specific killing of the tumor), then what indeed is the value of measurement of CEA levels in this case? It has become apparent that, along with a number of oncofetal antigens, CEA has significant value in monitoring early recurrence (before it becomes clinically detectable). These measurements can be made in a very sensitive and cost-effective manner, saving use of other more expensive (and often less sensitive) imaging procedures. The case of another oncofetal marker (β-human chorionic gonadotropin [β-hCG] in choriocarcinoma) is a prime example of the value of such measurements. This tumor is normally treated effectively with high doses of methotrexate. However, the sensitivity of a rising β-hCG level in the presence of methotrexate therapy is sufficiently convincing of failure of therapy that such a measurement alone is sufficient to demand an alteration in therapy.

THERAPY

Colon resection, chemotherapy, internal radiation, or external radiation are all potential therapies. In internal radiation therapy a radioisotope is injected or implanted directly into the tumor; in external radiation high levels of radiation are emitted by a machine and directed at the tumor.

Tumor-Associated Antigens

The driving thesis behind the concept of tumor immunology is that tumors have cell surface molecules that are preferentially expressed (with respect to the normal tissue) and that can be recognized by the host immune system. As such, they are referred to as antigens. Antigens may be tumor specific (TSA) or tumor associated (TAA). (See Tumor Immunology, Section IV.) TAAs can be used to characterize tumors but are not necessarily unique to the tumor as opposed to other (normal) host tissues.

Oncofetal Antigens

TAAs are often molecules (antigens) that are expressed at stages of normal cell differentiation, although the tumor cell expression is either qualitatively or quantitatively different from normal cells at that particular stage of maturation/differentiation. An important class of TAAs is the so-called oncofetal antigens (OFAs). Oncofetal antigens, of which CEA is an example, are not unique to tumor cells but are in general not expressed at high levels in perfectly normal adult tissue. They tend to be, as the name implies, molecules expressed preferentially during normal fetal development but molecules for which transcriptional silencing of gene expression occurs during adult life. However, it has become apparent as we understand more about these OFAs that there are a number of *nonmalignant* conditions (for different tissues) in adulthood in which re-expression does occur. In addition to CEA, α-fetoprotein and β-hCG are also recognized oncofetal antigens (Fig. 34–1).

Carcinoembryonic Antigen

CEA itself is thought to be one of a family of cell:cell/matrix adhesion molecules. It probably thus subserves an essential role in normal tissue development during embryogenesis, ensuring that the appropriate cellular architecture develops in the gut. In adult (malignant) tissue, re-expression of this molecule may have profound effects on altering the manner in which cells interact with one another and with their environment, and thus expression on tumor cells is likely important in the regulation of metastatic spread.

Re-expression of CEA

As an example of other conditions in which high levels of CEA are found, in addition to in patients with gas-

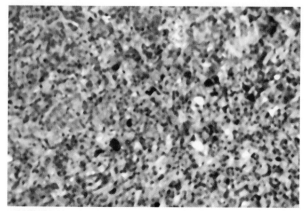

FIGURE 34–1 Oncofetal antigen, β-human chorionic gonadotropin (β-hCG). Choriocarcinoma, showing typical neoplastic syncytial cells and cytotrophoblast cells stained reddish brown using immunoperoxidase staining for hCG (the hormone synthesized in the syncytiotrophoblast of the placenta). (Immunoperoxidase for hCG, ×200.)

trointestinal malignancies (of the colon), increases have been observed in cigarette smokers and in alcoholic cirrhosis. Increased levels have also been described in nongastrointestinal malignancies (e.g., breast cancer). It is because of these numerous exceptions (false-positive results) that simple marked increased expression of CEA cannot be used as a specific marker for the detection of colon cancer.

Anti-CEA Antibodies

In the early stages after CEA was discovered it was hoped that the molecule could be used to develop a so-called magic bullet (anti-CEA antibody) to kill tumor cells. The principle behind this (and essentially any case in which expression of a molecule exists, against which a specific antibody can be made) is that infusion of "tagged" antibodies could now be used both to detect and even eliminate the tumor specifically (without affecting normal tissue). Labeling of antibodies with radioactive tracers (e.g., ^{125}I) should enable use of a gamma camera to "see" tumor in the intact patient. Labeling with a toxin (e.g., diphtheria toxin) would serve as a specific way to deliver a high dose of toxin (too toxic if given systemically to all cells in the body) only to tumor cells.

Cell-Mediated Assays to Detect CEA Expression

There is to date no well-described cell-mediated immune assay used for the detection of CEA on a cell surface. This is not surprising, given its postulated cell surface expression and its putative role thereby in regulating cell/cell and cell/matrix interactions. It may be instructive, nevertheless, to consider what immune responses might be measured to study the effect of CEA expression on a particular function? Development of assays to examine whether the immune response of antigen-challenged T (or B) cells (reactive with a conventional antigen) is altered in the presence of overexpression of CEA might be of interest. The assumption here is that CEA may play an auxiliary role in regulating a primary stimulus delivered to the lymphocyte-specific receptor. Increased CEA expression might also result in altered histopathology assessment of a tumor biopsy, altering both evidence for tumor cell/matrix interactions and also the incidence of, or interaction with, other immune cells within the tumor.

CW is a 30-year-old woman in your practice whose recent annual "Pap" smear results have just come to your attention. The diagnosis reads CIN type II (CIN = cervical intraepithelial neoplasia), which indicates inflammatory change and abnormal preneoplastic cells. You arrange a biopsy for her with your referring gynecologist, who confirms this result. In the meantime you order a serologic study for measurement of human papillomavirus 16 (HPV-16) antibody titers and a cervicovaginal lavage specimen to test for the presence of HPV-16 DNA. HPV-16 is implicated as a causative agent in cervical cancer. Based on recent findings in the literature, you wonder whether this woman could be considered for HPV-16 immunization. What other recommendations should you make?

QUESTIONS FOR GROUP DISCUSSION

1. What is a "Pap" smear?
2. Human papillomavirus is transmitted sexually. Most infections are benign, despite the fact that there are more than 50 types that can infect the genitalia. Which type has been isolated from over 50% of cancers of the cervix?
3. Explain why a serologic test is performed even though it is not diagnostic for a present infection.
4. What is the rationale for performing a DNA test for HPV-16? Why is an amplification test (e.g., polymerase chain reaction [PCR]) more likely to detect HPV than other types of DNA tests?
5. What is the generally accepted form of treatment for a CIN type II?
6. Where does the immunogenicity of papillomaviruses reside?
7. Explain how "empty viral capsids" are generated and why they have been considered as potential vaccines for women at high risk for cervical malignancy.
8. Discuss the results of a double-blind randomized study using this vaccine.
9. How would you advise the women in the study who experienced seroconversion but who did not have any evidence for cervical changes?
10. Explain the role of the HPV transformation proteins E6 and E7.

RECOMMENDED APPROACH

Implications/Analysis of Family History

No family history is provided and this is not particularly relevant at this time. Although there are a number of non-HPV factors that contribute to subsequent malignancy, among them being genetic predis-

position, the particular contributing gene has not been identified. One could speculate that genetic alterations in any one of a number of immune components could impact on the individual's ability to eliminate viral infections and hence susceptibility to progression to malignancy. However, at this time, these are not well enough defined to be included in the assessment of the patient.

Implications/Analysis of Clinical History

CW's clinical history is consistent with the majority of cases of CIN type II in that she did not have any clinical manifestations and this was only detected with the Papanicolaou (Pap) smear, a screening test that has substantially reduced the incidence of mortality resulting from cervical cancer, because of early detection. CIN type II typically indicates infections with HPV-16, one of the many types of HPV that infect the genital tract. A different HPV type is associated with a more common clinical manifestation, condylomata (warts), which are associated with infection with HPV types 6 and 11.

We are not provided any information regarding CW's immunologic status, which is a significant negative because drug therapies that lead to immunosuppression, and HIV is included in the list of non–HPV-related risk factors for HPV-induced malignant progression.

Implications/Analysis of Laboratory Investigation

A Pap smear is a cytologic test performed on a sample of cells from the uterine cervix. This is a screening test to identify patients with premalignant lesions/cellular changes that could progress to malignancy. The quality of the specimen obtained and degree of accuracy with which the cytology is interpreted play a key role in correct diagnosis. When abnormal cells are identified on a Pap smear a colposcopy may be performed for a magnified look at the cervix (Fig. 35–1).

Pap smears that are not normal are graded on a classification system. CIN type I lesions often revert spontaneously, but CIN type II lesions require treatment to prevent transformation to cervical cancer. CW's Pap smear indicated CIN type II lesions. She was referred to the gynecologist who performed a biopsy that confirmed the Pap smear results. CIN type III lesions are considered malignant and are classed as stages 1 through 4, with stage 4 indicating metastasis.

Additional Laboratory Tests

At least 50 different types of HPV have been shown to infect the genital tract. Of these, HPV-16 has been detected in about 50% of cervical cancers. Other types that play a prominent role in cervical cancer include types 18, 31, and 45. Genital warts are caused by HPV types 6 and 11.

Serologic testing is generally done using an enzyme-linked immunosorbent assay (ELISA) to determine the presence of IgG antibodies. The presence of antibodies is an indication that CW has been infected with HPV-16, but it does not provide information regarding a present infection. To confirm a current infection, a test to detect HPV DNA in the cervical sample was requested.

A number of different tests are commercially available to detect HPV DNA in a clinical sample, but amplification techniques (e.g., PCR) increase the likelihood of detecting HPV in a sample. CV's serology and DNA test for HPV-16 were both positive.

DIAGNOSIS

CW was diagnosed with HPV-16 infection as the likely cause of the CIN type II Pap smear result.

THERAPY

Therapy for CIN type II lesions includes laser vaporization or cryotherapy, a process that uses liquid nitrogen to freeze the tissue. Although a vaccine for HPV may soon be available, there is no evidence for a role for postexposure vaccination of HPV-16–positive individuals. CW should be counseled regarding the use of condoms to avoid transmission to her partner(s).

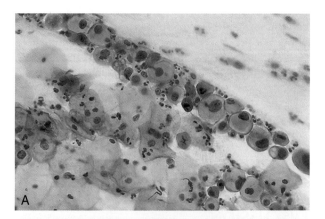

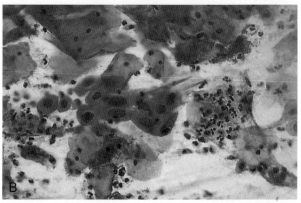

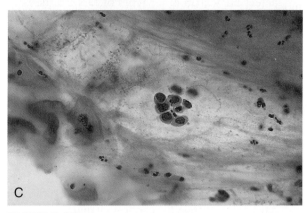

FIGURE 35–1 Cervical smear cytology showing CIN I (**A**), CIN II (**B**), and CIN III (**C**). Micrographs are from preparations obtained by Papanicolaou methodology. CIN I (low-grade squamous intraepithelial lesion) shows normal squamous cells and clumps of mildly dysplastic cells with large dark-stained nuclei, irregular contour, and coarse nuclear chromatin. CIN II shows abnormal epithelial cells with larger nuclear:cytoplasmic ratio and coarser hyperchromatic nuclei. Normal epithelial cells are also seen. In CIN III the nuclear:cytoplasmic ratio is greater, although cells are smaller.

ETIOLOGY: HUMAN PAPILLOMAVIRUS INFECTION

HPV is a sexually transmitted disease. Most infections are benign, but certain serotypes are implicated in cervical and other anogenital cancers, with HPV-16 the most highly linked, being present in about 50% of cervical cancers and high-grade CIN changes and about 25% of low-grade CINs.

Papillomaviruses are small, nonenveloped double-stranded DNA particles. The capsid consists of 360 copies of the major capsid protein L1. Small amounts of capsid protein L2 are also present. The immunogenicity of papillomaviruses involves antigen presentation of conformational epitopes displayed on viral capsids composed of L1 protein. Expression of recombinant L1 and L2 in an expression system results in self-assembly of a virus-like particle (VLP) that is similar to the capsid structure of the native particles (empty viral capsids). As such, these have been used in place of papillomavirus as antigen source for a vaccine.

Vaccine

Vaccination with L1 virus-like particles in animal model systems has led to evidence for protection from disease. This has formed the basis for consideration of use of such treatment for women at high risk for cervical malignancy. In a recently reported double-blind randomized study, HPV-16–negative women received three such vaccinations and were followed over an 18-month period for evidence of seroconversion and altered cervical pathology. Essentially all vaccinated individuals seroconverted, and only subjects in the control (nonvaccinated) group developed any evidence for CIN. The level of antibody seen in vaccinated individuals was about 60-fold higher than in women naturally seroconverting (evidence for HPV-16 infection and disease). None of the vaccinated females showed evidence for HPV-16 DNA in cervical tissue after vaccination.

Pathogenesis

Two proteins encoded by the HPV genome play an important role in malignant transformation of epithelial cells by HPV. These are the E6 and E7 proteins, which are expressed in malignant tissues. E6 and E7 interact with TP53 and RB, respectively, and this interaction leads to the degradation of both TP53 and RB. Because these proteins are tumor suppressors, their degradation plays an important role in the process of malignant conversion of infected cells.

You are looking after a 60-year-old male patient with renal carcinoma. The patient is due for surgery in 2 days, and you are investigating follow-up immunotherapies you might offer this patient, besides conventional chemotherapy. Discuss some of the options.

QUESTIONS FOR GROUP DISCUSSION

1. Explain the differences between sporadic and inherited renal cell carcinoma.
2. Describe the clinical presentation of renal cell cancer and general approach leading to diagnosis.
3. Describe the general procedure for tumor-infiltrating lymphocyte (TIL) therapy. What is the rationale for this approach?
4. TIL therapy has met with limited success. List at least two reasons why this approach may not work.
5. Attempts to enhance the efficacy of TIL therapy have led to changes in the protocol to include exogenous cytokines. Discuss the negative side effects associated with this modification. Describe an alternative approach to overcome this side effect and yet still benefit from intervention of cytokines.
6. Provide a rationale for introduction of each of the following cytokines in the TIL protocol: interleukin (IL)-2, interferon gamma (IFNγ), and granulocyte-macrophage colony-stimulating factor (GM-CSF).
7. Discuss the pros and cons (regarding tumor killing) of enhanced class I MHC on the tumor cells.
8. Discuss the general approach for treatment of tumors using antigen-pulsed dendritic cells.
9. What is the advantage of this approach compared with the tumor-infiltrating cell approach? What is the potential problem to this approach? How might this be addressed?
10. Describe, in general terms, the tetramer biology approach. Explain why this approach holds out more hope for treatment than the other two approaches (TILs, or pulsed dendritic cells).

RECOMMENDED APPROACH

Implications/Analysis of Family History

Renal cell carcinoma may be sporadic or inherited. Sporadic renal cancer typically develops in the elderly and is much more frequent in males. In contrast, hereditary renal cancers may develop much earlier in life, even in teenagers, and occur in equal frequency in females and males. There are a number of different hereditary renal cell cancers, the most common being von Hippel-Lindau (VHL) disease, a familial multiple cancer syndrome that includes renal cell cancer. The von Hippel-Lindau gene is now known to be a tumor suppressor gene.

Given that our patient is a 60-year-old man, it is likely that this patient has sporadic renal cell cancer.

Implications/Analysis of Clinical History

Clinical presentations generally include hematuria (blood in urine), abdominal pain, and mass in the abdomen. Some patients will also experience weight loss, night sweats, and a general listless feeling. However, incidental detection often occurs before these clinical symptoms appear when patients receive ultrasonography, computed tomography (CT), or magnetic resonance imaging (MRI) for other reasons.

Implications/Analysis of Laboratory Investigation

Diagnosis may involve urography (radiography of the urinary tract that is preceded by intravenous injection of a dye that is excreted by the kidney) and renal angiography (imaging of arteries that bring in blood to the kidneys) in the presence of the clinical symptoms described.

Additional Laboratory Tests

To characterize the mass, however, ultrasonography, CT, and MRI are more accurate than urography or renal angiography. Sporadic renal cell cancers are generally unilateral with (frequently) only one tumor mass, whereas inherited renal cell cancers are most likely to be bilateral with several tumors.

DIAGNOSIS

To confirm a diagnosis of renal cell carcinoma, it is essential to examine tissue, which is generally obtained during surgery. Surgery is the mainstay of treatment of renal cell carcinoma. In the United States, two different staging systems are used for prognosis: the modified Robson system and the American Joint Committee on Cancer.

THERAPY

For the most part, first-line therapy for renal cell carcinoma is surgery. However, adjunctive therapies are under investigation.

Tumor-Infiltrating Lymphocytes

One alternative therapy includes isolation of natural killer (NK) cells from the patient's peripheral blood lymphocytes or isolation of TILs from within the resected tumor mass and expanding these *ex vivo* (with IL-2 or other growth factors for NK cells). When these NK cells are cultured under these conditions, so-called lymphokine-activated killer (LAK) cells are produced. LAK cells are re-infused into the patient. This therapy has been used in renal carcinoma patients but with very limited success.

Potential Problem: Homing

A potential problem might be that the cells re-infused to the patient never "home" to the right locale *in vivo* to eradicate the tumor. In addition, there is no *a priori* evidence to document that TILs are necessarily the important cells (*in vivo*) for eliminating tumor. They

may locate to the tumor as a means of regulating immune responses directed against the tumor *in vivo!*

Potential Problem: Cytokine Toxicity

Both cell infusions (LAK cells or TILs) have also been used in the presence of additional exogenous cytokine infusion, although this has been often accompanied by toxicity from high-dose cytokine use (in particular, inflammation of the vascular bed, and a "capillary leak" syndrome). In other cases it has been suggested that we attempt further gene transfection into TILs, to circumvent the problem of infusion of cytokines separately. IL-2, IFNγ, and even GM-CSF (to attract dendritic cells for antigen presentation) have all been suggested as auxiliary reagents for gene transfection.

Role of MHC in CD8+ T cell and NK cell in Tumor Cell Killing

Some tumors can evade host CTL (CD8) immunity by downregulating class I MHC. However, because NK cells have killer inhibitory receptors (KIRs, recognizing class I MHC), which are thought to play a role in regulating killing activity by NK cells, one would predict that loss of class I MHC, while rendering a tumor less susceptible to killing by CD8+ CTL, would leave it *more* susceptible to NK cell lysis.

Pulsed Dendritic Cells Using Crude Extracts

Another current experimental therapy for treatment of some tumors consists of pulsing cultured dendritic cells with tumor cell antigens, and/or genes encoding the antigens, before re-infusing these dendritic cells into patients as a means of boosting host tumor cell antigen recognition.

Technique

Peripheral blood lymphocytes are obtained from the patient, and CD34+ cells (dendritic cell precursors) can be isolated using antibodies specific for CD34 antigen. These CD34+ cells are grown in bulk *in vitro* in the presence of GM-CSF and IL-4, which are potent dendritic cell growth factors. After 9 to 10 days, the dendritic cell population is "pulsed" *in vitro* with a crude extract of tumor antigen (e.g., a tumor cell lysate) and the mixture is re-infused *in vivo* alone, or again in the presence of additional cytokines. In some variants of this therapy, dendritic cells are first transfected with genes for additional cytokines.

Advantage

The clear advantage of this approach is that it makes no assumptions about what the relevant tumor antigen (for immunization) is, only that it is present in the tumor lysate. This may also be the problem with such an approach! Perhaps the lysate contains a more abundant source of tumor tolerogens, rather than immunogens.

Pulsed Dendritic Cells with Tumor-Specific Antigens

A variant of this theme attempts to use more defined tumor antigens to pulse the dendritic cells. These are preselected by screening (e.g., with antibodies or cultured T cells from patients with homologous tumors) for purified proteins/molecules that bind antibodies and/or induce proliferation in T cells. Such purified antigens can then be used for pulsing the tumor. Alternatively, the gene(s) encoding the tumor antigen may be cloned and used for transfection of enriched dendritic cells (again with/without genes encoding cytokines).

Tetramer Biology Approach

Finally, there is growing interest in an approach that is essentially a variant of both of the above. This uses a so-called tetramer biology approach to first enrich for T cells specific for the antigen under consideration (which must therefore be known). Artificial (tetramer) complexes of MHC proteins and antigen are made using fluorescence-marked MHC proteins. This combination is mixed with patient peripheral blood lymphocytes to allow binding of antigen-specific T cells (class I restricted CD8+) to the tetramers, which can be purified (>80% pure) by flow cytometry cell sorting. These are then cultured *in vitro*, with purified dendritic cells (obtained from CD34+ precursors) pulsed with tumor antigen. (*Note:* although the dendritic cells can endocytose antigen into vacuoles for subsequent presentation to MHC class II restricted T cells, dendritic cells can also pinocytose soluble antigens. Pinocytosed antigens enter the cytosol, not the endosome, and so the antigen can be processed for subsequent presentation to class I restricted CD8+ T cells).

This experimental approach has been used to generate large numbers ($>10^{10}$) purified antigen-specific CD8+ cytotoxic T cells, which can be infused for patient therapy. Although still in its experimental phase, this newer technology holds out hope of providing an important means of treating at least some human cancers in the future.

WT has been a "sun worshipper" all his life. Over the past several months he has noticed some worrisome changes in some freckles on his legs and arms, and one in particular seems to have grown substantially, with a significant change in coloration and an irregular contour. You recognize all of these signs as being potentially indicative of malignant melanoma and send him to a local dermatologist for biopsy. The results come back positive. WT has heard about some recent positive data using immunotherapy in melanoma and asks your advice.

QUESTIONS FOR GROUP DISCUSSION

1. Melanoma is one of the cancers for which "spontaneous" remissions are reported. Discuss possible mechanisms for this remission.

2. Tumor-specific antigens (TSAs) derived from melanoma DNA libraries have been cloned. What is the TSA on melanoma cells?

3. Immunity directed to melanoma can often be monitored by following evidence for anti-melanocyte reactivity. Explain how this would present clinically. What is the clinical term for this reaction?

4. Explain why normal melanocytes are destroyed after supposedly targeting of TSAs on the melanoma.

5. Discuss the rationale for therapy using dendritic cells that have been pulsed with cloned melanocyte-associated epithelial antigens (MAGE) proteins (referred to as vaccines).

6. Explain why granulocyte-macrophage colony-stimulating factor (GM-CSF) and interleukin (IL)-4 are used to culture CD34+ peripheral blood cells in question 5.

7. What approach could one use to ensure that the re-infused dendritic cells receive a constant supply of cytokines, without putting the patient at risk for complications normally experienced when administering cytokines?

8. Provide a rationale for these steps in generating a therapeutic vaccine for melanoma: culture of tumor infiltrating lymphocytes *ex vivo* with (a) MAGE-pulsed dendritic cells and (b) IL-2 before re-infusion.

9. Explain the rationale for introducing IL-2, tumor necrosis factor (TNF) or interferon gamma (IFNγ) as sole therapy (or adjunctive therapy) in melanoma patients.

10. In extension of the work on melanoma, breast cancer therapies have also been developed. What tumor antigens would one target in breast cancer patients?

RECOMMENDED APPROACH

Implications/Analysis of Family History

Low-risk alleles (e.g., melanocortin 1 receptor gene [MC1R]) may increase the risk of melanoma in the general population, when that population has a high sun exposure. These individuals have enhanced sun sensitivity, and so their risk of developing melanoma is increased.

We are not provided with any family history, but hereditary melanoma is rare. In such cases, melanoma transmission occurs along either the paternal or the maternal lineage but not both. Mutations in two genes—CDKN2A (cell cycle regulator) and CDK4 (cyclin-dependent protein kinase 4)—are associated with hereditary melanoma. CDKN2A is a cell cycle regulator that is often mutated or deleted in cancer, particularly melanoma. (Patients with a defect in CDKN2A also have an increased risk of developing pancreatic cancer.) Based on the information given in the case, this patient does not have hereditary melanoma but rather an idiopathic case of disease (related to environmental/behavioral risk factors).

Implications/Analysis of Clinical History

We need to consider the fact that no family history is provided as a significant negative. Although we have not determined that WW has one of the risk alleles for MC1R (see earlier), the fact that he has been a sun worshipper and that he has scattered freckles in sun-exposed areas puts him in a higher risk group than someone who has a low-risk sun exposure.

Implications/Analysis of Laboratory Tests

A biopsy specimen of the pigmented lesions indicated that WW has malignant melanoma.

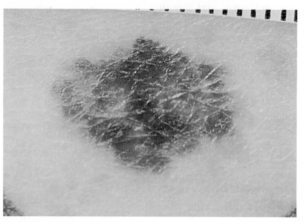

FIGURE 37–1   Skin lesion on patient with documented malignant melanoma.

Additional Laboratory Tests

To test for metastatic disease, a chest radiograph was requested but shown to be normal. Patients with malignant melanoma often show distant metastases (lungs, brain, kidney).

DIAGNOSIS

WW was diagnosed with malignant melanoma (Fig. 37–1). The most widely used measurement system (after skin biopsy) to predict 5-year survival is the "Breslow" measurement. In this system a defined melanoma thickness is associated with a 5-year survival in 97% of patients. At the other end of the scale a 10-fold increase in thickness is associated with a 5-year survival of only 32% of the patients. Another system, the "Clark Level of Invasion" can also be used to determine prognosis. There are five Clark levels of invasion, with level one indicating that the melanoma is confined to the outermost layer of skin and level five indicating penetration of the melanoma into fat cells beneath the dermis. This is then correlated with 5-year survival rate after surgical removal of the melanoma.

THERAPY

The lesion was excised with a large margin, and WW was shown how to perform routine self-examination and advised to seek professional examination every 6 months.

ETIOLOGY: MALIGNANT MELANOMA

Melanoma is indeed a bright spot on the horizon for those interested in the immunotherapy of cancer. It is indeed one of the cancers for which "spontaneous remissions" are reported, which may in turn reflect an autologous antitumor reaction (immunologically derived) in the natural host.

Tumor-Specific Melanocyte-Associated Epithelial Antigens

When laboratories first attempted to derive evidence for a host (human) antitumor response, and indeed for tumor antigens that could elicit these, melanoma was the first target used. The so-called MAGE antigens have been cloned from tumor-derived DNA libraries and represent molecules subtly different from the endogenous molecules. Because the MAGE antigen is different, albeit subtly, from normal melanocytes, it can function as a tumor-specific antigen and induce tumor-cell specific immunity. Interestingly, immunity directed to melanoma can often be monitored by following evidence for anti-melanocyte reactivity (which presents as patchy loss of pigmented cells in the normal skin, or "vitiligo").

Innovative Therapies

Current therapy in melanoma includes use of cloned MAGE proteins for pulsing dendritic cells (grown from autologous CD34+ peripheral blood lymphocytes *in vitro* in the presence of GM-CSF and IL-4) before infusion back into the patient as a tumor vaccine. Other vaccines have also been used, including these same cells (also transfected with GM-CSF/IL-4 to promote their growth *in vivo*) or tumor-infiltrating lymphocytes (TILs) cultured *ex vivo* with MAGE-pulsed dendritic cells and IL-2 before re-infusion *in vivo*.

IL-2 and other cytokines (TNF, IFNγ) have also been used as solo therapy (or adjunctive therapy) in melanoma patients, again with the express view of engaging the host immune response in protection against malignant growth.

Other Malignancies

In extension of the work on melanoma, other tumor antigens (e.g., BRCA [breast]; MUC-1 [breast/other adenocarcinomas]) have been used in similar trials in other human malignancies.

FURTHER READING

Bedrosian I, et al: Intranodal administration of peptide-pulsed mature dendritic cell vaccines results in superior CD8+ T cell-function in melanoma patients. J Clin Oncol 21:3826, 2003.

Berubstein N: Carcinoembryonic antigen as a target for therapeutic anticancer vaccines: A review. J Clin Oncol 20:2197, 2002.

Cameron EC, et al: Human papillomavirus-specific antibody status in oral fluids modestly reflects serum status in human immunodeficiency virus-positive individuals. Clin Diagn Lab Immunol 10:431, 2003.

Hensin T, et al: Case 7-2004: A 48-year-old-woman with multiple pigmented lesions and a personal and family history of melanoma. N Engl J Med 350:924, 2004.

Choyke PL, et al: Hereditary renal cancers, target for therapeutic anticancer vaccines: A review. Radiology 226:33, 2003.

Clarke MF: Chronic myelogenous leukemia—identifying the hydra's head. N Engl J Med 351:634, 2004.

Dighiero G, Binet JL: When and how to treat chronic lymphocytic leukemia. N Engl J Med 343:1799, 2000.

Druker BJ, et al: Efficacy and safety of a specific inhibitor of the BCR-ABL tyrosine kinase in chronic myeloid leukemia. N Engl J Med 344:1031, 2001.

Faderl S, et al: The biology of chronic myeloid leukemia. N Engl J Med 341:164, 1999.

Giannoudis A, et al: Variation in the E2-binding domain of HPV 16 is associated with high-grade squamous intraepithelial lesions of the cervix. Br J Cancer 84:1058, 2001.

Goldman JM, Melo JV: Chronic myeloid leukemia—advances in biology and new approaches to treatment. N Engl J Med 349:1451, 2003.

Hamblin TJ: Predicting progression—ZAP-70 in CLL. N Engl J Med 351:856, 2004.

Hausen HZ: Papillomaviruses and cancer: From basic sciences to clinical application. Nat Rev 2:342, 2002.

Hsueh EC, et al: Active specific immunotherapy of melanoma with a polyvalent vaccine and recombinant human GM-CSF: An immunogenicity study. Proc Am Soc Clin Oncol 22:176, 2003.

Igarashi T, et al: Effect of tumor-infiltrating lymphocyte subsets on prognosis and susceptibility to interferon therapy in patients with renal cell carcinoma. Urol Int 69:51, 2002.

Jamieson CHM, et al: Granulocyte-macrophage progenitors as candidate leukemic stem cells in blast crisis CML. N Engl J Med 351:657, 2004.

Karem KL, et al: Optimization of a human papillomavirus-specific enzyme linked immunosorbent assay. Clin Diagn Lab Immunol 9:577, 2002.

Kim CJ, et al: Immunotherapy for melanoma. Cancer Control 9:22, 2002.

Laughlin MJ et al: Outcomes after transplantation of cord blood or bone marrow from unrelated donors in adults with leukemia. N Engl J Med 351:2265, 2004.

Law TM, et al: Phase III randomized trial of interleukin-2 with or without lymphokine-activated killer cells in the treatment of patients with advanced renal cell carcinoma. Cancer 76:824, 1995.

Liu KJ, et al: Generation of carcinoembryonic antigen (CEA)-specific T cell responses in HLA-*0201 and HLA-A*2402 late stage colorectal cancer patients after vaccination with dendritic cells loaded with CEA peptides. Clin Cancer Res 10:2645, 2004.

Lode HN, Xiang R, Ursula P: Melanoma immunotherapy by targeting Il-2 depends on CD4+ T cell help mediated by CD40/CD40L interaction. Clin Invest 105:1623, 2000.

Margolin KA: Interleukin-2 in the treatment of renal cancer. Semin Oncol 27:194, 2000.

Mateo L, et al: An HLA-A2 polyepitope vaccine for melanoma immunotherapy. J Immunol 163:4058, 1999.

Matsukura T, Sugase M: Relationship between 80 human papillomavirus genotypes and different grades of cervical intraepithelial neoplasia: Association and causality. J Virol 283:139, 2001.

Menzies HP, et al: Phase I/II study of treatment with dendritic cell vaccines in patients with disseminated melanoma. Cancer Immunol Immunother 53:125, 2003.

Nagayama H, et al: Results of a phase I clinical study using autologous tumour lysate-pulsed monocyte-derived mature dendritic cell vaccinations for stage IV malignant melanoma patients combined with low dose interleukin-2. Melanoma Res 13:521, 2003.

O'Brien SG, et al: Imatinib compared with interferon and low-dose cytarabine for newly diagnosed chronic-phase chronic myeloid leukemia. N Engl J Med 348:994, 2003.

O'Rouke MG, et al: Durable complete clinical responses in a phase I/II trial using an autologous melanoma cell/dendritic cell vaccine. Cancer Immunol Immunother 52:387, 2003.

Pfister DG, Benson AB, Somerfield MR: Surveillance strategies after curative treatment of colorectal cancer. N Engl J Med 350:2375, 2004.

Rai KR, Chiorazzi N: Determining the clinical course and outcome in chronic lymphocytic leukemia. N Engl J Med 348:1797, 2003.

Ravaud A, et al: Subcutaneous interleukin-2 and interferon alpha in the treatment of patients with metastatic renal cell carcinoma—less efficacy compared with intravenous interleukin-2 and interferon alpha. Results of multicenter Phase II trial from the Groupe Francais d'Immunotherapie. Cancer 95:2324, 2002.

Rocha V, et al: Transplants of umbilical-cord blood or bone marrow from unrelated donors in adults with acute leukemia. N Engl J Med 351:2276, 2004.

Russo P: Renal cell carcinoma: Presentation, staging, and surgical treatment. Semin Oncol 27:160, 2000.

Saeterdal I, et al: Frameshift-mutation–derived peptides as tumor-specific antigens in inherited and spontaneous colorectal cancer. Proc Natl Acad Sci U S A 98:13255, 2001.

Sawyers CL: Chronic myeloid leukemia. N Engl J Med 340:1330, 1999.

Smith IIJW, et al: Immune effects of escalating doses of granulocyte-macrophage colony-stimulating factor added to a fixed dose, in patient interleukin-2 regimen: A randomized phase I trial in patients with metastatic melanoma and renal cell carcinoma. J Immunother 26:130, 2003.

Ullenhag GJ, Frodin JE: Durable carcinoembryonic antigen (CEA)-specific humoral and cellular immune responses in colorectal carcinoma patients vaccinated with recombinant CEA and granulocyte/macrophage colony-stimulating factor. Clin Cancer Res 10:3273, 2004.

SECTION V

Transplantation

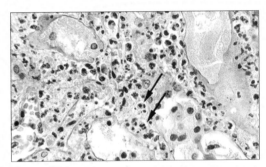

One of the major problems associated with transplantation medicine is of the same nature, though opposite in direction, as that of tumor immunity. How can we manipulate the immune system to accept a foreign graft as "self" (in the case of cancer we want to improve its recognition that this is "non-self")? Much has been learned about this problem from studies of autoimmune disorders, and we recognize how much more successful nature is than ourselves in formulating a systematic resolution to this problem. Another feature needs to be acknowledged, however. Even if we are not as successful as we would like, we are sufficiently capable of preventing graft rejection acutely now that transplantation is a recognized primary treatment modality for a number of diseases of end-organ failure. As a result, we are "victims of our own success," and major limitations in transplantation therapy now center around organ donor supply.

While there are subtle organ-specific differences among the problems facing the transplant surgeon, in general there is a commonality to the immunologic hurdles that need to be overcome. Acute and chronic rejection are well-recognized clinical phenomena and are highlighted in individual cases here (Cases 41 and 40, respectively). In addition, multiple long-term complications are often seen associated with the immunosuppressive therapy used to maintain the grafts, either drug toxicity (Case 43) or (opportunistic) infection (Cases 38 and 44), and even malignancy. Note that there has been interest in the possible use of organs from other species (in particular the pig) as an option in transplantation, both for recognizable medical reasons as well as in response to organ shortage. Rejection in this case (xenorejection) can represent novel immunologic problems not normally seen in transplantation within the species (allotransplantation), and are discussed in more detail in one of the cases here (Case 39).

Transplantation refers to the process of grafting cells or tissues from one individual (donor) to another (recipient); transfusion is a special case (blood cells). In genetically identical individuals, the grafted tissue (isograft) will survive with no other manipulations. In other cases of transplantation within a species (allograft), immune rejection of the graft survival is a function of the degree of genetic similarity between individuals and the immunosuppressive treatment used.

Graft rejection occurring early (days/weeks) is referred to as *acute* rejection and is generally reversed by increasing immunosuppression. Rejection occurring over the period weeks/months/years after transplantation is referred to as *chronic* rejection; this is less easily reversed by immunosuppressive therapy. Both acute and chronic rejection are believed to reflect recognition/operation of different components of cell-mediated immunity. However, it is clear that other features are of importance in chronic rejection (e.g., the dramatic increase in levels of non–T cell–derived nonspecific growth factors, such as fibroblast growth factor).

Grafts across a species (xenografts; e.g., pig into human) are still highly experimental. Rejection in this case occurs in minutes to hours (*hyperacute* rejection) and is probably a function of natural antibody (in humans) to pig carbohydrates on the transplanted organs, with subsequent complement activation. Similar rejections can sometimes be seen in allografts if the recipient has previously been immunized against the donor tissue and these antibodies were not detected before grafting (e.g., multiparous women; re-transplantation after graft failure).

GENETICS OF TRANSPLANTATION

Major Histocompatibility Complex

In general, the term *major histocompatibility complex (MHC) antigens* refers to the gene products of the gene loci that code for the MHC class I (HLA-A, -B, and -C) and MHC class II (HLA-DP, -DQ, -DR) antigens. HLA antigens are highly polymorphic in the population, with several alleles encoded for by each gene locus. Because genetic differences at any locus contribute to the immunologic rejection of a graft, in principle the fewer the number of mismatched loci, the greater the likelihood that the graft will be accepted. Consequently, MHC antigen matching is an important step for clinical transplantation of tissues. In the case of living-related donors it is possible to

match not only by serology/DNA typing but also by immune functioning (assayed in culture between the potential recipient and donor), thus ensuring that only donors whose MHC incompatibilities are least recognized (immunologically) by the recipient are used. This is especially the case in bone marrow transplantation.

Minor Histocompatibility Complex

Minor histocompatibility antigens represent molecules that have allelic forms and can induce variable degrees of graft rejection. Studies initially performed with rodents have shown that differences in minor histocompatibility antigens can sometimes lead to as vigorous a graft rejection as MHC differences. This has been confirmed in human bone marrow transplantation (when only MHC-matched grafts were used). However, as yet there are no easy methods to measure minor histocompatibility differences between donor and recipient, and thus clinical transplantation often occurs in the presence of significant immunologic minor histoincompatibility. A major unresolved problem in transplantation is how to produce unresponsiveness (in recipients) to foreign histocompatibility antigens without rendering the individual totally crippled immunologically, that is, how can graft-specific tolerance be produced?

Histocompatibility Matching Between Recipient and Donor

Until recently, matching by serologic techniques (for both MHC class I and class II antigens) was considered the method of choice. However, detecting "goodness of fit" was limited by the number of antibodies available (initially derived from multiparous females who have thus been immunized "naturally"). Mismatches at the MHC class II loci, which induce intense proliferation and cytokine production from CD4 cells, can also be measured using the mixed lymphocyte reaction (MLR). However this technique (which takes 72 to 96 hours) is impractical to apply in selection of suitable organ grafts, which must generally be used within 24 hours of availability. It does retain clinical use for bone marrow grafts and other cases of living-related donors (see earlier). More recently, tissue matching has been greatly improved by the use of technologic advances in molecular biology, such as restriction fragment length polymorphisms (RFLPs) and the polymerase chain reaction (PCR) using allele-specific primers for known genes. The problem of minor antigen mismatches (in unknown genes) remains.

IMMUNOLOGY OF GRAFT REJECTION

Evidence for Role of T Cells

A role for T cells in graft rejection is supported by the fact that neonatally thymectomized mice, and children with DiGeorge syndrome, tolerate grafts well. In addition, adoptive transfer of alloreactive CD4+ or CD8+ T cells causes graft rejection in a number of experimental models. Finally, a conventional approach (in experimental and clinical transplantation) to treat graft rejection is to use anti-CD4 or anti-CD8 antibodies.

Allo-MHC Recognition

Genetic differences at the MHC loci between the donor and recipient lead to the most vigorous rejection of grafts. The initial step of this rejection phenomenon is the recognition of the allogeneic graft as antigenically foreign by host T cells. *In vitro* studies with rodents to determine the molecular basis for the "strength" of allogeneic immune responses suggested that cell-mediated responses to allo-MHC antigens induce a vigorous response because there is a higher frequency of T cells recognizing allo-MHC antigens than recognizing nominal (conventional) antigens. It has been shown that 1% to 2% of the total T cell population may be reactive with any one allo-MHC antigen, whereas only about 1 in 10 (to 100) thousand T cells of the total T cell population is reactive to a nominal protein antigen. One popular hypothesis to explain this intense reactivity to alloantigens has been that allo-MHC mimics self-MHC plus foreign antigen(s), that is, allo-MHC = self-MHC + antigen x, plus self MHC + antigen y, etc.

Graft Invasion by CD4+ T Cells

Although the majority of naive T cells home to secondary lymphoid tissues, some naive T cells do recirculate and enter peripheral tissues via postcapillary venules, migrating to lymph capillaries and reentering the lymphatics. This migratory route of T cells from the circulation to the lymphatics in tissues (including grafted tissues) permits the activation of alloreactive CD4+ T cells when they come in contact with grafted cells expressing allo-MHC class II (dendritic cells, B cells, mononuclear phagocytes, and vascular endothelial cells); this has been called "direct allorecognition." Host (CD4) T cells may also be activated after recognition of "shed" donor-derived MHC antigens taken up by host antigen-presenting cells; this, in turn, is referred to as "indirect allorecognition." Both direct and indirect recognition are now believed to be important in graft rejection, with the latter (indirect recognition) taking on a more important role with time after engraftment.

Role of Alloreactive CD4+ T Cells

Activated CD4+ T cells secrete a number of cytokines. Discrete subsets of cells may be involved in production of different cytokines. Thus, so-called CD4+ Th1 cells produce interferon gamma (IFNγ), tumor necrosis factor (TNF), and interleukin (IL)-2, whereas CD4+ Th2 cells produce IL-4, IL-10, and IL-13. CD4+ Th0 cells produce a mixture of all of these cytokines. IFNγ and IL-10 are mutually antagonistic to Th2 or Th1 development, respectively; the mechanism involved is unclear but may operate at the level of the antigen-presenting cell (e.g., by regulation of expression of MHC antigens), or at the T cell level itself, altering expression of important transcription factors that regulate Th1/Th2 cell development. IFNγ is a potent nonspecific stimulator of both monocytes and macrophages. Other cytokines (e.g., IL-2, IL-4) seem to play important roles in development/differentiation of lymphocyte responses (e.g., IL-2 is an important growth factor for CD8 cells with IL-4 more so for B cells).

Role of Macrophages

The activation of macrophages leads to nonspecific enhancement of the inflammatory response and destruction of the donor tissue. Activated macrophages secrete a number of products, including IL-1 and TNF that cause subsequent bystander tissue injury. Most importantly, activated macrophages secrete IL-12, a molecule critically involved in stimulating ongoing IFNγ secretion and CD4+ Th1 activation. IL-1 and TNF also induce expression of adhesion molecules by vascular endothelial cells and enhance their secretion of the chemokines, IL-8 and monocyte chemotactic protein (MCP-1).

These secreted chemokines, in turn, augment the extravasation of leukocytes that occurs after cytokine-induced changes in the expression of a number of cell surface molecules on both endothelium and leukocytes. These molecules are important in leukocyte-endothelium adhesion and the transmigration of cells across the vascular endothelial barrier.

Role of Alloreactive CD8+ T Cells

Although there is clear evidence for a noncytolytic mechanism of graft destruction (delayed-type hypersensitivity–like response), it is also acknowledged that CD8+ cytotoxic T cells (CTLs) are important in graft destruction. *In vitro* studies of the mechanism of T cell–mediated cytotoxicity against allogeneic target cells have shown a requirement for IL-2, a cytokine produced primarily by CD4+ Th1 cells, for optimal CD8-mediated killing. This is consistent with *in vivo* studies in which graft rejection correlates with the number of donor MHC class II–bearing cells. These MHC class II donor cells would stimulate CD4+ Th1– cells to produce IL-2 *in vivo*, the cytokine required for the differentiation of precytotoxic CD8+ T cells to CTLs.

Analysis of effector cells generated in response to allogeneic cells in culture indicates that most of the CTLs recognize allo-MHC class I *directly*, suggesting that allo-MHC class I mimic self-MHC class I antigens plus foreign antigens. However, *in vivo*, some CD8+ T cells are activated after recognition of self-MHC class I with donor-derived peptide; thus indirect allorecognition is probably much more important than was previously realized for graft destruction. As anticipated, vigorous graft rejection can occur in the total absence of CD8+ T cell activation, in the presence of prominent CD4+ T cell activation, presumably via the activation of the nonspecific mechanisms referred to earlier.

Role of Vascular Endothelial Cells

Vascular endothelial cells become adhesive for neutrophils, monocytes, and lymphocytes under the influence of cytokines such as TNF and IL-1. This increased adhesion, along with changes in permeability, promotes the extravasation of leukocytes from the circulation into the graft bed.

Role of B Cells

Because B-cell activation generally requires CD4+ T cell–mediated immune responses, it is difficult to demonstrate a unique role for antibodies in graft destruction. However, the presence of preformed antibodies will initiate complement-mediated tissue destruction minutes to hours after transplantation in so-called hyperacute rejection.

IMMUNOSUPPRESSION IN TRANSPLANTATION

Nonspecific Immunosuppression

Drugs

The amount of immunosuppression required for effective long-term survival of any given graft differs between individuals. However, the use of high doses of immunosuppression leads to significant adverse side effects, including an inability to control infection (sepsis), development of lymphoid/skin malignancies, and toxicity from the drugs themselves (Fig. V–1). The following drugs are currently in clinical use: cyclosporine, corticosteroids, azathioprine, tacrolimus, rapamycin, mycophenolate mofetil, and anti-CD3 antibodies.

Mechanisms of Drug Action

Cyclosporine and tacrolimus block the transcription, and hence production, of IL-2 by CD4+ Th1 cells. These drugs bind calcineurin in the cytoplasm and thus interfere with delivery of the IL-2 gene-activating stimulus to the nucleus. Rapamycin inhibits a later stage in the promotion of IL-2 gene transcription, and thus its effect is synergistic with tacrolimus or cyclosporine. Corticosteroids are nonspecific anti-inflammatory agents. They probably inhibit rejection by interfering with the process of antigen presentation.

Azathioprine, an antimetabolite, is an analog of 6-mercaptopurine. It acts by inhibiting purine metabolism and therefore blocking cell division (and clonal expansion of activated cells). In humans, anti-CD3 antibodies transiently suppress the activity of all T cells (CD3+). However, interaction of CD3 with anti-CD3 often initially causes transient activation of T cells before downregulation of the expression of CD3 occurs. In addition, anti-CD3 is a murine antibody to which the patient frequently generates an immune response, rendering further treatments less effective.

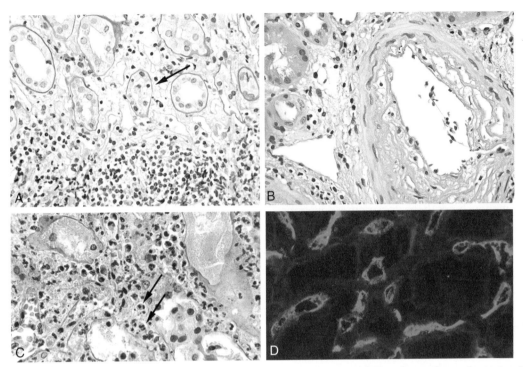

FIGURE V–1 Histology showing renal allograft with acute cellular rejection (**A** and **B**) and acute humoral rejection (**C** and **D**). **A,** Interstitial mononuclear infiltrate. The *arrow* points to an area with tubulitis. **B,** Arteritis. Note the accumulation of inflammatory cells beneath the intima, which is characteristic of acute cellular rejection type 2 (Banff criteria). **C,** Acute humoral rejection. The peritubular space is occupied by an inflammatory infiltrate with the presence of polymorphonuclear neutrophils *(arrows).* **D,** Positive C4d staining in the peritubular capillaries by immunofluorescence, a hallmark of humoral rejection. (From Goldman L, Ausiello D: Cecil Textbook of Medicine, 22nd ed. Philadelphia, Saunders, 2004.)

SPECIFIC IMMUNOSUPPRESSION (TOLERANCE INDUCTION)

This represents an as yet unrealized goal for human transplantation. One of the seminal observations made in early clinical transplantation was that prior exposure to donor antigens can surprisingly lead to prolonged survival of grafted organs. Typically, exposure was in the form of blood transfusion and the process was most well characterized for renal graft recipients. Some of these patients even developed antidonor antibodies, which nevertheless did not seem to promote accelerated graft rejection. (In these cases transplantation was initially avoided because of the fear of hyperacute rejection.)

One hypothesis to explain this increased survival after transfusion was that there had been a preferential activation of CD4+ Th2 cells, leading to increased production of IL-10 (or IL-13) which then suppressed the activation of CD4+ Th1 cells (secreting IL-2 and IFNγ), thus decreasing rejection. However, this notion

that graft rejection is correlated with CD4+ Th1 activation and graft survival with CD4+ Th2 activation is known to be overly simplistic, and there are likely as yet unknown mechanism(s) in operation.

Chimerism

Debate also continues surrounding the need for persistent donor hematopoietic chimerism in long-term graft recipients to explain graft survival. If tolerance is a passive process, tolerance might be expected from persistent presentation of allo-MHC, itself, on the grafted tissue. However, if tolerance is an active process associated with host CD4+ Th2 activation, one might expect that persistent donor antigen-presenting cells (hematopoietic cells: bone marrow–derived) might be needed for maintenance of tolerance. This proposal underlies some of the newer trials incorporating introduction of small numbers of donor bone marrow cells to recipients of solid organs.

CLINICAL TRANSPLANTATION

Tissue Differences

Liver Transplants

Liver transplants seem to be surprisingly resistant to subsequent rejection episodes, once the early phase of acute rejection is passed. Long-term graft survival is similar for either well-matched or unmatched tissues. At least 80% of patients can expect to survive at least 1 year.

Understanding the biology and immunology for this phenomenon holds hope for progress in transplantation in general. One model suggests the liver preferentially induces long-term tolerance because it is itself a lymphohematopoietic organ and induces chimerism in recipients.

Heart Transplants

Heart transplants have recently become standard clinical "treatments." Eighty-five to 90 percent of the patients who have a heart transplant survive at least 1 year. A major problem with heart transplants is the high incidence of atherosclerotic disease in the recipients (including within the donor heart itself), a result of either the drug treatments used to avoid rejection and/or the long-term immunologic effects of subclinical rejection episodes).

Bone Marrow Transplants

Bone marrow transplants are used to treat aplastic anemia, leukemia, and lymphomas. There are major problems unique to bone marrow transplantation. Not only do we see rejection of allogeneic donor stem cells by immunocompetent hosts (host versus graft rejection), but, because many recipients of bone marrow transplants are themselves immunologically compromised by chemotherapy, radiation, or genetic disease, there is also a potential for the graft to attack the host immunologically, so-called graft versus host disease (GvHD).

Corneal, Bone, Kidney, Lung, and Pancreas Transplants

Corneal transplants survive without immunosuppressive drug treatment because they are in privileged sites (not "seen" by host cells). Bone transplants are essentially used to provide an inert "scaffold"—they are avascular and again immune rejection is generally not a problem. One-year patient survival after kidney transplantation is about 90%. However, patients have to take immunosuppressive drugs for the rest of their lives. Lung and pancreas transplants have long-term success rates that are less favorable than for heart, liver, and kidneys, and ongoing production of insulin (for pancreatic grafts) decreases, with patients returning to a requirement for insulin for diabetes treatment. Lung grafts remain beset by chronic rejection, with fibrosis and graft failure (bronchiolitis obliterans).

GRAFT VERSUS HOST DISEASE

GvHD is a reaction in which alloreactive donor T cells initiate rejection of host tissue. Skin sloughing, diarrhea, and inflammation of the lungs, liver, and kidneys are common problems associated with this disease. This would suggest that the removal of T cells from the donor tissue would facilitate graft acceptance. Attempts to include removal of donor T cells as part of the protocol for the relevant transplants (bone marrow) abolished not only GvHD but also engraftment of the donor tissue. This is because cytokines, which can be donor T cell derived, are required for engraftment. Relatively standard procedures now recommend administration of T cell–produced cytokines in clinical bone marrow transplantation.

Graft versus Leukemia Effect

A further issue, which has yet to be resolved, is that donor T cells are often extremely effective in killing residual host cancer cells (the so-called graft versus leukemia effect [GvL]), the very reason for which the graft is often used. Again removal of donor T cells resolves GvHD but simultaneously abolishes GvL.

FG is a 62-year-old man who had received a renal transplant 12 years earlier after a period of 5 years during which he had undergone both peritoneal dialysis and later hemodialysis. The underlying cause of his chronic renal failure was believed to be a combination of diabetes (he had been insulin dependent since the age of 16) and long-standing hypertension (>25 years), which had been refractory to simple therapy and required triple therapy for adequate control. He has been on maintenance therapy (rapamycin and azathioprine) for immunosuppression, having been weaned from an earlier regimen of cyclosporine and prednisone at the suggestion of his transplant team, who thought this would be a simpler regimen for him.

FG lives at home with a daughter and son-in-law. He was referred by his general practitioner for admission to the hospital to investigate both a progressive jaundice of some 4 to 6 weeks' duration, along with a scaling erythematous rash on both legs, which his physician had initially thought to be a simple cellulitis but that has failed completely to respond to oral antibiotics (he has received both cloxacillin and later ciprofloxacin without any significant impact on his symptoms).

QUESTIONS FOR GROUP DISCUSSION

1. In the early post-engraftment phase, the most frequent early complication is acute graft rejection. Given that 10 years have passed since transplantation, the likelihood that we are dealing with a manifestation of an acute rejection response is low. Review the etiology of acute graft rejection. Explain the rationale for immunosuppressive therapy (and cell target) in this therapeutic intervention.

2. Chronic graft failure, which is more insidious than acute rejection and more difficult to treat, is not a likely possibility. How would you rule out chronic rejection in the case of kidney transplants?

3. Infection is a leading cause of death in immunosuppressed patients. Cytomegalovirus (CMV/ human herpesvirus 6) and Epstein-Barr virus (EBV/human herpesvirus 4) are common infections in post-transplant patients. These patients may present with hepatitis, elevated liver enzymes, but rarely jaundice. Yet, these may not be *de novo* infections. Explain.

4. Explain why hepatitis C infection would be high on your list of considerations for this patient.

5. CMV and EBV have evolved immunoevasive strategies that allow them to remain in a latent phase even in the presence of a healthy immune system. Describe these immunoevasive strategies.

6. Virally infected cells are destroyed by natural killer (NK) cells and cytotoxic T cells. Despite this, patients develop anti-CMV and anti-EBV antibodies when infected. Explain.

7. A number of infectious agents (e.g., hepatitis C) and some malignancies induce the production of cryoglobulins, abnormal antibodies that precipitate at temperatures below 98.6°F (37°C) and become soluble again at normal body temperatures. Discuss how the production of cryoglobulins could be the stimulus for processes that cause the rash.

8. Although there is some evidence that complement activation can lead to lysis of enveloped viruses, this is not considered one of the main effector mechanisms in host immunity to viral infections. Therefore, it is unlikely that this would lead to a low C4 level in serum as observed in this patient. Provide a rationale for the low levels of C4 (and C3) complement proteins.

9. In this patient, polymerase chain reaction (PCR) detected high levels of hepatitis C in the blood, indicative of active viral infection. Given this information, what would you expect to be the cause of the rash on this patient's legs? Explain how this would manifest. How would you treat the hepatitis C infection?

10. Discuss other possible causes of the leukocytoclastic vasculitis and how you would treat this even in the absence of confirmation that this was the cause of the rash.

RECOMMENDED APPROACH

Implications/Analysis of Family History

Although we are not provided with any family history, this patient has had insulin-dependent diabetes and hypertension for decades. Disease susceptibility for type 1 diabetes mellitus depends on the degree of genetic similarity that an individual has with the proband (see Case 24). Hypertension is known to have a strong genetic association, but the genes have not been identified. There are a number of risk factors for development of hypertension, one of which is diabetes.

Implications/Analysis of Clinical History

There is a case history of multiple medical problems, along with the specific ones potentially related to engraftment and immunosuppression.

Complications Associated with Graft Rejection

Note that in the early phases after engraftment the most frequent early complication seen is acute graft rejection. Given that this patient's problems started 10 years after transplantation the likelihood that we are dealing with a manifestation of an acute rejection response is unlikely. Even chronic rejection, which is more insidious and results in chronic graft failure, is doubtful. In this case, a hint that this was a problem would appear in the form of a slow and inexorable increase in serum creatinine levels over time, an indication that the kidney was slowly losing its major filtration functional capacity. If, indeed, the disease processes we are seeing are related to the transplant itself, they are more subtly related than these two obvious scenarios.

Complications of Immunosuppressive Therapy

Complications of the immunosuppressive therapy used to ensure graft survival are unfortunately quite common and include malignancy (lymphoma and melanoma), infection, and drug toxicity. Recrudescence of earlier infections or opportunistic infections can also cause problems in immunosuppressed individuals. Opportunistic infections that could certainly be of concern include *Pneumocystis carinii* (*jiroveci*) pneumonia (PCP) and infection with *Cryptosporidium, Mycobacterium tuberculosis*, as well as the opportunistic species *M. avium*. Indeed, a variety of pathogens seen in another population of immunosuppressed individuals (e.g., acquired immunodeficiency syndrome; see Case 13) is of more than passing interest as we remember that this patient first came to attention with evidence of liver disease (jaundice).

A number of viral infections are also prevalent in immunosuppressed individuals. These include cytomegalovirus (CMV/human herpesvirus 6), hepatitis C, Epstein-Barr virus (EBV/human herpesvirus 4), and human herpes simplex virus (HSV/human herpesvirus 1/2), although the latter two are less likely to cause this hepatitis. Recrudescence of chickenpox (herpes zoster) may also occur in immunosuppressed individuals (Fig. 38–1).

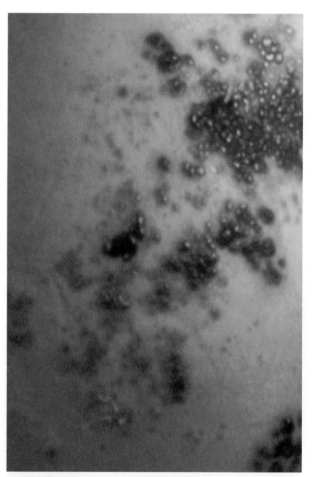

FIGURE 38–1 Disseminated herpesvirus infection such as can occur in immunocompromised (post-transplantation) patients on chronic prednisone therapy. (From Fireman P, Slavin R: Atlas of Allergies, 2nd ed. St. Louis, Mosby, 1996.)

Implications/Analysis of Laboratory Tests

To determine where to focus laboratory investigations we should keep in mind that the risk of malignancies is in fact quite restricted, with lymphomas and skin malignancies (especially epithelial cancers) quite common. Infections are more common. CMV can cause hepatitis, but jaundice is rare with infection with this virus. A more appropriate test to learn if infection is the cause of this patient's symptoms is to determine if this patient is infected with hepatitis C.

Malignancy

Investigation for lymphomas (abdominal ultrasound/computed tomography [CT]; head CT) proved negative. Biopsy of the rash (see later) indicated this was *not* the cause of either difficulty.

Viral Infections

Serologic investigation to test for anti–hepatitis C antibodies using the enzyme-linked immunosorbent assay (ELISA) revealed a high anti–hepatitis C antibody titer. To further investigate this, a request was made for a viral load measure.

Additional Laboratory Tests

Polymerase Chain Reaction

PCR was used to access hepatitis C viral load. Results indicated high levels of hepatitis C in the blood, indicative of active viral proliferation.

Complement

Chronic antibody production to hepatitis C could lead to immune complex deposition disease and a vasculitis reaction (which may be what the skin lesion is all about!). To assess the role of immune complex–mediated activation of complement in the etiology of the vasculitis, serum levels of complement proteins C3 and C4 were measured. Both were decreased relative to controls.

Biopsy of the Skin

A biopsy of the skin (rash) on the legs showed marked infiltration with neutrophils and some lymphocytes, along with other activated monocytes. The picture was described by a pathologist as being typical of leukocytoclastic vasculitis, in which deposition of immune complexes plays an important role (e.g., hepatitis C/anti–hepatitis C antibody complexes). After immune complex deposition and complement activation, the subsequent inflammatory reaction results in impairment in the circulation in small vessels in the skin and damage to blood vessels, with resultant bleeding into the skin often manifesting as a rash.

Finally it is worth remembering that included among the potential complications of immunosuppression is toxicity of the drugs themselves, which can cause both hepatotoxicity reactions and hypersensitivity reactions. Therefore, the vasculitis could, in fact, be the result of a hypersensitivity reaction to the drugs, subsequent formation of antigen-antibody complexes, and associated inflammatory processes involving both complement and neutrophil activation.

Kidney Biopsy and Serum Creatinine

A renal biopsy suggested extensive immunoglobulin deposition in the glomerulus and parenchyma, with some mononuclear cell infiltration. Serum creatinine levels were mildly elevated, reflecting damage to the glomeruli as a result of immune complex–mediated activation of complement and neutrophils with associated inflammatory processes.

DIAGNOSIS

This patient is infected with the hepatitis C virus and should be treated accordingly (see Therapy). The rash, diagnosed as leukocytoclastic vasculitis, is the result of immune complex deposition and subsequent inflammatory processes. Whether the antigen-antibody complexes are the result of a drug/anti-drug antibody interaction or hepatitis C/anti–hepatitis antibody interaction would require further testing.

THERAPY

In FG's case, a prudent course of action would be to treat the acute hepatitis C infection (with interferon alpha [IFNα]) and to modify further the rejection therapy FG is receiving, presuming that the relatively new addition of some drugs may be a cause of the hypersensitivity.

ETIOLOGY: ANTIBODIES IN CHRONIC GRAFT REJECTION

In the absence of hyperacute rejection, it is accepted that early after transplant there is little evidence for antibody-mediated rejection processes. There is, however, a growing realization that with time anti–donor-specific antibodies are present in graft recipients. What is not altogether clear is whether this has beneficial (blocking) effects or is a contributor to the pathology of rejection.

FD, a 3-month-old HIV-positive patient who is stable on triple therapy with essentially normal CD4 counts, is referred to your transplant team with fulminant hepatitic failure (FHF). A complete blood cell count with differential was requested. Rapidly progressing liver failure has been apparent over the past 2 days, during which laboratory tests (bilirubin, aspartate aminotransferase [AST], alanine aminotransferase [ALT], albumin, international normalized thromboplastin ratio [INR], prothrombin time [PT], and activated partial thromboplastin time [aPTT]) were ordered. Hepatitis B infection was confirmed when enzyme-linked immunosorbent assay (ELISA) revealed anti-HBc IgM antibodies. Following the results of these tests, abdominal computed tomography [CT] and ultrasonography were also requested.

Despite appeals to the organ-sharing network (UNOS), FD is not deemed a candidate for high placement on their list. After discussion with his mother, who is a chronic Epstein-Barr virus (EBV) carrier, you agree to consider him a candidate for experimental transplantation with a pig liver, even if only potentially as a bridging solution until a human organ becomes available. You are made aware of a newly derived, pathogen-free colony of so-called decay accelerating factor (DAF) pigs and arrange to obtain one. Why this choice? Why a pig liver?

QUESTIONS FOR GROUP DISCUSSION

1. Transplantation is the primary treatment of choice for many diseases. What problems has this created?
2. What are some of the causes of fulminant hepatitic failure (FHF) in infants?
3. What is the sole intervention for FHF?
4. Explain why the pig is a good choice for organ transplantation into humans (at least three reasons).
5. One of the problems arising in transplantation across species is the presence of a carbohydrate structure Galα1-3-Galβ1-4GlcNAc-R (α-galactosyl epitope) in pigs (and many other animals). Explain why humans do not express this carbohydrate structure on cell surfaces.
6. Explain why humans have IgM antibodies specific for this carbohydrate structure, despite the fact that we have not been exposed to pig (or other animal) tissues that express this antigen.
7. Describe the immune response that follows when the transplant recipient's (host) antibodies bind to the surface of xenografts expressing the α-galactosyl epitope on the surface that leads to hyperacute rejection of the tissue.
8. Explain why transgenic pigs expressing the human form of decay accelerating factor (DAF) have been designed to overcome this problem of hyperacute rejection.
9. There is evidence that any time cells from different species are mixed, a zoonotic infection is possible. What is a zoonotic infection? Explain why

attempts to eliminate the immunologic response to the α-galactosyl epitope on pig tissues using DAF transgenic pigs may result in an increased risk of infection with the porcine endogenous retroviruses (PERV).
10. Extrapolate the ideas just discussed to *in vitro* fertilization egg cultures that are grown on a "feeder" layer of animal cells (e.g., bovine kidney) before reimplantation into the mother.

RECOMMENDED APPROACH

Implications/Analysis of Family History

FD's mother is a hepatitis B virus (HBV) carrier who was identified during maternal screening and was found to have anti-HBc and anti-HBe IgG antibodies specific for the HBV core and HBe (pre core) antigens (HBcAg and HBeAg, respectively). HBeAg is associated with HBcAg (Fig. 39–1). Additional enzyme-linked immunosorbent assays (ELISAs) revealed that the mother was positive for the HBs antigen (HBsAg) but negative for HBeAg. Had the mother been HBeAg positive, the infant would have been given gamma globulin (anti-HBV antibodies) and the first of the three required HBV vaccine antigens. Because the mother was negative for HBeAg, the child had not been given either therapy, according to the regulations in place. HBsAg may also be detected in liver biopsies (Fig. 39–2).

In some regions, however, different regulations are in place and infants born to mothers who are HBsAg

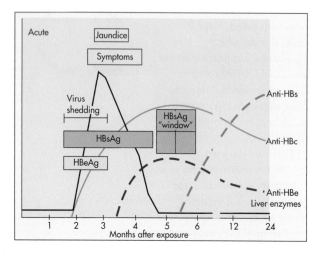

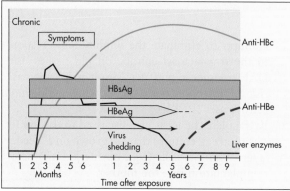

FIGURE 39–1 Serologic and clinical patterns observed during acute and chronic hepatitis B infection. (From Murray P, Rosenthal K, Kobayashi Y, Pfaller M: Medical Microbiology, 4th ed. St Louis, Mosby, 2002; redrawn from Hoofnagle JH: Annu Rev Med 32:1–11, 1981.)

positive are immunized at birth. Otherwise, the first dose of the HBV vaccine is deferred until the infant is 2 to 6 months of age. There are reported cases when vertical transmission has occurred in the first months post partum if the mother becomes infected during this time or if she is a chronic carrier. Additionally, development of FHF in infants, despite appropriate prophylaxis, has been documented.

The mother had been prescribed interferon alfa (IFNα) and a nucleoside analog. Both of these therapeutic agents have been approved by the U.S. Food and Drug Administration (FDA) for treatment of chronic EBV infection.

Analysis/Implications of Clinical History

For many children the etiology of FHF cannot be identified; however, common causes include viruses,

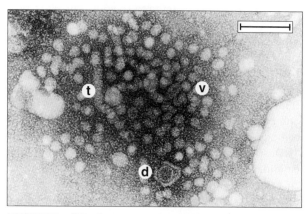

FIGURE 39–2 Negative-stain electron micrograph of plasma from a patient with acute hepatitis B virus infection. The complete virus (Dane) particles (d) have a lipid envelope with a loop containing the double-stranded DNA genome in a cuboidal nucleocapsid. The tubular (t) and vesicular (v) particles comprise only viral lipid envelope. (bar =100 nm.) (From Hart CA, Shears P: Color Atlas of Medical Microbiology, 2nd ed. St Louis, Mosby, 2004.)

toxins, congenital abnormalities (e.g., biliary atresia), metabolic diseases, and hepatotoxic drugs (e.g., acetaminophen overdose). Included in the list of viruses that can cause FHF are herpes simplex virus, adenovirus, cytomegalovirus, and EBV. Hepatitis A and hepatitis B are common causes of FHF in children and infants, but hepatitis C is not. Patients with hepatitis non–A-E infections and FHF have a higher fatality rate. Symptoms of severe liver failure include jaundice, fever, bleeding, abdominal distention and pain, fatigue, and vomiting.

Implications/Analysis of Laboratory Tests

The infant's blood cell count indicated a leukocytosis (see Appendix for normal reference values) and thrombocytopenia. Biochemical tests revealed high serum bilirubin, increased ALT and AST levels, decreased albumin, an increased INR (>4; normal ~1.0), and an increase in PT (normal: 12 to 14 seconds) and aPTT (normal: 25 to 38 seconds). Overall, the results of these tests indicated severe liver damage. Patients with severe FHF have an increased PT because the liver makes the majority of the clotting factors. Consequently, bleeding is common. A diagnosis of HBV infection was confirmed when the ELISA revealed anti-HBc IgM antibodies in FD's serum, as well as anti-HBc IgG antibodies, transferred via the placenta ELISA. On the basis of the results of these tests, abdominal CT and ultrasonography were requested.

Note: The PT refers to the time required for thrombin to convert plasma fibrinogen to fibrin. The aPTT measures the clotting time of plasma as a result of the activation by factor XII after serum contact with a negatively charged surface (e.g., silica).

DIAGNOSIS

Results of the CT and ultrasonography indicated evidence for an enlarged liver with abdominal ascites but no evidence for biliary atresia. Subsequent needle biopsy confirmed FHF likely due to overwhelming viral hepatitis.

THERAPY

The only intervention option at this stage is a liver transplant. Consideration is given to living-related donor transplant (of one of the hepatic lobes) but none of FD's relatives is either willing or deemed medically suitable as a donor.

Outcome of the Xenograft

The porcine liver transplant itself goes well. There is, in fact, no evidence of early graft loss (hyperacute rejection, see later). The team is also aware of potential problems with the so-called delayed hyperacute rejection response, occurring several days later and also believed to be associated with antibody-mediated immune activation, this time at the (graft) endothelial bed, resulting again in thrombosis and graft failure. Once again this, too, seems not to play any part in the events occurring postoperatively for this transplant. The anti-HBc IgM antibody titer does fall in the early days post transplant, which it was hypothesized may have reflected the failure of pig liver to support HBV replication.

Complications

The physicians treating the infant acknowledge to the parents that there is some concern over the functioning of other organs, in particular the kidneys, and the child has been anuric (no urine output) for 3 days in the second postoperative week. He is receiving dialysis. Possible causes are thought to be drug-related toxicity, because the levels of drug used were extrapolated from those used in adults, with little real-life information to go by. Biopsy of the kidneys has failed to show

any evidence for infiltration by mononuclear cells suggestive of an immune rejection process.

Several days later the infant suffered a cardiac arrest and died approximately 30 minutes later. An autopsy again revealed no evidence for immune rejection events, and drug toxicity is thought to be a major cause.

OVERVIEW OF XENOTRANSPLANTATION

Xenotransplants have become an interesting option in an era where we are, in many ways, a victim of our own success (as transplant biologists and clinicians). Our ability to treat a number of acute and chronic disorders in many patients has improved such that these patients no longer contribute to a donor organ pool. Moreover, the success of treating rejection is such that transplantation is now the primary treatment of choice for a number of diseases associated with end organ failure. The resulting mismatch between supply and demand forces us to consider other sources of viable organs for transplantation. The pig is in many ways a good choice for human transplantation. The organ size of the mature animal is on a par with humans. The ethical problems are not perceived to be as great as those for use of nonhuman primates. Furthermore, pig liver coagulation proteins (among others) seem to work well in human biologic processes. Another potential advantage in this case is that there is reason to believe that pig liver may not support growth and proliferation of HBV in the same manner as human liver cells, so this transplant may help clear this disease.

Challenges of Xenotransplants: Hyperacute Rejection

Transplantation across species barriers (xenotransplantation) is fraught with risks not seen in allotransplants. The first problem that arises from major species barriers is a ubiquitously expressed carbohydrate structure Galα1-3-Galβ1-4GlcNAc-R (α-galactosyl epitope). Humans and Old World monkeys do not express in their genome the gene encoding α1-3-galactosyltransferase (α1-3GT), an enzyme that synthesizes α-galactosyl epitopes on glycoproteins and glycolipids (using uridine diphosphate galactose [UDP-Gal]). Hence we, unlike multiple other species, including pigs, cats, dogs, horses, and New World primates, do not link Galα1-3 to the ends of carbohydrates expressed at the surface of cells. Accordingly, lacking tolerance to this α-galactosyl epitope, we have abundant antibodies (anti-Gal) that target this particular epitope (induced in response presumably to exposure from commensal bacteria, expressing this on their cell walls). Transplantation of organs expressing the α-galactosyl epitope on the surface leads to rapid antibody deposition at the cell surface, complement fixation, and thrombosis, with graft loss. Consequently, it has been thought that if complement activation could be controlled, this form of rejection (hyperacute rejection) would be minimized.

Transgenic Pigs: A Solution to Hyperacute Rejection

DAF pigs (overexpressing human decay accelerating factor CD55) have been designed to help overcome this problem. Interestingly, as noted in FD's case, there is some rationale for the belief that if the first phase of hyperacute rejection is overcome, accommodation may take place with no further production of anti-Gal antibodies (for presumably the reasons given earlier, including perhaps an unexplained tolerance induction in the relevant B cell population). Attempts to eliminate the immunologic response to this epitope, however, may result in an increased risk for zoonosis, particularly for infection from porcine endogenous retroviruses (PERV, see later). Zoonosis refers to the establishment of pathogens from one species in another.

Zoonosis: Increased Risk of Porcine Endogenous Retrovirus Infection with DAF Pigs

There is evidence that any time cells from different species are mixed a zoonotic infection is a potential problem. Consequently, the use of porcine tissues for xenografts also increases the potential for the transmission of PERV. Although heterografts using pig aortic heart valves have been used for years, these valves were sewn into a cloth-covered frame and therefore somewhat inaccessible to the immune system. Additionally, the valve recipients were not immunosuppressed.

As described earlier, one of the major problems with the use of porcine tissues has been hyperacute rejection because these tissues express α-galactosyl epitope to which humans have natural antibodies (anti-Gal). The presence of DAF proteins within the membranes of porcine cells should disrupt the formation of C3 convertase enzymatic complexes on the cell surface. These complexes form after activation of complement—in this case, by anti-Gal antibody-α-galactosyl epitope immune complexes.

Attempts to eliminate this immunologic reaction, however, may contribute to the transmission of PERV because the DAF proteins will be incorporated into the viral envelope when the virus buds from the DAF pig cells. Consequently, the PERV will be as resistant to complement-mediated destruction after formation of immune complexes on their envelopes as the porcine cells.

Note: In vitro studies have shown that human anti-Gal antibodies inactivate retroviruses released from animal cells by triggering the activation of the classical pathway of complement.

Other Approaches That Also Increase Risk of PERV

In another approach, the gene that encodes the enzyme α1-3GT has been knocked out and so the α-galactosyl epitope is not expressed in the porcine tissues. The absence of this epitope in these tissues would eliminate the hyperacute rejection problem. However, in the transgenic porcine infected cells, the PERVs that bud from these cells would not express this epitope either. Therefore, the anti-Gal antibodies would not be able to target these viral particles, thereby eliminating what may be an effective mechanism for viral elimination. The extent to which complement plays a role in viral immunity *in vivo* is not clearly defined. However, *in vitro* studies have shown that anti-Gal antibodies inactivate retroviruses released from animal cells. The same argument has been used for the removal of human anti-Gal antibodies from the transplant recipient.

Other Scenarios for Zoonosis

The potential for zoonotic infection is not limited to xenografts. In many *in vitro* fertilization (IVF) centers, human eggs and preimplantation embryos are cultured on animal feeder cells, most commonly bovine kidney cells, before reimplantation to the mother. Whether this poses a long-term hazard is not known. To eliminate the risk of zoonosis, some IVF centers use only cells derived from one of the embryo's biologic parents.

Bill has cystic fibrosis and received a double-lung transplant approximately 8 months ago. When you see him in your follow-up clinic today he looks far more short of breath than on his last appearance. Your nurse measures his oxygen saturation at rest on room air (normal, nonsmoker: 97%-100%), and you are disturbed to find his level only 88%. He becomes quite cyanotic (low oxygen supply to peripheral tissues) with minimal exertion in your office. He has diffuse wheezes throughout the lung fields and is afebrile. There has been no recent change in immunosuppressive therapy. You admit him to a hospital for further investigation.

QUESTIONS FOR GROUP DISCUSSION

1. What is the genetic defect in cystic fibrosis? To what types of infections are these patients particularly prone?
2. Explain why patients with cystic fibrosis are prone to infection with *Staphylococcus aureus* and *Pseudomonas aeruginosa*.
3. One of the first considerations in a patient with a relatively recent transplant is acute rejection. However, evidence of acute rejection typically occurs in the first 2 months, and so one would have expected some earlier indication that this was occurring. What is the accepted therapy for a patient who is undergoing acute rejection of the transplanted tissue? (See Introduction to Transplantation and Case 42.)
4. This patient had received a double-lung transplant (instead of a single lung). This is a generally accepted procedure for patients with cystic fibrosis. Explain.
5. What is your primary concern in a patient who is immunosuppressed? Explain why immunosuppressive therapy would predispose an individual to viral and fungal infections, in particular.
6. To which viral infections are immunosuppressed patients particularly prone? Describe the immunoevasive strategies that are protective for these viruses and explain why they hinder destruction of the virally infected cells.
7. The wheezing probably reflects generalized airway irritation/hyperreactivity and not a type I hypersensitivity reaction in that no change in medication is reported. Type I hypersensitivity reactions are associated with the production of IgE, mast cell degranulation, histamine and leukotriene release, and eosinophilia. As a review, discuss the mechanisms by which each of these occurs with emphasis on the role of interleukin (IL)-4 and IL-5.
8. A bronchoscopy sample of this patient's lung revealed a chronic inflammatory/fibrosing picture referred to as bronchiolitis obliterans (loss of small airways and chronic graft loss). Explain why increasing immunosuppressants would not help this patient yet would help a patient experiencing acute rejection. (Bronchoscopy is a diagnostic technique in which a tiny camera, within a tube, is inserted into the lungs via the nose or mouth. In addition to generating a "picture" of the airways, it is possible to obtain samples of the lung tissue and secretions.) (See Introduction to Transplantation and Case 42.)
9. Treatment measures are still in their infancy, among which is the administration of IL-10 in aerosolized fashion. Explain the rationale for this approach. Include in your discussion each of the following: antigen-presenting cells; natural killer (NK) cells; Thp, Th0, and Th1 cells; and type 1 cytokines.
10. Explain the rationale for considering anti-integrin antibodies as therapeutic agents for chronic rejection. (*Hint:* inflammation is a component of chronic rejection.) What is the "down side" to this type of approach?

RECOMMENDED APPROACH

Implications/Analysis of Family History

Cystic fibrosis is an autosomal recessive disorder resulting from mutations in a gene that encodes the cystic fibrosis transmembrane regulator (CFTR), an epithelial chloride channel expressed in a number of tissues, including airways, testis, and pancreas. Depending on the mutation, CFTR may function abnormally or not be expressed at all. Although we are not given a family history, Bill's parents would both have been carriers (heterozygotes) for the mutated CFTR. In the general population the frequency of heterozygosity is 1:40, with the incidence of CF about 1:2000.

Implications/Analysis of Clinical History

Patients with cystic fibrosis represent the highest group receiving double-lung transplants for end-stage lung disease. These patients generally receive a double-lung transplant instead of a single lung because *Staphylococcus aureus* and *Pseudomonas aeruginosa* infections are common in this patient population. Given that Bill had a double-lung transplant, a bacterial infection as a result of cross-contamination from the donor lung is unlikely, particularly since he is afebrile.

The fact that Bill is short of breath with minimal exertion suggests that his peripheral tissues are not receiving sufficient oxygen. In addition, the wheezes throughout the lung fields probably reflect generalized airway irritation/hyperreactivity and should be treated with bronchodilators and/or corticosteroids (which is temporizing therapy until we find the cause). There is no change in medications reported. Thus, it is (in general) unlikely to be a new hypersensitivity reaction to a medication. Such a reaction would likely be associated with predominant IL-4/IL-5 and leukotriene mediator release, along with hypereosinophilia.

The fact that Bill is receiving immunosuppressive therapy, a viral infection, particularly with cytomegalovirus (human herpesvirus 5) or Epstein-Barr virus (human herpesvirus 4) as a causative agent for pneumonitis is plausible.

These viruses sabotage the expression of the peptide/class I MHC complexes on the cell surface. This effectively protects the virus and the infected cells can serve as veritable "factories and reservoirs" for viruses.

Implications/Analysis of Laboratory Tests

Your nurse measures Bill's oxygen saturation at rest on room air (normal, nonsmoker: 97%-100%), and you are disturbed to find his level only 88%. Oxygen saturation is a measure of the amount of oxygen bound to hemoglobin and hence carried by circulating red blood cells. This can be measured using a pulse oximeter, which is a noninvasive technique in which a probe is attached to a patient's finger. The probe is linked to a computerized unit that displays the value as a percentage. An oxygen saturation value of less than 90% puts the patient at risk for chronic hypoxic damage to end organs (e.g., brain, heart, lungs, kidney). Alternatively, the amount of oxygen in a sample of arterial blood can be measured directly.

Additional Laboratory Tests

It is most likely that you will want a sputum sample; however, a bronchoscopy sample will be more diagnostic. This sample is obtained using a thin, flexible instrument called a bronchoscope, through which air passages in the lung can be examined directly. The advantage of a bronchoscopy sample is that it enables you to make more informed judgment about the pathology, based on the histologic and cytologic examination of the sample. Moreover, it allows for concomitant biopsy of the lung tissue with the same investigation. In Bill's case, no microbial pathology was seen, but pathologic reports of the biopsy suggest the diagnosis.

DIAGNOSIS

In the absence of a defined etiology, the clinical picture described already suggested a diagnosis of bronchiolitis obliterans, a syndrome in which small airways and alveolar sacs become partially or completely blocked by scar tissue formed when healing processes are activated to repair the damage caused by nonspecific inflammatory processes. Bronchiolitis obliterans (besides acute rejection graft loss) is the most common cause of chronic rejection and failure of lung transplants today. In Bill's case there is no other etiology and all evidence points toward a chronic inflammatory/fibrosing picture, a fact confirmed by biopsy.

THERAPY

Treatment measures are still in their infancy, but an experimental approach generating a great deal of interest involves gene transfer of IL-10 as a potent anti-inflammatory cytokine (to the transplanted organ and/or to the recipient post transplantation in aerosolized fashion). Additional regimens include measures directed toward prevention of infiltration of the graft bed with host leukocytes capable of causing damage (e.g., anti-integrins), although recognizing that this may increase susceptibility to airway microbial pathogens.

ETIOLOGY: CYSTIC FIBROSIS

Cystic fibrosis is an autosomal recessive disorder resulting from mutations in a gene that encodes the cystic fibrosis transmembrane regulator (CFTR), an epithelial chloride channel expressed in a number of tissues, including airways, testis, and pancreas. A mutation in this protein disrupts the normal homeostasis (ion exchange) across the lung epithelium, and a thick, sticky mucus accumulates in the airways, resulting in airway obstruction and an inability to clear inhaled pathogens. In the normal state, a thin, moist mucus layer overlies the epithelial cells such that pathogen binding is hindered while cilia that line the airways expel microbes that enter the airways.

For most patients, a diagnosis of cystic fibrosis is made after two elevated sweat chloride measures on separate days or by identification of a mutation using molecular techniques.

Chronic airway infections with *S. aureus* and *P. aeruginosa* are common in patients with cystic fibrosis and lead to vigorous inflammatory responses characterized by the migration of neutrophils to this region. In fact, most deaths from cystic fibrosis result from complications associated with infections. One of the factors contributing to infection with these pathogens is the increased numbers of asialolated glycolipids (e.g., asialoGM$_1$) present on epithelial cells that express a mutated CFTR (or that are regenerating). AsialoGM$_1$ functions as a receptor for pili present on both *S. aureus* and *P. aeruginosa*. This receptor/ligand interaction leads to the activation of NFκB, a transcription factor for IL-8, which is a chemokine specific for neutrophils. The activated epithelial cells secrete IL-8, which recruits more neutrophils to the site; however, they are unable to clear these infections. Neutrophils in patients with cystic fibrosis have been shown to spontaneously secrete IL-8, with airway neutrophils secreting more than blood neutrophils in the same patient. Additionally, neutrophils release a number of inflammatory products that can cause damage to the lung tissue.

The chronic inflammatory state that characterizes cystic fibrosis may, in fact, represent a defect in immunoregulation in that cystic fibrosis airways are deficient in IL-10, a cytokine that is known to downregulate inflammatory responses. *In vitro* studies have shown that T cells expressing a mutated form of CFTR secrete less of the anti-inflammatory cytokine IL-10 than controls. (*Note:* IL-10 inhibits secretion of IL-12 by antigen-presenting cells. In the absence of IL-10, IL-12 activates NK cells to secrete interferon gamma (IFNγ), which plays a role in the differentiation of CD4+ T cells to Th1 cells secreting inflammatory cytokines (e.g., IFNγ, tumor necrosis factor).

Geoffrey is a 14-month-old child born with biliary atresia (absence of the biliary tree). His parents are advised that the only possibility of cure and a normal life is a liver transplant. Given the shortage of donors, the surgeon discusses the risk/benefit of living related transplants. Both parents are eager to consent, although the best match is deemed to be the father. Surgery involves transplantation of the left lobe of the father's liver to his son. Both surgeries go well, and both patients make excellent recoveries, returning home within a week after surgery. There are no further complications of the father's care. Some 4 weeks after the transplant, Geoffrey develops a desquamating, erythematous rash over his trunk, legs, and arms, a low-grade fever, and some diarrhea. His parents return him to the transplant center and are very concerned.

There has been no dramatic change in Geoffrey's post-transplant immunosuppressive regimen. Blood work looks relatively normal, with some moderate elevation of liver function tests. The diarrhea is quite profuse, although stool cultures are negative for infectious organisms. In fact, blood cultures, urine, induced sputum, and even a lumbar puncture fail to identify an infectious cause of disease, despite evidence for a continuing low-grade fever. During the third hospitalization day he actually becomes quite tachypneic (short of breath), although again a chest radiograph fails to document any obvious pathologic process. He is holding reasonable oxygen saturation only when receiving high-flow 100% oxygen. Of particular concern, you have not been able to discern the cause of the rash, and he is only maintaining normal urine output with vigorous fluid resuscitation. The nurse in the intensive care unit comments that only in burn patients has she seen a rash this bad.

QUESTIONS FOR GROUP DISCUSSION

1. Acute and chronic rejection of a graft by a host is referred to as host-versus-graft disease (HvGD). Compare these two types of HvGD with respect to effector cells, time of onset, and treatment (see Case 42).

2. Explain why immunosuppressive therapy is essential for all transplants except for those from an identical twin.

3. Patients on immunosuppressive therapy have risk factors that are unrelated to the graft itself. Discuss these factors.

4. None of the risk factors (see question 3) will present as a desquamating rash (shedding of the outer layer of skin/epidermis). Furthermore, this complication occurs only with intestinal, bone marrow, and liver transplants. What do these tissues have in common?

5. Graft versus host disease (GvHD), as the term implies, refers to the immunologic assault of the host tissues by the graft. Given that one of the prominent features of GvHD is the desquamating rash, to what host antigens is this immunologic response directed?

6. Immunologic responses in HvGD and GvHD involve the same components of the immune system. In HvGD the host is targeting the graft, whereas in GvHD the graft is targeting the host tissues. In both these scenarios, CD4+ Th1 cells play a significant role. Review immunologic responses that require Th1-derived cytokines. (Begin by listing the type 1 cytokines.)

7. With reference to question 6, how would you treat GvHD?

8. For liver transplants, GvHD is a recognized complication; but once this is overcome, graft acceptance by the host occurs more readily than for other types of graft. One explanation is that the liver establishes microchimerism. Explain the term *microchimerism* and discuss how this might contribute to tolerance of a foreign tissue.

9. Assuming that the microchimerism model proposed is indeed the mechanism by which liver allograft tolerance is induced, explain why vigorous immunosuppression immediately after trans-

plantation would condemn a patient to life-long immunosuppressive therapy.

10. Acceptance of a liver graft can itself facilitate acceptance of a later (different) organ allograft from the same donor. Discuss the potential implications of this for organ transplantation.

RECOMMENDED APPROACH

Implications/Analysis of Family History

Biliary atresia is a disorder characterized by the absence or obstruction of bile ducts that normally transport bile to the small intestine or to the gallbladder for storage. The retention of bile within the liver leads to cell damage and subsequent scarring that can lead to cirrhosis.

No family history is provided, and for a clinical presentation of biliary atresia this is not critical in that there is no evidence of a genetic link for this disorder. Therefore, this disorder usually presents in only one child in a family or in only one child of a pair of twins. The incidence of this disorder is low, occurring in only 1:1500 to 1:2000 members of the general population. Interestingly, Asians and African Americans are more likely to be affected than whites.

Implications/Analysis of Clinical History

Patients with biliary atresia generally appear normal at birth and initially show normal weight gain. By the time they are 2 or 3 weeks of age, they develop jaundice, become irritable, and show weight loss. Urine samples are dark; stool samples become light colored. When a diagnosis of biliary atresia is made before the infant is 3 months of age, surgical intervention may reestablish bile flow. When this intervention is not successful, or if the infant is not diagnosed within the time frame that allows surgery, the only option is a liver transplant. Although we are not given the early clinical history, we are told that Geoffrey received a liver transplant when he was 14 months of age. This would necessitate immunosuppressive therapy even though we are not provided with this information. Four weeks after the liver transplant, Geoffrey was brought back to the transplantation center because he had developed a desquamating, erythematous rash over most of his body, a low-grade fever, and some diarrhea.

Given this clinical history, our immediate concern is acute rejection of the graft or a complication of immunosuppressive therapy that would include infection, malignancy, or drug toxicity.

Implications/Analysis of Laboratory Testing

Graft rejection (host versus graft disease [HvGD]) is our first concern. However, liver function tests revealed only moderate elevation of liver function tests. Whereas complications of immunosuppressive therapy include malignancy and drug toxicity, as well as infection, the fact that Geoffrey has a fever and profuse diarrhea puts infection at the top of this list. However, stool cultures, blood cultures, urine, induced sputum, and lumbar puncture were all negative for any infectious agent. Although a viral diagnosis could have explained the profuse diarrhea and fever, it would not account for the rash. An idiosyncratic drug hypersensitivity reaction could present as a desquamating rash, but this would not present as a fever and diarrhea.

We need to consider the fact that transplantation of liver, bone marrow, and intestinal grafts is unique in that these grafts contain major donor lymphoid elements. A complication of grafts that have major lymphoid donor cells is graft versus host disease (GvHD), which occurs when donor immune cells attack host tissues.

Additional Laboratory Tests

A biopsy of skin was examined histologically, and these findings were characteristic of changes occurring in GvHD. Consistent with such a diagnosis, there was evidence for lymphoid infiltration with death of basilar epidermal cells, vacuolization of more superficial epidermal cells, and eosinophilic bodies. Polymerase chain reaction was used to determine if the human leukocyte antigens present in the skin tissue and peripheral blood lymphocytes obtained by biopsy (phlebotomy) was predominantly of donor (father) or recipient origin.

DIAGNOSIS

On the basis of these laboratory results and the clinical presentation, Geoffrey was diagnosed with GvHD. In GvHD, donor cells of allograft origin target host antigen present on the epithelia of the gut, lung, and biliary tree. Inflammation, edema, and increased vascular permeability to both fluid and cells characterize these reactions.

THERAPY

Immunosuppression should be increased.

ETIOLOGY: TOLERANCE OF LIVER ALLOGRAFTS

Many different mechanisms have been put forward to explain the observation that allograft tolerance occurs more often with transplanted livers than with other organs. Some of the proposed mechanisms include production of soluble MHC class I proteins, generation of immunoregulatory suppressor T cells, induction of regulatory cells, and microchimerism. The concept of microchimerism is particularly interesting in that it suggests that patients with stable microchimerism may eventually be able to be withdrawn from all immunosuppression without loss of the graft (stable graft-specific tolerance).

Microchimerism

In the world of transplantation, an ideal scenario would be one in which the patient becomes tolerant to the allograft without the need for long-term immunosuppressive therapy. Although still uncommon, there are documented reports of allograft tolerance after liver transplantation. The explanation may lie in the ability of the liver to establish cellular microchimerism. Within this context, microchimerism refers to the seeding of peripheral tissues with blood cells present in the graft. In one model, tolerance is induced because donor cells attack the host cells (graft versus host), which would cause graft versus host disease; whereas if host cells attack the donor cells (host versus graft), that would cause host versus graft disease. Following their activation, both populations of cells undergo apoptosis, resulting in tolerance. Support for this model comes from studies that have shown that prior acceptance of a liver graft can itself facilitate subsequent acceptance of a later (different) organ allograft from the same donor.

Multiple attempts have been made to document evidence for such microchimerism in patients with long-standing grafts on minimal (or often no) immunosuppressive therapy. To date there has been no consistent evidence that microchimerism represents the common theme explaining tolerance in these cases, and this remains an intellectually attractive, although still unproven, explanation.

Elizabeth is a 19-year-old girl with severe Crohn's disease. In the course of this disease characterized by diarrhea, pain, loss of appetite, and weight loss, the associated inflammatory processes led to bowel obstruction that necessitated resection of a large portion of the intestine. Unfortunately, so much of the small intestine was removed that the remaining segment could no longer absorb the required nutrients. Consequently, Elizabeth began receiving total parenteral nutrition, which is intravenous feeding. As such, she was an ideal candidate for a pilot intestinal transplant program and had received a small intestinal transplant 1 month earlier. In this procedure, the surgeon transplants a segment of a cadaver's small intestine into the patient. The patient was also prescribed a regimen of immunosuppressive drugs to overcome the rejection, but this also increases the risk of infection.

After 27 days, Elizabeth returned to the hospital showing evidence of weight gain, but with a diffuse "weeping" rash covering her body, abdominal cramps, and a fever of 5 days' duration. As you begin to consider this problem, think of issues related to transplantation in general, of the side effects of transplantation, and of small intestinal transplantation in particular.

QUESTIONS FOR GROUP DISCUSSION

1. What is Crohn's disease? Families of patients with Crohn's disease have shown a strong association with mutations in the NOD2 gene. What is NOD2?

2. *Ex vivo* studies have repeatedly shown that macrophages isolated from diseased intestinal segments of Crohn's disease patients produce more interleukin (IL)-12 compared with macrophages isolated from control patients. Explain how IL-12 production would lead to an increase in interferon gamma (IFNγ), tumor necrosis factor (TNF), and IL-2 but a decrease in IL-4.

3. IFNγ, TNF, and IL-2 play a significant role in various aspects of the immune system. Discuss these and how each might play a role in destruction of the intestine.

4. T cells isolated from Crohn's disease patients also produce more IFNγ and decreased amounts of IL-4. Both IL-12 and IFNγ play an important role in inflammation, and this is supported by studies in which Crohn's disease patients treated with antibodies that block the IL-12 receptor showed a significant decrease in inflammation.

5. Acute graft rejection by the host's immune system is the most frequent early complication of transplantation. What is acute graft rejection, and what is the primary underlying cause? How do we try to avoid this problem clinically?

6. Evidence for acute rejection would be nonspecific (e.g., fever) as well as physiologic "failure" of the graft. Explain the role of cytokines in nonspecific graft rejection and how cytokines play a role in the induction of fever.

7. Rejection of an intestinal graft would manifest as a loss of weight with cramping. Explain what is causing the cramping.

8. Acute rejection episodes are best treated by increasing nonspecific immunosuppression. However, the side effects of immunosuppression itself are often the cause of the patient's main complaints. CD4+ T cells are usually the target for immunosuppression. Review the role of CD4+ T cells in immune responses and in acute rejection.

9. What organs and tissues are particularly susceptible to drug (cyclosporine and tacrolimus) toxicity? In addition to the drug toxicity, to what malignancies and types of infections are immunosuppressed patients particularly prone?

10. A peculiarity to intestinal transplantation is that we generally transplant donor lymphoid tissue here (as well as the intestinal graft itself). In fact, the intestine is a source of some 50% of the total body lymphoid pool and can lead to graft versus host disease (GvHD). Discuss how a diagnosis of GvHD would explain the cramps, fever, and weeping rash.

RECOMMENDED APPROACH

Implications/Analysis of Family History

Crohn's disease is a disorder that develops from an unregulated mucosal immune response in the gastrointestinal tract. This disease is, in part, genetically determined because studies with identical twins indicate that there is a 58% to 67% concordance. Whole genome screens of families of patients with Crohn's disease have shown a strong association with mutations in the NOD2 gene, also known as CARD15. NOD2, an intracellular receptor for peptidoglycan present in various bacteria, is expressed by epithelial cells as well as by phagocytes and antigen-presenting cells. Several hypotheses have been put forward regarding the mechanism by which NOD2 mutations could contribute to unregulated mucosal immunity; however, more studies are required to provide a solution to this problem. No specific pathogen from the normal resident flora has been identified as a stimulus for the inflammatory process.

Implication/Analysis of Clinical History

Elizabeth's clinical presentation includes a weekend-long fever, abdominal cramps, and a diffuse "weeping" rash covering her body. In a patient who is 1 month post transplant, the first considerations are acute rejection and infection to account for a fever of 5 days' duration.

Infection

Infection could certainly be a cause of the fever. Viral infections, particularly cytomegalovirus (CMV), are particularly prominent early after transplantation because the primary target of immunosuppressive therapy is the T cell. T cells play a key role in many aspects of the immune system, including activation of the cytotoxic T cell, a key player in viral immunity.

In intestinal transplant patients, immunosuppressive drugs and/or graft rejection may disrupt the mucosal barrier such that bacteria can enter the lamina propria and from there access the mesenteric lymphatics and, ultimately, the circulation. Sepsis is a common cause of death after an intestinal transplant.

Acute Rejection

The most frequent early complication of transplantation is acute graft rejection by the host immune system. This is a function of, among other things, the degree of MHC incompatibility between donor and host. Pretransplant MHC "matching" of donor and recipient is an attempt to minimize acute rejection.

Fever in Acute Rejection

Acute rejection triggers an inflammatory response as activated macrophages secrete tumor necrosis factor (TNF) and interleukin-1 (IL-1) that alter the vascular endothelium to facilitate the transmigration of leukocytes from the circulation to the tissue.

When host CD4+ T cells are activated, they release cytokines (e.g., IFNγ/TNF) that enhance the cytotoxicity of macrophages, as well as their secretion of IL-1 and TNF. At high concentrations, TNF and IL-1 act on the hypothalamus, which triggers a cascade of events that lead to a febrile response, associated with elevated endogenous production of prostaglandin E_2. (Acute rejection also includes destruction of the graft as a result of CD8+ T cell activation.)

The abdominal cramping could be caused by histamine released from mast cells during an inflammatory response. Mast cell degranulation leads to the release of histamine, which can act on histamine receptors present on the mesenteric musculature, causing increased contractions with concomitant cramping.

Other Possibilities

Elizabeth has some, but not all, of these findings, which might serve to alert you to other possibilities!

Implication/Analysis of Laboratory Tests

How might you measure directly evidence for graft failure in this case? Various measures have been tried. *Note:* we need some specific assay for intestinal function (e.g., serum creatinine for the kidney). Accordingly, measuring the absorptive function of the intestine is currently the best approach.

Assessing Intestinal Absorption

The D-xylose absorption test may be used to assess absorption of carbohydrates. D-Xylose is a carbohydrate that is absorbed normally by the small intestine but is not utilized by the body. This test measures the amount of D-xylose in the blood or urine about 2 hours after swallowing a drink containing the sugar. Because D-xylose is normally absorbed by the intestine, this test can be used to assess absorption of carbohydrates.

Fat absorption can be assessed with the fecal fat test in which dietary intake of fat during a defined period (e.g., 3 days) is compared with the amount of fat in feces in the same period of time. The fat content in the feces will be higher than normal in patients who are unable to absorb fats.

Additional Laboratory Tests

There is one key feature that none of these explanations has addressed, however, namely the rash. Endoscopy and colonoscopy with tissue biopsy of the intestine are used to obtain tissue samples to establish an unequivocal answer. In general, pathologic and histologic assessment is more definitive than endoscopy (visual inspection alone), which only diagnoses rejection about two thirds of the time. The pathologic report indicates evidence for villous blunting, a significant mononuclear cell infiltrate with edema of the lamina propria, inflammation of crypts (cryptitis), and increased cell death (crypt cell apoptosis). All are findings consistent with intestinal GvHD.

DIAGNOSIS

A peculiarity in intestinal transplantation for Crohn's disease is that we generally transplant donor lymphoid tissue here (as well as the intestinal graft itself). In fact, the intestine is a source of some 50% of the total body lymphoid pool. GvHD is thus a distinct problem in this form of transplantation. Massive cytokine production (now from both activated host and donor CD4 cells) often leads to the severity of the symptoms (a so-called cytokine storm). This would also account for the "weeping rash" (elevated permeability of vessels after cytokine release) and the cramps (and fever).

THERAPY

As in all cases, we have to weigh the pros and cons of different treatments. Acute rejection episodes are best treated by increasing nonspecific immunosuppression. Increased (or different) immunosuppression would be a first step. However, increased infection (a consequence of immunosuppression) and increased evidence of malignancy are two of the "big" side effects. Interestingly, the incidence of malignancy is relatively restricted to two problems: lymphomas and skin malignancies.

Another complication of immunosuppressive treatment is often the toxicity of the drugs themselves. Hypersensitivity reactions are included as possibilities but are rare because the drugs themselves are immunosuppressive. However, toxicity to other tissues is common, such as renal toxicity and neurotoxicity, which is particularly common with cyclosporine and tacrolimus.

Depending on the patient's response to increased immunosuppression, graft removal may be the only remaining option.

ETIOLOGY: CROHN'S DISEASE

Crohn's disease is a chronic inflammation of the intestine. For most patients, this disease requires extensive bowel resections and a need for total parenteral nutrition. Often patients are unable to maintain a satisfactory nutritional status or fluid and electrolyte balance. Consequently, weight loss becomes a problem.

Before bowel resection, inhibition of cytokines that play a role in an unregulated immune response may be successful. In recent years, monoclonal antibodies that bind TNF have been used for some patients with Crohn's disease with varying degrees of relief. For this patient, blocking cytokine activity was not an option because a substantial length of the small intestine had already been removed and so intestinal transplantation had been her only remaining option.

Models for Unregulated Immune Response

Although no genetic susceptibility genes have been identified that would result in an unregulated immune response, two models have emerged. The first is that unregulated mucosal inflammatory response arises as a result of a predominance of inflammatory cytokines (e.g., IL-12, IFNγ, TNF); the other is that unregulated responses could occur if patients have a defect in the regulatory T cells that would normally dampen this response.

Ex vivo studies have repeatedly shown that macrophages isolated from diseased intestinal segments of patients with Crohn's disease produce more IL-12 compared with macrophages isolated from control patients. Additionally, T cells isolated from patients with Crohn's disease also produce more IFNγ and decreased amounts of IL-4. Both IL-12 and IFNγ play important roles in inflammation, and this is supported by studies in which patients with Crohn's disease treated with antibodies that block the IL-12 receptor showed a significant decrease in inflammation.

Ms. Bell received cardiac transplantation approximately 6 years earlier for a cardiomyopathy that developed after she received chemotherapy (doxorubicin [Adriamycin]) for breast cancer. She has had routine endomyocardial biopsies each year, the last being 1 year ago. At that time the pathologist read the biopsy as normal, with no signs of rejection. The only change in her anti-rejection therapy over the past 2 years was a reduction in the prednisone dose (now 7.5 mg/day) and replacement of cyclosporine (which she had received for nearly 5 years since the time of transplantation) with tacrolimus. You (her son) were told that the advantage of tacrolimus was a slightly improved toxicity profile. You arrived home for a visit this afternoon to find your mother confused and with a droop on the left side of her face/mouth. You immediately call an ambulance and arrange transport to the local hospital.

QUESTIONS FOR GROUP DISCUSSION

1. Tissue rejection is of concern for any transplant patient. Explain why this patient's symptoms are unlikely to be caused by hyperacute rejection.
2. Review the immunology of acute rejection and why this is unlikely the cause of the clinical presentation. In general terms how is acute rejection treated? Provide a rationale for the use of each of the following as therapy for acute rejection: (a) intravenous anti-CD3 antibodies and (b) anti-CD25 antibodies.
3. Explain how you would determine whether the clinical symptoms are the result of tissue (heart) damage.
4. Chronic rejection is still a possibility. What is the underlying cause of chronic rejection? Describe how (a) numerous, but minor, acute rejection episodes and (b) chronic immunostimulation against minor antigens in the graft could lead to chronic rejection. Discuss how this would affect heart function and how it might lead to generalized neurologic deficits. What aspect of this patient's clinical presentation cannot be explained by a diagnosis of chronic rejection?
5. A diagnosis of "rejection" seems unlikely in this patient as discussed in the previous questions. What three potential problems should we consider given that this patient is on immunosuppressive therapy?
6. Discuss the three types of malignancies to which this patient may be susceptible and how these could account for the neurologic symptoms.
7. Why would you want to include Ms. Bell's original breast cancer as a risk, in addition to the three

that you have just described? What is the proposed mechanism underlying this increased risk of malignancies?
8. How would you rule out a new immune response in a patient known to be (a) infected with a virus prior to the transplant and (b) uninfected before the transplant?
9. Direct drug toxicity reactions are also a major consideration. Discuss how toxicity reactions secondary to therapy with tacrolimus and cyclosporine would manifest in (a) the kidney and (b) nervous tissue?
10. Discuss the possible complications of prednisone therapy. Explain how this would account for this patient's clinical symptoms.

RECOMMENDED APPROACH

Implications/Analysis of Family History

At this stage we are not provided with any family history. Family history regarding cardiac problems is likely irrelevant in that Ms. Bell's heart problems were related to chemotherapy after she was diagnosed with breast cancer.

Implications/Analysis of Clinical History

Ms. Bell received a cardiac transplant 6 years ago, and all the evidence we are provided with indicates that this was a successful graft in that the yearly endomyocardial biopsies have all been normal. In fact, the only change in her anti-rejection therapy has been a reduction in immunosuppressive therapy and change from cyclosporine to tacrolimus, which is slightly less toxic.

Chronic Rejection

Chronic rejection, most readily correlated with release of nonspecific "growth factor"-like mediators (e.g., fibroblast growth factor, endothelial growth factor) tends to take the form of an insidious fibrosing/proliferative reaction, which is relatively refractory to immunosuppressive treatment. (*Fibrosis* refers to the excessive accumulation of connective tissue in an organ.) Note that a fibrotic (noncompliant) heart would not pump as efficiently. Therefore, the resulting inability to oxygenate the tissues might cause some generalized neurologic deficits (e.g., the confusion referred to in the case description). Thus, one might consider the neurologic deficits as one possible manifestation of chronic rejection. However, the history suggests a more sudden onset, which does not fit this picture.

Organ-Specific Damage

Organ-specific damage is high on the list of possible diagnoses. Whenever we look for organ-specific damage (from T cell-mediated "attack") we think of organ-specific "markers" for the damage. Thus, in kidney grafts, you would measure creatinine. For the heart you can look at the electrocardiogram and also measure specific cardiac muscle enzymes in the blood (see Implications/Analysis of Laboratory Investigation).

Implications/Analysis of Laboratory Investigation

Routine blood work, physical examination, electrocardiogram, and serum levels of cardiac enzymes should be initiated at this time. A number of cardiac enzymes (e.g., troponin I, creatine phosphokinase, creatine kinase) are released when heart tissue is damaged. Although an increase in the level of these enzymes occurs after heart damage, some of these enzymes are present in other tissues, as well. Therefore, results of these tests must be interpreted in light of the electrocardiographic findings. Measurement of cardiac muscle enzymes was normal, as was the ECG, ruling out killing (lysis) of heart cells as the cause of this patient's problem.

Side Effects of Drug Therapy

You must consider the fact that this disorder could represent one of a possible number of side effects of the treatment she received for the transplant. In general, the chronically immunosuppressed populations show an increased frequency of three major problems: (1) malignancy, (2) infections, and (3) drug toxicity.

Additional Laboratory Tests

Impaired tumor immunosurveillance, as a result of the immunosuppression she has received, could make this patient more susceptible to a secondary metastasis (to the brain) from her original breast cancer. A new-onset central nervous system (CNS) lymphoma might also be a concern. Both lesions might cause confusion, as might a viral encephalopathy.

To address these concerns, computed tomography (CT) was requested along with viral antibody titers for herpes simplex virus (human herpesviruses 1 and 2) and cytomegalovirus (human herpesvirus 6). CT was normal and the viral antibody titers were negative, ruling out both a CNS lymphoma and viral encephalopathy.

Having ruled out graft rejection, infection, and a CNS lymphoma we need to consider drug toxicity as the cause of this patient's clinical presentation.

DIAGNOSIS

Toxicity, directly and indirectly from the drugs themselves, can cause severe complications. The drugs she is receiving as part of the post-transplant immunoprophylaxis, tacrolimus (and indeed the cyclosporine she received earlier) are nephrotoxic (damage the kidney) and have also been reported to show toxicity to nervous tissues (neurotoxic). Most of the neurotoxicity reported tends to reflect damage to peripheral nerves (peripheral neuropathy) rather than to reflect toxicity within the CNS.

Prednisone has been shown to leave patients at increased risk of atherosclerotic disease, both within the vessels of the grafted organs (here, the heart) and elsewhere in the body (e.g., the brain). This narrowing of the blood vessels, in turn, results in increased risk of ischemic damage to the central organs (heart attack and, in the brain, a stroke). Most of the evidence points to prednisone toxicity as causing narrowing of the blood vessels, which, in turn, led to ischemic damage in the brain. This manifested as a stroke.

THERAPY

Treatment of stroke has been revolutionized in the past few years. Now instead of reliance on anti-thrombotic drugs such as aspirin (or the newer clopidogrel [Plavix]), there is intense interest in the acute use of "clot dissolving therapy" (tissue plasminogen activator therapy) such as that used for heart attacks and stroke. This is not without considerable risk (increased risk of bleeding with intracerebral hemorrhage and death), so risk-benefit considerations are crucial.

ETIOLOGY: TRANSPLANTATION COMPLICATIONS

Graft rejection, infections, malignancies, and drug toxicity are all possible complications after transplantation and immunosuppressive therapy

Graft Rejection

For the most part, grafts are allografts. That is, they are donated from another person who is genetically dissimilar. The rejection of an allograft reflects a composite of both antigen-specific and antigen-nonspecific inflammatory processes that include activation of (1) the intrinsic coagulation pathway; (2) T cells and B cells; and (3) macrophages, neutrophils, mast cells/basophils, and the vascular endothelium. Cytokines, chemokines, and inflammatory products secreted by antigen-specific and antigen-nonspecific cells all contribute to graft rejection.

Hyperacute Rejection

Hyperacute rejection, as the name implies, occurs in the immediate aftermath of transplantation—it is antibody (and complement) mediated. When hyperacute rejection occurs after an allograft, it is an indication that the recipient has previously been sensitized to the antigens on the donor tissue and these antibodies were not detected before the transplant. This could happen when the recipient is a multiparous woman or is receiving a transplant after a previous graft failure.

Acute Rejection

Acute rejection is a function of, among other things, the degree of MHC incompatibility between donor and host and is minimized both by "matching" of donor and recipient at the MHC before engraftment and by judicious use of immunosuppressive drug therapy after engraftment to decrease the likelihood of sensitization. Despite immunosuppressive therapy, some degree of cell activation can (and generally does) occur, marked both by development of killer CD8+ T cells (CTLs) specific for graft antigen/MHC and by activated CD4+ cells, able to release a variety of molecules capable of engaging other elements of the immune recognition process.

ROLE OF CD4+ T CELLS Activation of CD4+ T cells during acute graft rejection occurs after both direct and indirect recognition of allo-MHC. In direct recognition, donor peptides are displayed within the groove of MHC molecules on the surface of host antigen-presenting cells. That is, T cells are recognizing self-MHC/donor peptide complexes. The number of T cells responding to this form of antigen recognition is comparable to that of other T cell responses against nominal antigen. In contrast, direct allorecognition of donor MHC molecules (donor MHC) expressed on donor cells leads to the activation of large numbers of T cells and vigorous immune response against the donor tissue.

Activated CD4+ cells release both interleukin (IL)-2 (a T cell growth factor) as well as interferon gamma (IFNγ) and tumor necrosis factor (TNF), both potent inflammatory mediators, which can trigger activation of cells of the innate immune system (e.g., macrophages/neutrophils) to cause damage. Although CD4+ cells both augment differentiation of CD8+ killer T cells and provide "help" for B cell recognition (and conventional immunoglobulin production in response to foreign antigen), antibody-mediated damage itself is generally not thought to contribute in an important fashion to early graft alloreactions and loss.

ROLE OF SOLUBLE MEDIATORS AND NONSPECIFIC IMMUNE CELLS Chemokines, produced by a number of cells in the inflammatory milieu (including fibroblasts/endothelial cells) attract other cells to the site of rejection, further propagating the process. Along with endothelial cell activation, engagement of the serum-derived plasminogen and thrombotic cascade occurs, as well as thrombosis mediated both

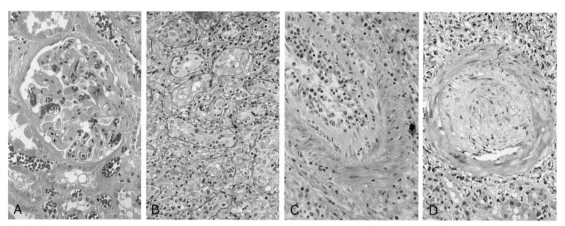

FIGURE 43–1   Histopathology of different forms of graft rejection. **A,** Hyperacute rejection of a kidney allograft with endothelial damage, platelet and thrombin thrombi, and early neutrophil infiltration of a glomerulus. **B,** Acute rejection of a kidney with inflammatory cells in the interstitium and between epithelial cells of the tubules. **C,** Acute rejection of a kidney allograft with inflammatory reaction destroying the endothelium of an artery. **D,** Chronic rejection in a kidney allograft with graft arteriosclerosis. The vascular lumen is replaced by an accumulation of smooth muscle cells and connective tissue in the vessel intima. (Courtesy of Dr. Helmut Rennke, Department of Pathology, Brigham and Women's Hospital and Harvard Medical School, Boston.)

by tissue factor and a novel prothrombinase discovered comparatively recently and referred to as fibroleukin. This procoagulant activity (a product of endothelial cells and macrophages) is distinct from previously described ones and occurs after immune-mediated activation of an inflammatory event.

REGULATORY T CELLS Several types of immune cells have been shown to downregulate T cells that play a role in acute graft rejection. Of these, the CD4+, CD25+ regulatory T cells (Treg) have been most widely studied. Treg cells have been shown to inhibit CTL proliferation, cytokine production, and B cell activation. Furthermore, Treg cells appear to induce phenotypic change in some cytopathic cells such that they become IL-10–secreting T cells. IL-10 downregulates IL-12 secretion by antigen-presenting cells. IL-12 plays a key role in the differentiation of immature CD4+ T cells to mature T cell–secreting proinflammatory type 1 cytokines. The role that these IL-10-secreting cells play in immunoregulation of transplants is underscored by the fact that (in *in vitro* systems) neutralization of IL-10 abrogates its immunosuppressive effect on acute rejection during skin grafts. In allograft rejection, it seems that the contribution of Treg cells, while present, is overwhelmed by the vigorous immune response generated by direct alloantigen recognition by T cells.

THERAPY FOR ACUTE REJECTION Acute rejection is mediated primarily by T cells, and so these cells are the target of immunosuppressive therapy. This would

be done only after consultation with the transplant team and would almost certainly necessitate obtaining a biopsy (to document evidence for rejection). Medication that would likely be used in such a scenario would include intravenous OKT3 (anti-CD3 antibodies, directed at all T cells) and/or anti-CD25 antibodies (directed at activated T cells expressing IL-2 receptor as a marker of their activation/proliferation).

Chronic Rejection

Chronic rejection may reflect the net outcome of numerous (even unidentified) minor acute rejection episodes and/or a chronic immunostimulation directed against minor incompatibilities (minor antigens) between graft and recipient. Like acute rejection, chronic rejection involves components of cell-mediated immunity; however, chronic rejection also involves the dramatic increase in non–T cell–derived growth factors (e.g., fibroblast growth factor), which leads to the production of fibrosed tissue that does not function well (Fig. 43–1). Note, too, that chronic rejection is generally not easily treated.

Infections

Complications of the immunosuppressive therapy used to ensure graft survival are unfortunately quite common. An increased incidence of (opportunistic) infection is observed in these patients. Recrudescence of earlier infections that were previously cleared can also cause problems.

Individuals who are immunosuppressed are particularly prone to viral infections. This likely represents a consequence of suppressed CD4/CD8-mediated T cell immunity. In general, immunoglobulin levels, essential for resistance to bacterial infection, are unaffected.

When infection is suspected, determination of antibody titers for the suspect infection should include assays for both IgM and IgG. IgM antibodies would indicate a new immune response in a person known to be seronegative before transplantation. IgG antibodies would indicate a previous infection.

Malignancy

An increased evidence of malignancy is a risk factor for transplant patients. It is worth noting that although they are immunosuppressed, this patient population (the transplant population) does not seem to be at risk for increases in *all* solid tumors but predominantly those of viral etiology, lymphomas, and skin tumors (especially epithelial cancers). This is thought to indicate a risk involvement caused by direct action of drugs on the immune system and/or specific body tissues, rather than an indirect effect on immunosurveillance itself.

Toxicity

Toxicity, directly and indirectly from the drugs themselves, can cause severe complications. Tacrolimus (and indeed cyclosporine) can damage the kidney (nephrotoxic) and have also been reported to show toxicity to nervous tissues (neurotoxic). Most of the neurotoxicity reported tends to reflect damage to peripheral nerves (peripheral neuropathy) rather than to reflect CNS toxicity. Reactions are important side effects to consider.

FG, a 42-year-old patient with fulminant cardiac failure secondary to acute viral myocarditis, receives a heart (via UNOS) from a trauma victim. You are aware incidentally that the lungs, liver, and kidneys of the same donor have been used in other transplants around the globe.

The postoperative course for this patient is essentially unremarkable, and he is discharged home at 10 days after transplantation on a conventional immunosuppressive drug regimen. He returns through the emergency department 7 days later in acute respiratory distress, with oxygen saturation less than 85% and febrile. What are your thoughts, and what will you do?

QUESTIONS FOR GROUP DISCUSSION

1. Tissue rejection is of concern for any transplant patient. Explain this patient's workup to investigate whether his symptoms are caused by hyperacute/acute rejection.

2. Review the immunology of acute rejection and consider whether the kinetics suggest this is a likely cause of the clinical presentation. How is acute rejection generally treated? Would a biopsy help here? Discuss the rationale for the use of each of the following as therapy for acute rejection: (a) intravenous anti-CD3 antibodies and (b) anti-CD25 antibodies.

3. Early chronic rejection is a (less likely) possibility. How would the pathophysiology of chronic rejection help us understand a presentation of acute respiratory failure?

4. If a diagnosis of "rejection" is not supported by the results obtained, what other considerations come to mind in patients on potent immunosuppressive therapy?

5. Malignancies and drug toxicity are important considerations. Are these likely to account for the predominant symptoms seen at this time after transplantation? How might this patient develop such an early appearing malignancy (consider donor origin)?

6. Direct drug toxicity reactions are certainly a consideration. Often an idiosyncratic drug (hypersensitivity) reaction, independent of common drug toxicities, will lead to respiratory complications. Is this likely with a patient on high doses of corticosteroids?

7. You should consider (early) the likelihood of infectious complications. Discuss the type of infections to which this patient is susceptible and the potential source of these infections.

8. Transplant patients are at increased risk of death from severe acute respiratory syndrome (SARS) compared with the normal population. Explain. Also, why is SARS of particular concern for this particular patient?

RECOMMENDED APPROACH

Implications/Analysis of Family History

We are not provided with any family history for the patient.

Implications/Analysis of Clinical History

The myocarditis as the cause of his cardiac failure is a potential issue. Could this infection have recurred causing failure of the transplanted organ with resultant respiratory failure (secondary to cardiac failure)? History regarding possible CMV (cytomegalovirus/human herpes virus 5) status before the transplant is worth knowing, as is the patient's drug history (any risk factors for HIV [human immunodeficiency virus] or other unsuspected pathogens?).

Acute and Chronic Rejection

Acute rejection is certainly the most likely initial explanation readily correlated with symptoms and presentation. However a biopsy failed to find any evidence for this: there were no signs of lymphocyte infiltration into the organ, no biochemical markers of cardiac cell death (elevated cardiac enzymes), and no changes in the electrocardiogram.

Chronic rejection occurs with release of a variety of mediators, including fibroblast growth factor and endothelial growth factor, which can cause an insidious fibrosing/proliferative reaction relatively refractory to immunosuppressive treatment. This could affect the heart, causing secondary lung failure

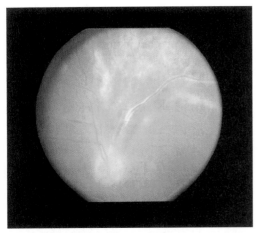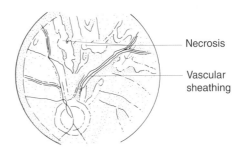

Necrosis

Vascular
sheathing

FIGURE 44-1   Vascular sheathing, edema, necrosis, and hemorrhage of the retina, characteristic of cytomegalovirus retinitis. (From Fireman P, Slavin R: Atlas of Allergies, 2nd ed. St. Louis, Mosby, 1996.)

(and the respiratory distress). However, the kinetic picture (<4 weeks after transplant) does not suggest this as a likely explanation.

Organ-Specific Damage

The most likely organ-specific damage to be seen in this patient (4 weeks after transplant) is the heart. However, all markers of cardiac biochemistry/function look normal. The organ affected is the lung (not transplanted). Moreover, this patient has a fever not yet explained.

While we treat symptoms (urgent provision of respiratory support; workup of infectious causes) it is time to "expand our net" to include other diagnoses.

Implications/Analysis of Laboratory Investigation

Routine blood work, physical examination, electrocardiogram, and serum levels of cardiac enzymes should be initiated at this time. As noted, a number of cardiac enzymes (e.g., troponin I, creatine phosphokinase, creatine kinase) are released when heart tissue is damaged. Measurement of cardiac muscle enzymes was normal, as was the electrocardiogram, ruling out killing (lysis) of heart cells as the cause of this patient's problem. You were unable to maintain this patient's oxygen saturation above 90% without providing artificial breathing support (intubation and ventilation). A chest radiograph shows "patchy" infiltrates throughout the lung fields.

Side Effects of Drug Therapy

Could this disorder represent one of a possible number of side effects of the treatment he received for the transplant? In general, we know that chronically immunosuppressed populations show an increased frequency of malignancy, drug toxicity, and infections (Fig. 44-1).

Malignancy is unlikely (too early post transplant), unless the tumor was "transferred" with the donor organ. Drug toxicity (particularly idiosyncratic hypersensitivity reactions to drugs) are a consideration. You should certainly be considering the risk of infection, both common (community acquired), opportunistic (e.g., *Pneumocystis carinii (jiroveci)*, CMV), and others that are more individual specific (e.g., transferred with the transplant).

Additional Laboratory Tests

Impaired tumor immunosurveillance, as a result of immunosuppression, would be unlikely to cause fulminant growth of an endogenous tumor so early but could result in rapid proliferation of one inadvertently transferred from the donor. A biopsy (lung) would be helpful. At this stage you might consider contacting UNOS to find out about the status of other recipients (from this donor) and more about the donor's history.

The chest radiograph was consistent with an infiltrate, but biopsy showed no signs of malignancy.

Drug toxicity (or idiosyncratic drug effects) remains a possible explanation of this patient's clinical presentation. Tacrolimus has been associated with fibrotic reactions, but this is very early for such an effect. Moreover, checking his file, you find he is not on tacrolimus as immunosuppressant!

There is no eosinophilia, which is often seen in the case of hypersensitivity reactions.

You request viral antibody titers (IgM and IgG) for herpes simplex virus (human herpesviruses 1 and 2), CMV, and influenza viruses (asking whether this might be a primary infection or recurrence). You should begin treatment with broad-spectrum antibiotics.

DIAGNOSIS

UNOS reports back that all of the recipients of this donor's organs are in intensive care units, with the exception of the lung recipient who died 2 days ago. All have a fever, with marked respiratory distress. There is no evidence of opportunistic malignant cell transfer in any case.

The donor was a businessman who had recently traveled to Southern China and Hong Kong on a sales mission. UNOS tells you that his wife was also recently admitted to the local hospital with respiratory distress and fever of unknown origin, although she seems to be recovering. Serologic tests from his wife have just become available, showing evidence for SARS coronavirus infection.

THERAPY

Transplant patients are at a highly increased risk of death from SARS compared with the normal population. Exact figures are still quite preliminary, but an estimate of a 10-fold increased mortality rate seems reasonable. Transplant patients have an enormous viral load compared with nontransplant patients ($>10^5$ more) and shed virus at high levels, putting care

workers at increased risk. Viral polymerase chain reaction (PCR) and serology can be used to confirm infection. Therapy is in its infancy. There is evidence that combination use of corticosteroids (anti-inflammatory) and interferon alpha (IFNα) can be an effective treatment, although use of other antiviral agents (e.g., ribavirin) has been ineffective to date.

ETIOLOGY: TRANSPLANTATION COMPLICATIONS

The transplant cohort is at increased risk of infection as a result of immunosuppression through endogenous reactivation, transfusion, community-acquired infection, and transplant-related infection (from organ), with a resulting marked elevation in mortality. Although we have become cognizant of the risk of Epstein-Barr virus infection (lymphoproliferative disease in transplant patients) and polyomavirus infection (especially in renal cohorts, since this virus is endogenous to the urinary tract) with resultant increased graft loss (and often distant disease, e.g., leukoencephalopathy in some patients), emerging infectious complications of equal importance are related to CMV, HIV, hepatitis C and B, West Nile virus, and SARS. All can also be transferred by transfusion, with marked decrease in risk by screening the blood pool (HIV and hepatitis C, <1 in 10^6; West Nile [pre 2003] 1 in 10^3; now with screened blood, 1 in 10^5), but it is important to note that even a screened blood pool does not detect the infection from a recent mosquito bite (hence we should ask blood donors about recent history). PCR (on a transplanted organ) is a sensitive assay for virus but again will not detect low copy numbers (from recent infection). If there is a risk, the organ should be declined.

FURTHER READING

Aldallal N: Inflammatory response in airway epithelial cells isolated from patients with cystic fibrosis. Am J Respir Crit Care Med 166:1248, 2002.

Araujo MB, et al: Development of donor specific microchimerism in liver transplant recipient with HLA-DRB1 and -DQB1 mismatch related to rejection episodes. Transplant Proc 36:953, 2004.

Arul A, Murday AJ, Jackson R: Natural killer-like T cell lymphoma, CD56+, following cardiac transplantation. J Heart Lung Transplant 23:783, 2004.

Blusch JH, et al: Infection of nonhuman primate cells by pig endogenous retrovirus. J Virol 74:7687, 2000.

Chalasani G, et al: The allograft defines the type of rejection (acute versus chronic) in the face of an established effector immune response. J Immunol 172:7813, 2004.

Chantranuwat C, et al: Sudden unexpected death in cardiac transplant recipients: An autopsy study. J Heart Lung Transplant 23:683, 2004.

Chen HL, et al: Pediatric fulminant hepatic failure in endemic areas of hepatitis B infection: 15 years after universal hepatitis B vaccination. Hepatology 39:58, 2004.

Cho JH: Advances in the genetics of inflammatory bowel disease. Curr Gastroenterol Rep 6:467, 2004.

Conese M, et al: Neutrophil recruitment and airway epithelial cell involvement in chronic cystic fibrosis lung disease. J Cyst Fibros 2:129, 2003.

Corvol H, et al: Distinct cytokine production by lung and blood neutrophils from children with cystic fibrosis. Am J Physiol Lung Cell Mol Physiol 284:L997, 2003.

D'Haens G, Hlavaty T: Advances in medical therapy for Crohn's disease. Curr Gastroenterol Rep 6:496, 2004.

De Hertogh G, Geboes K: Crohn's disease and infections: A complex relationship. MedGenMed 10:14, 2004.

Dransfield MT, Garver RI, Weill D: Standardized guidelines for surveillance bronchoscopy reduce complications in lung transplant recipients. J Heart Lung Transplant 23:110, 2004.

Fateh-Moghadam S: Cytomegalovirus infection status predicts progression of heart-transplant vasculopathy. Transplantation 76:1470, 2003.

Galili U: Interaction of the natural anti-Gal antibody with α-galactosyl epitopes: A major obstacle for xenotransplantation in humans. Immunol Today 14:480, 1993.

Gardner R, et al: Gamma/delta T-cell lymphoma as a recurrent complication after transplantation. Leuk Lymphoma 45:2355, 2004.

Grazia TJ, et al: A two-step model of acute CD4 T-cell mediated cardiac allograft rejection. J Immunol 172:7451.

Halloran PF: Immunosuppressive drugs for kidney transplantation. N Engl J Med 26:2715, 2004.

Helmi M, et al: *Aspergillus* infection in lung transplant recipients with cystic fibrosis: Risk factors and outcomes comparison to other types of transplant recipients. Chest 123:800-808, 2003.

Hoercher KJ, et al: Cardiac transplantation at the Cleveland Clinic. Clin Transpl 17:267, 2003.

Huo TI, et al: Long-term outcome of kidney transplantation in patients with hepatitis C virus infection. Hepatogastroenterology 48:169, 2001.

Kaufman DB, et al: Immunosuppression: Practice and trends. Am J Transpl 4:38, 2004.

Kaufman SS, et al: Discrimination between acute rejection and adenoviral enteritis in intestinal transplant recipients. Transplant Proc 34:943, 2002.

Lacouture ME, Hsieh FH: Skin rash in a transplant patient receiving multiple drugs. Cleve Clin J Med 70:1071, 2003.

Lin KW, Kirchner JT: Hepatitis B. Am Fam Physician 69:75, 2004.

Loinaz C, et al: Bacterial infections after intestine and multivisceral transplantation. Transplant Proc 35:1929, 2003.

Ludwiczek O, et al: Imbalance between interleukin-1 agonists and antagonists: Relationship to severity of inflammatory bowel disease. Clin Exp Immunol 138:323, 2004.

Magre S, et al: Reduced sensitivity to human serum inactivation of enveloped viruses produced by pig cells transgenic for human CD55 or deficient for galactosyl-α(1-3) galactosyl epitope. J Virol 78:5812, 2004.

Mahmond IM, et al: The impact of hepatitis C virus on renal graft and patient survival: A 9-year prospective study. Am J Kidney Dis 43:131, 2004.

Mazariegos GV, et al: Graft versus host disease in intestinal transplantation. Am J Transpl 4:1459, 2004.

Meloni F: Bronchoalveolar lavage cytokine profile in a cohort of lung transplant recipients: A predictive role of interleukin-12 with respect to onset of bronchiolitis obliterans syndrome. J Heart Lung Transplant 23:1053, 2004.

Neff GW, et al: Outcomes in liver transplant recipients with hepatitis B virus: Resistance and recurrence patterns from a large transplant center over the last decade. Liver Transplant 10:1372, 2004.

Nigen S, Knowles SR, Shear NH: Drug eruptions: Approaching the diagnosis of drug-induced skin diseases. J Drugs Dermatol 2:278, 2003.

Paul LC, et al: Antibodies and chronic organ graft rejection. Ann Transplant 2:46, 1997.

Piazza A, et al: Impact of donor-specific antibodies on chronic rejection occurrence and graft loss in renal transplantation: Post-transplant analysis using flow cytometric techniques. Transplantation 71:1106, 2001.

Quinn G, et al: Porcine endogenous retrovirus transmission characteristics of galactose α1-3 galactose deficient pig cells. J Virol 78:5805, 2004.

Rosen HR, et al: Cutting edge: Identification of hepatitis C virus–specific CD8+ T cells restricted by donor HLA alleles following liver transplantation. J Immunol 173:5355, 2004.

Schwartz KB, et al: Viral hepatitis. J Pediatr Gastroenterol Nutr 35:S29, 2002.

Schwartz KB: Pediatric issues in new therapies for hepatitis B and C. Curr Gastroenterol Rep 5:233, 2003.

Starzl TE, et al: Chimerism and tolerance in transplantation. Proc Natl Acad Sci U S A 101(Suppl 2):14607, 2004.

Starzl TE, Zinkernagel RM: Antigen localization and migration in immunity and tolerance. N Engl J Med 339:1905.

Thomas AR, et al: Hepatitis B vaccine coverage among the infants born to women without perinatal screening for hepatitis B virus infections: Effect of the joint statement of thimerosal in vaccines. Pediatr Infect Dis J 23:313, 2004.

Treem WR: Fulminant hepatic failure in children. J Pediatr Gastroenterol Nutr 35:S33, 2002.

Vanclaire J, Cornu Ch, Sokal EM: Fulminant hepatitis B in an infant born to a hepatitis Be antibody positive, DNA negative carrier. Arch Dis Child 66:983, 1991.

Verkman AS, Song Y, Thiagarajah JR: Role of airway surface liquid and submucosal glands in cystic fibrosis lung disease. Am J Physiol Lung Cell Mol Physiol 284:C2, 2003.

Weiner SM, et al: Impact of in vivo complement activation and cryoglobulins on graft. Clin Transpl 18:7, 2004.

Wy AU, et al: Graft versus-host disease after liver transplantation: Documentation by fluorescent in situ hybridization and human leucocyte antigen typing. Clin Transpl 14:174, 2000.

Zheng HX, et al: Interleukin 10 production genotype protects against acute persistent rejection after lung transplantation. J Heart Lung Transplant 23:541, 2004.

Zhong R, et al: Improvement in human decay accelerating factor transgenic porcine kidney xenograft rejection with intravenous administration of GAS914, a polymeric form of alpha GAL. Transplantation 75:10, 2003.

SECTION VI

Immunization

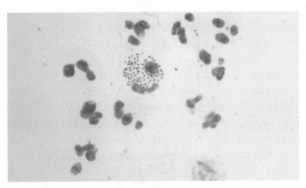

Immunization represents the *sine qua non* of modern immunology. Long before any rational cell/molecular-based understanding of the immune system was in place, human populations had been accidentally or deliberately immunizing themselves or others for protection against disease. The name Jenner springs to everyone's lips when we discuss vaccination against smallpox (from seminal observations that milk-maids exposed to [cross-reactive] cowpox failed to develop the lethal disease), and Pasteur when we consider rabies vaccination. But in North Africa it was known for some time that bites by the phlebotomine sand-fly often left disfiguring lesions in the affected area, without other long-term complications. Accordingly, mothers often sat their infants on sand-hills to be bitten by the fly, carrying the infectious leishmania organisms, in areas of their anatomy where only the "nearest and dearest" would ever see the lesion. How long this vaccination strategy has been practiced is difficult to evaluate.

What we have said above refers obviously to artificial active immunization processes. When mothers breast-feed their infants, Nature ensures that a passive immunization process affords the young mammal protection (whose immune system has not developed to a stage to provide full protection from pathogens in the environment) with a resistance mechanism adequate for immunity to the major significant pathogens present early in life. Some clinical problems can represent examples of pathology in passive immunization (*hydrops fetalis*). We discuss problems of a general interest, which are important to consider to understand the pathology associated with a failure to overcome chronic infection (e.g., complement defects—Case 46), and immunization prophylaxis of patients who represent at-risk populations for infectious disease (Case 45). The final cases we discuss place more emphasis on our growing interest in the need to consider vaccines to recognized viral pathogens (hepatitis—Case 47) and the so-called emerging infectious diseases, such as SARS, West Nile Virus, and so forth (Case 48).

Protection from infectious diseases is a momentous achievement and represents a major success story for clinical immunology. Emerging diseases, however, still present a challenge on this front, and much research is focused on bringing these diseases under control through unique approaches for immunization.

IMMUNIZATION

Immunization is a deliberate effort to protect individuals from disease. Immunization may be active or passive and natural or artificial. Active immunization is also referred to as vaccination. Unintentional immunization may occur when an individual is inadvertently exposed to an infectious agent.

The type of immunization that is administered will depend on the type of protection that is required for a particular pathogen. For example, for antibacterial immunity (extracellular bacteria), IgG and IgM antibodies are required to activate the classical pathway of complement; IgG can serve as an opsonin. For intracellular bacteria, cell-mediated immunity and cytokines are required. For optimal anti-viral immunity, cytotoxic T cells are required, although for some viruses high antibody titers may be protective.

Passive Immunization

In passive immunization the individual's immune response is not activated. Rather, protection requires the transfer of immune cells or molecules that have been generated by active immunization in another individual.

Natural Passive Immunization

Passive immunization may be natural as occurs during placental transfer of IgG antibodies or via transfer of IgA antibodies and leukocytes in breast milk. Whereas placental transfer of IgG antibodies provides antiviral and antibacterial protection, IgA and leukocytes are protective for enteric pathogens (e.g., *Escherichia coli*).

Artificial Passive Immunization

In general, artificial passive immunization refers to the administration of concentrated immunoglobulins (gamma globulins). Artificial passive immunization is administered to individuals who are unable to respond to active immunization or who need protection before active immunization will be effective.

HETEROLOGOUS, HOMOLOGOUS, AND HUMANIZED ANTIBODIES Artificial passive immunization may be homologous (human source) or heterologous (animal source). Heterologous antisera are only administered if antibodies from a human source are not available. Where commercially advantageous, heterologous antiserum has been replaced with humanized monoclonal antibodies. Humanized antibodies are genetically engineered so that the hypervariable regions are derived from an immunized animal but the remainder of the antibody is derived from a human antibody.

Gamma globulins may be isolated from pooled human plasma/serum of individuals who have recently recovered from disease or from volunteers who have been intentionally immunized. Alternatively, IgG antibodies of a particular specificity may be used for more specific intention. For example, RhoGAM consists of IgG antibodies that target the Rh antigen; VZIG is specific for the varicella-zoster virus immunoglobulin (chickenpox). Other immunoglobulin preparations are available that target hepatitis B virus or tetanus toxin. IgG antibodies are administered intravenously, whereas IgM antibodies are administered intramuscularly.

Active Immunization

In active immunization (intentional), individuals receive a modified antigen that may consist of attenuated or killed organisms, subcellular components, or detoxified toxins that trigger immunologic processes. (Active immunization is also referred to as vaccination.) The expectation in active immunization is that subsequent exposure to unmodified antigen will lead to rapid activation of the immune system and elimination of the pathogen before it can cause pathology. However, killed viruses (vaccine) may trigger different forms of immunity than live viruses. As well, protection afforded by killed vaccines is shorter lived than that from live viruses.

Different routes of administration are used, depending on the type of immunity that is desired (e.g., oral, intramuscular, subcutaneous). For example, the Sabin poliovirus (oral) is a live attenuated vaccine that generates IgA antibodies and provides mucosal immunity. In contrast, the Salk poliovirus (intramuscular) is a killed vaccine that provides protection after the virus has breached the mucosal barrier. In the United States, the Salk poliovirus vaccine is recommended for childhood immunization and the Sabin poliovirus vaccine is recommended only in regions where polio is endemic.

Antigens used in vaccines must be safe to administer, produce the appropriate immune response (e.g., cytotoxic T cells, antibodies) for the infectious agents, and be affordable for the target population. For vaccines that have a short incubation (2 to 4 days) it is important to maintain a high level of protective IgG, and this is achieved through repeated immunization.

Unintentional immunization may occur when an individual is inadvertently exposed to an infectious agent.

Age of Active Immunization

There are two major determinants in choosing the age of immunization; the first is that the child is protected for 3 to 6 months because maternal IgG antibodies cross the placenta. By this age, the IgG antibodies have decayed to about 50% of that present in adults. The second consideration is the age at which cell-mediated immunity is developed. As such, infants are at risk for a number of infectious agents that include *Mycobacterium tuberculosis*, human herpes simplex viruses, *Toxoplasma gondii*, and other pathogens that require cell-mediated responses. Consideration must be given to the effects of vaccination at too early an age. For example, does early immunization lead to tolerance rather than protection? Does the presence of maternal IgG block B cell activation?

Hazards of Active Immunization

Unfortunately, immunization is not without risk. This was certainly brought to focus during the swine flu epidemic in 1976 when there was a rush to vaccinate individuals who were at risk (infants and the elderly). Significant neurologic complications (e.g., Guillain-Barré syndrome) were seen in about 13.3%/million (vs. 2.6%/million), supposedly due to cross-reactive immunity induced against antigens present within the nervous system. Guillain-Barré syndrome is an autoimmune disorder characterized by loss of muscle control (see Case 28). Neurologic complications after immunization had been reported as early as the late 1950s.

Different types of vaccines present their own risks. For example, attenuated vaccines can cause disease in the immunocompromised or in individuals with immunologic deficiencies. As example, the bacillus Calmette-Guérin (BCG) vaccine, which is an attenuated form of *Mycobacterium bovis*, is recommended by the World Health Organization for protection against *Mycobacterium tuberculosis*. In children with defects in the interferon gamma receptor, or T cell–related dysfunction, this vaccine can result in disseminated infection. Attenuated vaccines can also pose a problem if they revert back to wild type or if they mutate to virulence, as has been documented for the Sabin poliovirus vaccine.

Other complications and hazards are associated more with the preparation of the vaccine or components, other than the organism. These can lead to local hypersensitivity reactions (e.g., diphtheria toxoid, tetanus toxoid) or more serious reactions if the patient is allergic to eggs (viruses grown in chick embryos) or preservatives in vaccines (e.g., neomycin).

Adjuvants in Vaccines

Adjuvants are substances that enhance the efficacy of the vaccine, and hence immunity, by prolonging antigen survival, stimulating antigen-presenting cell expression of co-stimulatory molecules, or secreting molecules that enhance the response. The most commonly used adjuvant in human vaccines is aluminum hydroxide. A relatively new development in adjuvants is MF59, which consists of a submicron oil-in-water emulsion (5% v/v squalene, 0.5% v/v Span 85, and 0.5% v/v Tween 80). For experimental use Freund's complete adjuvant (aqueous solution of antigen emulsified in mineral oil containing heat-killed mycobacterial organisms) is widely used and considered to be most effective.

New Approaches to Vaccines

In recent years several new strategies have been designed and tested to overcome some of the major limitations of particular vaccines.

Conjugate Vaccines

For example, conjugate vaccines (polysaccharide linked to protein) have been constructed to increase the efficacy of the polysaccharide vaccine. Polysaccharide vaccines are T cell–independent antigens, and as such the antibodies generated are primarily of the IgM isotype. In addition, memory B cells are not generated and so the vaccine is only effective for a limited period. When polysaccharides are linked to proteins, the immune response becomes one in which α/β T cells are recruited, which leads to isotype switching and memory cell formation. One of the first effective conjugate vaccines developed was the *Haemophilus influenzae* B conjugate vaccine, in which *Haemophilus* capsular polysaccharides are linked to a carrier protein (e.g., tetanus toxoid, diphtheria toxoid, meningococcal outer membrane protein). More recently, a conjugate vaccine has been developed as protection against *Streptococcus pneumoniae*.

Recombinant Vaccines

Recombinant vaccines are proteins that have been generated in the laboratory using recombinant DNA technology. One of the first recombinant vaccines developed was the hepatitis B vaccine. The advantage of these recombinant vaccines is that there is no risk of infection and so these can be given without negative side effects to the elderly and the immunocompromised, as well as to the general population. Additionally, these vaccines obviate the concern for contaminating infections, when the virus is isolated from human donors.

DNA Vaccines

DNA vaccines represent one of the most recent developments in vaccine technology. These vaccines are intended for immunization against pathogens that are too virulent for administration as attenuated or killed vaccines and for which recombinant proteins are ineffective in generating protection. One of the reasons that DNA vaccines are particularly attractive is that they can be used to generate CD8+ T cells, something which cannot be done with recombinant protein vaccines (e.g., hepatitis B vaccine).

"VACCINES" AS THERAPEUTIC AGENTS

Vaccines that are used as therapeutic agents are, in fact (but not always), antibodies that are specific for a particular receptor or molecule on a cell surface and so can be used to target that cell.

Anti-Idiotypic Antibodies

Anti-idiotypic antibodies are therapeutic vaccines and not intended for protection against a particular pathogen. These anti-idiotypic vaccines, as the name implies, are specific for idiotopes present in the variable region of antibodies. The target of anti-idiotypic antibody therapy is the B cell tumor (e.g., B cell chronic lymphocytic leukemia [CLL]) because the tumor cells express membrane immunoglobulin of a particular specificity, which is defined by the variable region. As such, antibodies that are specific for the variable region and to which a radioactive molecule or a toxin has been attached, can be generated. These can then be used as therapeutic interventions to destroy the tumor.

Antibodies to Target Receptors or Soluble Molecules

Anti-receptor antibodies can be used as therapeutic agents to block the interaction of a ligand or a virus with molecules for which they have a trophism. As example, anti-CD4 and/or anti-chemokine receptor (CXCR5) antibodies have been considered as potentially useful agents to block binding of HIV (gp120) to CD4/CXCR5, respectively, and hence block viral entry into the cell. In other examples, anti-CD3, anti-CD4, or anti-IL-2 receptor antibodies are used to target and destroy T cells in diseases where pathology is the result of T cell activation.

Antibodies are increasingly being used as therapeutic agents in clinical scenarios. As example, antibodies that "mop up" tumor necrosis factor (TNF), a cytokine that plays a key role in inflammation, are currently being used to treat a number of autoimmune disorders in which inflammation is a key factor.

Mary, a 3-year-old girl, had her spleen removed after a motor vehicle accident, in which both parents died. When she was transferred to the emergency department of a nearby hospital, it became apparent that her spleen had ruptured and the surgeon had no option but to remove it. Mary recovered well from the surgery, but her next of kin, who knows that the spleen is important in immune responses, wants to know how removal of the spleen will affect her immunologically, and so you arrange for a consultation with an immunologist.

C A S E

45

QUESTIONS FOR GROUP DISCUSSION

1. Mary has just received a splenectomy. What is the immunologic role of the spleen? To what types of infections will Mary be particularly susceptible?

2. Explain how a simple act such as brushing or flossing teeth could pose a problem for Mary now that her spleen has been removed.

3. Review the current recommended immunization schedule for the United States in 2005. See Figure 45-1.

4. Mary's record showed that she had received most of the vaccines that were recommended. The immunologist recommended immunization with the polysaccharide pneumococcal vaccine (Pneumovax 23). Explain why.

5. What would you recommend as daily prophylaxis for this patient? Explain why. Discuss circumstances under which you would increase this drug regimen.

6. Asplenia in this patient was the result of surgery; however, asplenia can also be a congenital defect. Congenital asplenia has an autosomal recessive mode of inheritance. Explain this form of inheritance. Under what circumstances would offspring be at increased risk for autosomal recessive disorders.

7. Describe how severe pneumococcal pneumonia would present clinically.

8. What would you expect a complete blood cell count to reveal in patients with severe pneumococcal pneumonia? What would you expect a chest radiograph to indicate?

9. Respiratory infections can be lethal in the elderly and in splenic individuals. As such, an influenza vaccine would be recommended for Mary. What are the limitations of these vaccines?

10. Discuss risks of immunization with the polysaccharide vaccine Pneumovax.

RECOMMENDED APPROACH

Implications/Analysis of Family History

Family history is insignificant here because the asplenia was surgery related. In cases of congenital asplenia family history is significant because this disorder has an autosomal recessive mode of inheritance. The parents of these offspring can be normal, with each carrying this recessive gene. The presentation of the gene is more common in offspring of consanguineous marriages, a setting in which autosomal recessive disease is encountered more frequently than in outbred people. Chance alone predicts that most likely one in four offspring can be affected in such a family (both parents carriers), because in each pregnancy there is a one in four chance of the fetus inheriting the abnormal gene from both parents. The actual genetic defect causing asplenia in this case has not yet been identified.

Implications/Analysis of Clinical History

Mary's growth and development have been normal. She suffered a middle ear infection (otitis media) at age 24 months, but otherwise she has had no other illnesses except for a common cold each winter. Having determined that Mary was a healthy child, your next consideration is her immunization record.

Childhood immunization is important, particularly if we are to maintain what is referred to as herd immunity (protection from spread of disease within a group because most members are immunized). However, in asplenic patients, immunization is recommended for their own protection. Mary's medical files indicated that she had received most of the recommended pediatric vaccines and boosters. These included vaccines for DTaP (diphtheria, tetanus toxoids, and acellular

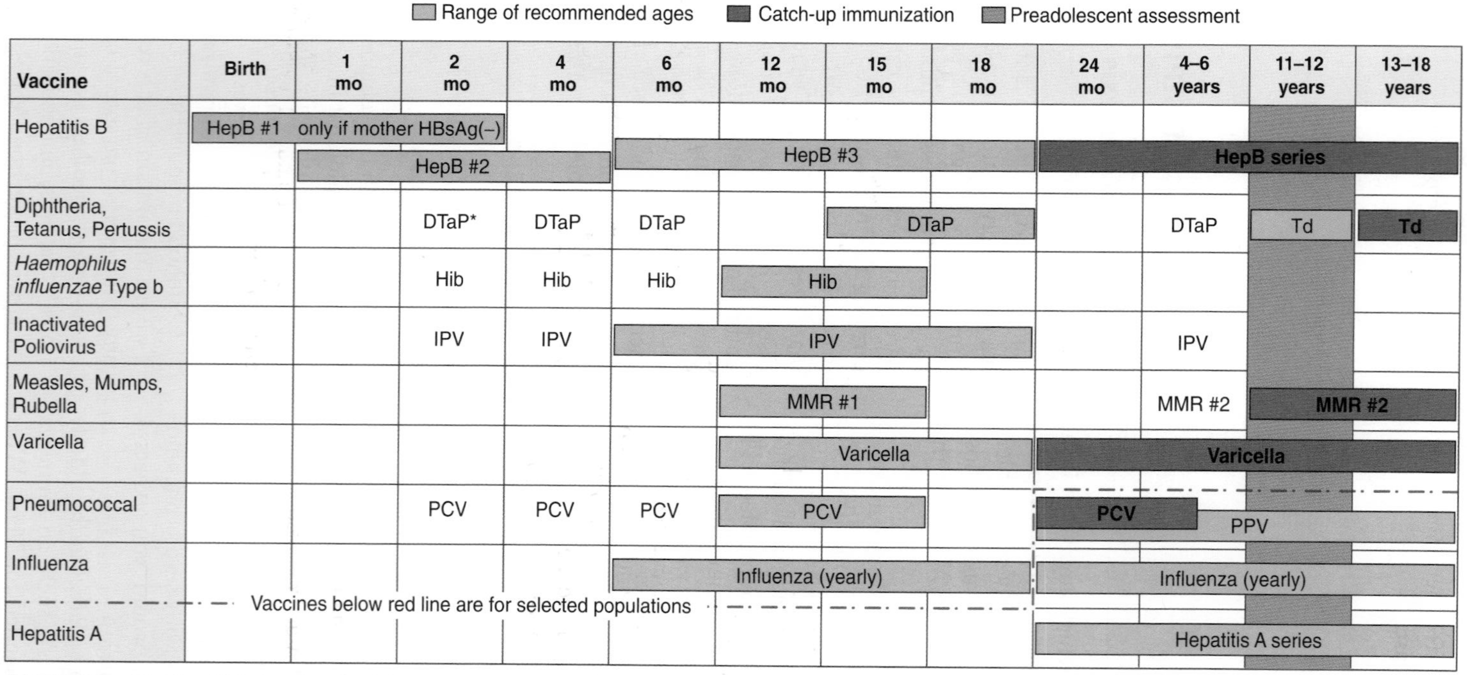

Legend: ▪ Range of recommended ages   ▪ Catch-up immunization   ▪ Preadolescent assessment

Vaccine	Birth	1 mo	2 mo	4 mo	6 mo	12 mo	15 mo	18 mo	24 mo	4–6 years	11–12 years	13–18 years
Hepatitis B	HepB #1 only if mother HBsAg(−)	HepB #2			HepB #3						HepB series	
Diphtheria, Tetanus, Pertussis			DTaP*	DTaP	DTaP		DTaP	DTaP		DTaP	Td	Td
Haemophilus influenzae Type b			Hib	Hib	Hib	Hib						
Inactivated Poliovirus			IPV	IPV	IPV		IPV	IPV		IPV		
Measles, Mumps, Rubella						MMR #1				MMR #2	MMR #2	
Varicella						Varicella	Varicella	Varicella			Varicella	
Pneumococcal			PCV	PCV	PCV	PCV	PCV		PCV		PPV	
Influenza						Influenza (yearly)				Influenza (yearly)		
Hepatitis A										Hepatitis A series	Hepatitis A series	

Vaccines below red line are for selected populations

Preadolescent assessment

FIGURE 45–1 Childhood and adolescent immunization schedule, by vaccine and age, recommended by CDC's Advisory Committee on Immunization Practices (ACIP), June 2004. (*Abbreviations:* HepB, hepatitis B; DTaP, diphtheria, tetanus toxoids, and acellular pertussis; Hib, *Haemophilus influenzae* type b conjugate; IPV, inactivated polio; MMR, measles, mumps, and rubella; PCV, pneumococcal conjugate; Td, tetanus and diphtheria toxoids. *DTaP (diphtheria, tetanus toxoids, and acellular pertussis) has replaced DTP/DPT (diphtheria, tetanus toxoids, and whole cell pertussis) vaccine. Products containing whole cell pertussis vaccines have been discontinued. (Modified from Centers of Disease Control and Prevention. Recommended Childhood and adolescent, immunization schedule—United States, 2005. MMWR 53(51–52): Q1–Q3, 2005.)

pertussis), MMR (measles, mumps, rubella), hepatitis, and the inactivated poliovirus (IPV).

Of significance is the fact that Mary had already received the Hib vaccine (a conjugated capsular polysaccharide vaccine for *Haemophilus influenzae* type b), as well as the pneumococcal conjugate vaccine (PCV) for *Streptococcus pneumoniae* (PCV7/Prevnar). *Haemophilus influenzae* (type b) and *Streptococcus pneumoniae* are encapsulated bacterial pathogens that can enter the bloodstream where, in a normal patient, they would be eliminated in the spleen by innate and adaptive immune responses. In the absence of a spleen, patients who become infected with these encapsulated bacteria are at risk for fulminant pneumococcal sepsis, which is associated with high mortality.

Implications/Analysis of Laboratory Investigation

Given the fact that Mary is now without a spleen, antibody titers to various pediatric vaccines were requested to ensure that Mary was sufficiently protected. Although laboratory results indicated normal antibody titers, and even though Mary has been immunized with the pneumococcal conjugate vaccine Prevnar, there is concern that Mary is at risk for pneumococcal disease caused by pneumococcal serotypes not included in the this vaccine. The Prevnar pneumococcal conjugate vaccine (PCV7) contains only seven purified capsular polysaccharides of *S. pneumoniae* serotypes. These serotypes have been selected because they cause the majority of pneumococcal disease in children. Consequently, the Pneumovax 23 polysaccharide vaccine, which consists of 23 pneumococcal capsular types, was administered.

Additional Laboratory Tests

No further laboratory testing was required at this time.

DIAGNOSIS

Mary had surgery-induced asplenia, resulting in a need for additional immunization and prophylactic antibiotics.

THERAPY

For broader protection, Mary was administered the Pneumovax 23 vaccine. Mary's guardian should be notified that there is a low risk of encephalomyelitis with the vaccine.

Antibiotics were prescribed to be taken at a low dose daily but at higher doses when Mary has any dental work done or undergoes any invasive surgical procedure. As well, "flu shots" should be recommended in that respiratory virus infection can be lethal in both the elderly and in asplenic individuals. However, the vaccine is generally made to previous year's agents and does not convey total resistance to current serotypes! Mary will still get a subclinical infection, but less severe than natural disease.

ETIOLOGY: STREPTOCOCCAL INFECTIONS AND IMMUNIZATION

Streptococcus pneumoniae, more commonly referred to as "pneumococcus," is the causative agent of pneumonia, acute otitis media, meningitis, and sinusitis, particularly in young children. This infection is spread via respiratory droplets during sneezing/coughing or directly from person to person contact. As such it may be inhaled into the lungs and spread to the blood. Bacteria enter the bloodstream all the time, including when we brush our teeth or when we have a local infection, for example of the middle ear. Normally these bacteria are disposed of efficiently by the spleen. When the spleen is not present, serious or even fatal infections occur.

Clinical Presentation

A typical presentation of severe pneumococcal pneumonia would include unrelenting fever, elevated white blood cell count, and a "left shift," indicating the presence of predominantly neutrophils, recruited to defend the body against bacterial infection. A chest radiograph would generally show infiltrates suggestive of consolidation.

Pneumococcal Polysaccharide Vaccines

The major components of the pneumococcal capsules are T cell–independent antigens. As the term implies, these antigens can activate B cells in the absence of cognate interaction with T cells. The predominant antibody isotype produced in response to T cell–independent antigens is IgM. As such the response is not long lasting and memory B cells are not generated. Therefore, protection is not long lasting. The Pneumovax 23 vaccine is a mixture of purified capsular polysaccharides from the 23 most prevalent *S. pneumoniae* serotypes causing infection in North America. Included in the vaccine are the seven serotypes in the Prevnar vaccine (see later). Protective antibodies are usually detectable 3 to 4 weeks after immunization. This vaccine is recommended for the elderly, the immunocompromised, and children older than the age of 2 who are congenitally asplenic or have had a splenectomy.

Responses to this vaccine have all the limitations of antibody responses to T cell–independent antigens. Furthermore, children younger than 2 years of age respond poorly to T cell–independent antigens because their immune system is immature. To overcome this limitation, a pneumococcal conjugate vaccine (Prevnar) was developed.

Pneumococcal Conjugate Vaccine

Conjugate vaccines are generally polysaccharide vaccines to which a potent T cell–dependent antigen is linked. The *S. pneumoniae* conjugate vaccine (Prevnar) consists of seven purified capsular polysaccharides each coupled to a carrier protein (nontoxic variant of diphtheria toxin). This conjugate vaccine triggers a T cell–dependent response that leads to the generation of IgG antibodies and memory B cells. As such, booster responses lead to enhanced antibody titers. Antibodies generated can serve as opsonins and facilitate the phagocytosis of *S. pneumoniae*.

Anne is 20 months of age and has been hospitalized with a fever, irritability, and moderate dehydration. Blood work suggests a bacterial infection, with elevated neutrophils (see Appendix for reference value), although chest radiograph and urinalysis are normal. A lumbar puncture taken yesterday showed an elevated white blood cell count, and preliminary culture results today suggest growth of *Neisseria meningitidis*. She has been receiving intravenous antibiotics for 30 hours, and there is some improvement in her condition. Physical examination indicated that Anne was below the 50th percentile for weight, had recurrent diarrhea, and had seborrheic dermatitis, more commonly referred to as "cradle cap." Detailed question of Anne's clinical history revealed that she had had recurrent infections, but none had ever been this bad. Detailed family history reveals that a distant male cousin and an aunt both died at an early age (<2 years) of meningitis. What further tests might you order? What is the significance of the history and findings?

C A S E
46

QUESTIONS FOR GROUP DISCUSSION

1. Bacterial infections characterize defects in B cells, complement, or phagocytes. Explain why a major B cell defect (e.g., agammaglobulinemia) is unlikely in this case. Discuss how you would test for defects in phagocytes. To test for complement defects you would measure overall complement activity using the CH50 test. Assuming that the results of this test show a complement defect, how would you proceed? What single test would allow you to determine if the defect is in the terminal pathway or the classical pathway?

2. Because preliminary culture results suggested growth of *Neisseria meningitidis*, Anne was diagnosed with systemic inflammatory response syndrome (SIRS), formerly referred to simply as "sepsis" during infection. Review the processes that are activated during inflammation (see Case 23), with emphasis on the role of interleukin (IL)-1 and tumor necrosis factor (TNF). Note that the current dogma states that SIRS leads to the excessive release of cytokines that produce fever, shock, and often death.

3. Infections with Gram-negative bacteria lead to their lysis, release of lipopolysaccharide (LPS/endotoxin) from the cell wall outer membrane, and subsequent secretion of TNF by monocytes and macrophages. Describe how these events are connected. Include in your discussion each of the following terms: lipopolysaccharide binding protein (LBP), soluble CD14, MD-2, and TLR-4. How would you explain the fact that in animal models of endotoxin-induced peritonitis and in human SIRS trials blocking both TNF and TNF antagonists increased mortality?

4. With respect to question 4, how would you explain the following: (a) in humans, mortality associated with meningococcemia correlates with high TNF levels; (b) in SIRS patients (infected with Gram-negative bacteria), antagonists of IL-1 receptor, TNF, and endotoxin do not improve outcome; and (c) mice that have mutations in the TLR-4 gene have increased mortality to SIRS induced by infection with Gram-negative bacteria.

5. Review the differentiation of Thp cells to Th1 or Th2 cells secreting type 1 and type 2 cytokines, respectively. List these cytokines. What factors influence the polarization of a response to either a Th1 or a Th2 cell? An increased level of IL-10 in SIRS patients is a predictor of mortality. What is the role of IL-10 in the regulation of Thp cell activation? What is the consequence of increased IL-10 on the production of type 1 cytokines by Th1 cells?

6. Antigen presentation by macrophages after phagocytosis of necrotic cells polarizes the Thp differentiation to that of a Th1 phenotype, whereas phagocytosis of apoptosed cells polarizes the response to that of a Th2 phenotype. Patients who died of SIRS have evidence for apoptosis-induced loss of immune cells. What cytokines would you expect to be increased in these patients? What effect would this have on the production of type 1 cytokines? Based on this information, why would apoptosis-induced death of immune cells be a predictor of mortality?

7. Explain why neutrophils are regarded as "double-edged swords" in SIRS. What is the rationale for the administration of the cytokine granulocyte colony-stimulating factor (G-CSF)? Explain the role of activated protein C in the extrinsic coagulation system. How do you reconcile the use of

recombinant protein C with studies in which G-CSF increased survival rates in patients with SIRS? How would you rationalize the use of this therapeutic agent with studies that showed that antigen presentation by macrophages that have ingested apoptosed cells leads to the induction of Th2 cells secreting type II cytokines (e.g., interleukin [IL]-10) and the fact that increased IL-10 is an independent predictor of mortality?

8. Intensive insulin therapy has been shown to result in lower morbidity and mortality in patients with SIRS. Although the mechanism of action is unknown, insulin prevents apoptotic death of cells. What effect would this have on IL-10 levels? Discuss the studies that could be used to rationalize the use of insulin therapy.

9. Newer therapies for SIRS that are under consideration include interferon gamma (IFNγ), IL-12, and C5a. Provide a rationale for each of these as potential therapeutic agents.

10. *Ischemic preconditioning* is a term used to describe a phenomenon in which a transient episode of myocardial ischemia subsequently protects the individual from severe myocardial ischemia. Extrapolate this concept to SIRS patients who survive SIRS sepsis.

RECOMMENDED APPROACH

Implications/Analysis of Family History

Detailed family history revealed that a distant male cousin and an aunt both died at an early age (<2 years) of meningitis. The fact that this disease susceptibility is so rare in the family suggests that we should be considering disorders with an autosomal recessive mode of inheritance.

Implications/Analysis of Clinical History

Anne's immediate problem is the *Neisseria meningitidis* infection, which is the cause of the overwhelming sepsis, now referred to as systemic inflammatory response syndrome (SIRS). Although deficiencies in B cells, phagocytes, and complement are considerations in patients with severe bacterial infections, the fact that this is a *Neisseria* infection suggests that we should be focusing our attention on possible deficiencies in the terminal pathway of complement. Patients with deficiencies in the proteins that compose the mem-

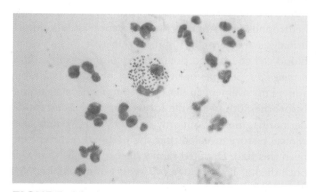

FIGURE 46–1 *Neisseria gonorrhoeae.* Gram stain of urethral pus from a patient with gonorrhea. Note that the diplococci occur mostly intracellularly. (×1000.) (From Hart CA, Shears P: Color Atlas of Medical Microbiology, 2nd ed. St. Louis, Mosby, 2004.)

brane attack complex are particularly susceptible to infections with *Neisseria* species (Fig. 46–1).

Note, however, that in addition to Anne's immediate problem of SIRS, she has a triad of symptoms—recurrent diarrhea, seborrheic dermatitis (which often manifests as cradle cap), and failure to thrive. Therefore, we should be attempting to determine if there is a defect that will account for both SIRS and the symptoms described.

Implications/Analysis of Laboratory Investigation

Results of blood work and culture were consistent with a strong inflammatory response to systemic infection with *Neisseria meningitidis*. Although the immediate problem facing Anne and her physician is SIRS, it is important to find the underlying problem for the uncontrolled spread of this infection. The most widely used test to screen for deficiencies in the classical or terminal pathway is the CH50 test. Low levels of CH50 indicate that there is a deficiency in either the classical or the terminal pathway. If the defect is in the terminal pathway, an AH50 test will indicate a deficiency as well.

In Anne's case both the AH50 and CH50 were low, indicating that the defect was in one of the proteins that make up the terminal pathway. Further laboratory tests would be required to identify the particular component that is defective. (*Note:* the AH50 test is only available in specialized laboratories.)

Additional Laboratory Tests

Although one could request a measure of each of the terminal pathway components, Anne's clinical history and results of the physical examination suggest that she may have a deficiency in C5. Patients with deficiencies in C5 present with Leiner's disease, which is characterized by recurrent diarrhea, seborrheic dermatitis (which often manifests as cradle cap), and failure to thrive. Anne's serum sample was sent to a specialized laboratory to test for a defect in C5. (C5 is only measured in specialized laboratories.)

DIAGNOSIS

Anne was diagnosed with a deficiency of C5, also referred to as Leiner's disease. A deficiency in C5 is a risk factor for infections with *Neisseria* species and SIRS. *Neisseria meningitidis*, a Gram-negative bacterium, is surrounded by a polysaccharide capsule whose composition defines the serogroup of the pathogen. This capsule prevents phagocytosis of this pathogen in the absence of opsonins. Five serogroups (A, B, C, Y, and W-135) cause most of the infections in North America. (*Note*: C5b, which is a proteolytic fragment of C5, is a component of the membrane attack complex.)

THERAPY

Anne was treated with antibiotics, along with symptomatic therapy as required. Additionally, Anne should be immunized, recognizing that immunization will only provide protection if the vaccine contains the same polysaccharide capsule serotype as that of the infecting pathogen.

Immunization: Polysaccharide versus Conjugate Vaccines

There are two types of meningococcal vaccines available: a polysaccharide vaccine and a conjugate vaccine. The polysaccharide vaccine (e.g., Menomune, Mencevax) consists of purified meningococcal polysaccharide from serogroups A, C, Y, and W135 but is only effective when administered to individuals over 2 years of age. Protection is relatively short term: 2 to 3 years. In contrast, the conjugate vaccine (e.g., Neis Vac-C, Menjugate) is effective even when administered to children 6 weeks of age, but it consists solely of meningococcal polysaccharide serotype C capsule chemically linked to tetanus toxoid.

Limitations of Meningococcal Vaccines

There is no effective vaccine for protection against serogroup B polysaccharide capsule, which is weakly immunogenic. Unfortunately, serotype B is the most common cause of meningococcal disease in young children and there is no cross-reacting protection from vaccines for other polysaccharide capsule serotypes.

ETIOLOGY: SIRS

Sepsis represents a leading cause of death/disability in the United States, affecting nearly a million people annually, with approximately one fourth of that number dying. Sepsis itself represents an uncontrolled inflammatory response, as witnessed in the Lewis Thomas notion that "the microorganisms that seem to have it in for us . . . turn out . . . to be rather more like bystanders. . . . It is our response to their presence that makes the disease. Our arsenals for fighting off bacteria are so powerful . . . that we are more in danger from them than the invaders." Accordingly, sepsis itself is now often referred to instead as SIRS, the systemic inflammatory response syndrome, which occurs during infection, particularly with Gram-negative bacteria. In essence, the immune system goes into overdrive, releasing a flood of cytokines that produce fever, shock, and often death.

Inflammation

Inflammation occurring in response to trauma or infection is complex, involves a number of cells, adhesion molecules, cytokines, chemokines, complement proteins, and coagulation proteins. Many of the processes occurring in inflammation are triggered following the release of tumor necrosis factor (TNF) and IL-1 from activated macrophages. Infections with Gram-negative bacteria lead to the activation of immunologic processes that lead to lysis of bacteria and release of lipopolysaccharide (LPS/endotoxin) from the cell wall outer membrane and subsequent release of TNF from activated macrophages. Release of TNF from activated macrophages occurs after binding of endotoxin-MD-2 complex with toll-like receptor-4 (TLR-4). Complex formation and signaling via TLR-4 occurs only if endotoxin undergoes interactions with, and transfer from, LPS-binding protein (LBP) and soluble CD14. Whether these sequential bindings and transfer modify endotoxin so that it is able to form a complex with MD-2 and TLR-4 is unknown. Signaling via TLR-4, however, activates biochemical pathways that lead to the synthesis and secretion of TNF. Therefore, it is not surprising that TLR-4 mutations in humans make individuals more susceptible to Gram-negative infection. (See Case 7)

Role of Inflammation in SIRS

An awareness of the role of TNF and IL-1 in inflammation has spawned a variety of trials destined to attempt to control the disorder, all including the use of agents that should block the inflammatory cascade, including, but not limited to, corticosteroids, anti-endotoxin antibodies, TNF antagonists, and IL-1 receptor blockage. In general, however, the results of such trials of anti-inflammatory mediators have been poor, leading clinicians to question whether death in patients with sepsis results from uncontrolled inflammation. However, exhaustive meta-analysis of clinical trials using anti-inflammatory agents in SIRS patients has shown that although high doses of anti-inflammatory agents can be harmful in such patients, there is at least a subgroup of patients (~10%) showing a clear benefit. It must be noted, however, that clinical trials of treatments for sepsis are difficult to interpret for many reasons, not the least of which is the heterogeneity of patients and the high rates of culture-negative sepsis.

Evidence Supporting a Role for TNF in SIRS

The theory that sepsis caused death after an uncontrolled stimulation of the immune system came essentially from animal studies, often using high doses of endotoxin or bacteria that induced levels of circulating cytokines (e.g., TNF) far higher in animals than those seen in patients with SIRS. And, in at least one sepsis syndrome in humans—meningococcemia—circulating TNF levels are high and do indeed correlate with mortality.

Evidence Challenging a Role for TNF in SIRS

There is confounding evidence now that cytokines can have beneficial effects in sepsis: (1) in animal models of peritonitis, blocking TNF worsened survival; (2) in a recent clinical trial, a TNF antagonist increased mortality; (3) a strain of mice, C3H/HEJ, is resistant to endotoxin because of a mutation in their TLR-4 gene, but, interestingly, despite their resistance to endotoxin, these mice have increased mortality from SIRS; and (4) recent evidence suggests that TLR-4 mutations in humans may similarly make individuals more susceptible to infection.

Differentiation of Thp to Th1 or Th2 Cells

CD4+ Thp cell differentiation is initiated when these cells interact with antigen-presenting cells that display major histocompatibility complex (MHC) class II antigen peptide and appropriate co-stimulatory molecules on their surface. Thp cells differentiate to either Th1 cells secreting type 1 cytokines or Th2 cells secreting type 2 cytokines. The factors controlling which type of Th cell is activated are complex, but the polarization in T cell cytokine synthesis is known to be influenced by (1) the type of pathogen, (2) the size of the bacterial inoculum, (3) the site of infection, and (4) the type of macrophage stimulation (see later). Type 1 cytokines, which include TNF, interferon gamma (IFNγ), and IL-2, have inflammatory properties; type 2 cytokines (e.g., IL-4 and IL-10) have anti-inflammatory properties.

Type of Macrophage Stimulation in Polarization to Th1 or Th2 cells

Macrophages, antigen-presenting cells, that ingest necrotic tissue release IL-12, a cytokine that promotes differentiation of Thp cells to Th1 cells. Th1 cells secrete type 1 cytokines, which are proinflammatory. In contrast, ingestion of apoptosed cells leads to the induction of Th2 cells secreting type 2 cytokines, which are anti-inflammatory cytokines. (Apoptosis is genetically programmed cell death in which the cells "commit suicide" after the activation of various proteases.)

Regulation of Type 1 and Type 2 Cytokines

Type 1 and type 2 cytokines reciprocally regulate cytokine secretion. Therefore, high levels of IL-10 would lead to a decrease in type 1 cytokine production (i.e., inflammatory cytokines), supporting studies in which anti-inflammatory agents did not rescue patients with SIRS. Further support for a positive role for proinflammatory cytokines comes from studies in which mononuclear cells from patients with sepsis (secondary to burns or trauma) have reduced type 1 and increased type 2 levels of cytokines and reversal of the dominant cytokine profile using IL-12 reduced mortality. IL-12 activates natural killer cells to secrete IFNγ, which promotes differentiation of Thp to Th1 cells secreting type 1 cytokines that downregulate IL-10 production.

Role of IL-10, a Type 2 Cytokine, in SIRS

Studies have shown that a high level of IL-10 in patients with SIRS is an independent predictor of mortality. Interestingly, autopsy studies in persons who died of SIRS sepsis showed evidence for apoptosis-induced loss of immune cells (B cells, CD4 cells, and follicular dendritic cells). Differentiation of Thp cells to Th2 cells predominates in responses in which macrophages that have ingested apoptosed cells are serving as antigen-presenting cells. Because Th2 cells secrete IL-10, this would be consistent with studies that showed that IL-10 was an independent predictor of mortality. Once again, studies in animals showed that prevention of lymphocyte apoptosis improved the likelihood of survival from SIRS. It is important to keep in mind, however, that decreases in cells that undergo apoptosis are likely to impair antibody production, macrophage activation, and antigen presentation.

Role of Neutrophils in SIRS

Neutrophils have been regarded as potential double-edged swords in SIRS, important both for the eradication of pathogens and for excessive release of neutrophil oxidants and proteases responsible for organ injury. Because of the intrapulmonary sequestration of neutrophils and the frequent complication of the acute respiratory distress syndrome (ARDS) in SIRS patients with sepsis, this link between neutrophil activation and organ injury was thought especially to affect the lungs. However, studies using G-CSF to increase the number of neutrophils and enhance their function showed improved survival among SIRS patients!

New Approaches to Therapy

Recombinant Human Activated Protein C

Activated protein C has a normal regulatory role in coagulation in that it inactivates factors Va and VIIIa, preventing the generation of thrombin, and thus decreasing inflammation by inhibiting platelet activa-

tion, neutrophil recruitment, and mast cell degranulation. Activated protein C also has direct anti-inflammatory properties, including blocking of the production of cytokines by monocytes and blocking cell adhesion, and in addition it has anti-apoptotic actions that may contribute to its efficacy.

Recombinant human activated protein C, an anticoagulant, is the first anti-inflammatory agent that has proved effective in the treatment of sepsis, showing, in a recent clinical trial, a 20% reduction in the relative risk of death and an absolute risk reduction of about 6%. Note that a major risk associated with activated protein C is hemorrhage (intracranial hemorrhage, a life-threatening bleeding episode, or a requirement for 3 or more units of blood), and thus at present activated protein C is approved only for use in patients with SIRS who have the most severe organ compromise and the highest likelihood of death.

Insulin Therapy

Intensive insulin therapy (blood glucose level of 5 to 6 mmol/L) was also reported to result in lower morbidity and mortality among critically ill patients than conventional therapy (maintaining blood glucose levels at 10 to 11 mmol/L) and was noted to decrease the risk of death in patients with multiorgan failure, regardless of whether they had a history of diabetes. The mechanism of action of insulin in SIRS is unknown, although the phagocytic function of neutrophils is impaired in patients with hyperglycemia and insulin prevents apoptotic cell death from numerous stimuli by activating distinct biochemical pathways (the phosphatidylinositol 3-kinase/Akt pathway). As noted earlier, ingestion of apoptosed cells by antigen-presenting cells leads to the differentiation of Thp cells to Th2 cells that secrete IL-10, as well as other anti-inflammatory cytokines.

Immunotherapy Regimens

A number of other immunologic therapies are under consideration. IFNγ is a potent macrophage activator and has been reported to improve survival in a subgroup of patients with SIRS, possibly by restoring macrophage human leukocyte antigen (HLA)-DR expression (induction of Th1 activation) and TNF production. Similarly, IL-12, another Th1 inducer, reduced mortality from subsequent sepsis when administered after burn injury. In a different approach, anti–complement-activation product (anti-C5a antibodies) decreased the frequency of bacteremia, prevented apoptosis, and improved survival in SIRS patients. Not unexpectedly, given the previous discussion, strategies that block apoptosis of lymphocytes or gastrointestinal epithelial cells (both profoundly increased in almost all models of SIRS and in patient populations) have improved survival in experimental models of sepsis. This is consistent with evidence that mice with sepsis that are deficient in poly-adenosine diphosphate-ribose polymerase 1 (PARP-1), a key molecule in the proapoptotic pathway, have improved survival and that administration of a PARP-1 inhibitor was beneficial in pig models.

Surviving SIRS: A Consequence of Preconditioning?

Ischemic preconditioning is a term used to describe a phenomenon in which a transient episode of myocardial ischemia subsequently protects the individual from severe myocardial ischemia. Similarly, it has been proposed that organ dysfunction in SIRS patients is best explained by "cell hibernation" or "cell stunning." That is, SIRS is presumed to activate defense mechanisms that cause cellular processes to be reduced to basic "housekeeping" roles. If we are to extrapolate the concept of ischemic preconditioning to SIRS, patients who survive and have secondary exposure to SIRS would fare well. Alternatively, we could use this concept to explain survival of patients with SIRS, saying that earlier infections preconditioned them so that they were able to survive this major infection.

These hypotheses have arisen as a consequence of intriguing findings from autopsy studies that there is discordance between histologic findings and the degree of organ dysfunction seen in patients who died of sepsis. Histologic findings in patients with sepsis and acute renal failure showed only focal injury with preservation of normal glomeruli and renal tubules, as predicted from evidence that patients who survive sepsis and acute renal failure recover baseline renal function.

ED is a 33-year-old man with a history of "globe-trotting" since the age of 18 and who has recently returned from a 4-month trip to Indonesia. He had declined all vaccinations before travel, with the exception of those (e.g., for yellow fever) demanded by the immigration authorities of the countries he wished to visit. Three weeks after his return his family noticed he was quite "yellow" about the face, and he felt listless and nauseated. His family physician ordered a variety of blood tests. Results of these show a picture of acute hepatitis, negative serology for hepatitis C or hepatitis A(E), but positive results for hepatitis B. You ask the laboratory for more detailed information on the immunoglobulin isotypes of the anti–hepatitis B antibodies. Why?

QUESTIONS FOR GROUP DISCUSSION

1. Obviously we can be wise with hindsight here and agree that ED should have received the standard hepatitis B vaccine at some time before he became naturally exposed. The big question now is whether he is a carrier of hepatitis B (infected a long time ago) or whether this is a new infection. Explain why testing for particular anti–hepatitis B isotypes would help you to determine this.
2. Draw a schematic of hepatitis B virus and show the following antigens: surface antigen HBsAg, core antigen HBcAg, and HBeAg, from which the HBcAg is derived.
3. During the course of hepatitis B infection, antibodies are generated that are specific for the antigens listed in question 2. Detection of antibodies to these various antigens plays an important role in determining the stage of infection. Explain why anti-HBs antibodies will not be detected until after the disappearance of HBsAg in serum, even though it is believed that these antibodies are produced early in the infection.
4. Study Figure 39-1. Discuss the role of anti-HBc IgM antibodies in the diagnosis of hepatitis B. How would you interpret a report in which the patient has anti-HBc IgG antibodies? Why would you not use anti-HBe antibody titers to diagnose an early infection?
5. Discuss how you would assess recurrent/novel infection with hepatitis B.
6. Discuss antiviral therapy for hepatitis B and hepatitis C.
7. The best treatment is avoidance (if possible) or immunization (for hepatitis B [not yet available for hepatitis C]).

RECOMMENDED APPROACH

Implications/Analysis of Family History

There is no evidence to indicate the susceptibility to hepatitis B infection had a genetic component. However, spontaneous recovery from hepatitis B infection versus persistent infection may in fact have a genetic basis in that it has been shown that some human leukocyte antigen (HLA) class II alleles confer protection against chronic infection.

Implications/Analysis of Clinical History

ED was listless and nauseated. As well, he was quite "yellow" about the face. These are typical symptoms of hepatitis A and hepatitis B infection. Clinical symptoms may also include rashes, joint pains, arthritis, and abdominal pain. Individuals infected with hepatitis C often have just a mild illness or no clinical symptoms. Obviously we can be wise with hindsight here and agree that ED should have received the standard hepatitis B vaccine at some time before he became naturally exposed. The big question now is whether he is a carrier of hepatitis B (infected a long time ago) or whether this is a new infection.

Implications/Analysis of Laboratory Tests

A number of automated tests (Abbott Laboratories) are available. In general, these are modified enzyme-linked immunosorbent assays (ELISAs) that permit large numbers of samples to be processed in a short time period. In essence, the patient's serum is allowed to react with immobilized antibody in a reaction vessel, and then (after several washings to remove unbound antibody) some indicator system is added to detect and quantify the signal. Results of ED's tests showed a picture of acute hepatitis: negative serology for hepatitis C and hepatitis A(E) but positive results for hepatitis B. On request for antibody isotype information, you are told that both IgM and IgG anti-HBc antibodies were present, indicating that this is a new infection. Antibody tests to HBsAg and HBeAg were negative.

Additional Laboratory Tests

To further assess the stage of hepatitis B infection, tests were requested for the hepatitis antigens HBsAg and HBeAg. When testing for hepatitis B antigens, the same general procedure and principle is used as that described earlier for anti–hepatitis B antibodies, except that the patient's serum is allowed to react with immobilized antigen. Results were positive for HBsAg and HBeAg. (There are no commercially available tests for HBcAg.)

DIAGNOSIS

ED was diagnosed with acute hepatitis B infection. Based on the fact that he is positive for HBsAg and HBeAg and is seropositive for anti-HBc IgM antibodies, we know that this is a recent infection. HBeAg is released into the bloodstream when hepatitis B virus is actively replicating, and so these patients are highly infectious. The incubation period for hepatitis B ranges from 45 to 160 days, suggesting that ED was infected long before he returned home.

Discrepancy?

As you think about this apparent discrepancy in the data you realize that the anti-HBs antibodies are binding to HBsAg to form complexes (and HBeAg with anti-HBe antibodies). HBsAg detected in serum represents intact virion antigen as well as shed particles that consist primarily of aggregated HBsAg. In the face of high antigen in plasma and low antibody titers, immune complexes form so that the antibodies to these two antigens cannot be detected. These antigen-

antibody complexes may precipitate in the joints and skin to cause joint pain, arthritis, and a rash (type III hypersensitivity reaction). Consequently, the negative result for anti-HBs antibody and anti-HBe antibody (see earlier) were false negatives.

THERAPY

HBV-infected persons should be evaluated by their doctor for liver disease. ED should be monitored for liver disease. Drugs licensed for the treatment of chronic hepatitis B infection include lamivudine and adefovir dipivoxil. Both of these drugs are nucleoside reverse transcriptase inhibitors that block (DNA polymerase) and in doing so stop the replication of the virus. Both of these drugs are used for HIV therapy.

Interferon Alfa

A more recent development in antiviral drug therapy is interferon alfa (IFNα), which is administered by intramuscular or subcutaneous injection. IFNα is a cytokine secreted by virally infected cells during a normal immune response. When this cytokine is secreted, it binds to cognate receptors on neighboring cells, functioning in a paracrine fashion. Receptor-ligand interaction activates a signaling cascade that leads to the production of 2′5′-oligoadenylate synthetase, an enzyme whose activation triggers processes that result in the inhibition of viral replication. Additionally, IFNα leads to the upregulation of cell surface expression of members of the class I major histocompatibility complex, which enhances target cell recognition by cytotoxic T cells.

HEPATITIS B AND IMMUNIZATION

Hepatitis B infects the parenchymal cells of the liver, although it is also found in body fluids, including saliva, semen, breast milk, and blood. Transmission is by direct contact with these fluids. Consequently, health care workers are at risk for acquiring hepatitis B infection. Other individuals who are at high risk for infection are those who have unprotected sex with infected partners, as well as those who are intravenous drug users. Infected mothers can transmit the virus to neonates.

The hepatitis B vaccine (HBsAg) is a recombinant protein (Engerix B and Recombivax). Typically, the schedule of vaccination consists of three doses of vaccine administered intramuscularly on a 0-, 1-, and 6-month schedule. Slight modifications of this schedule are possible, depending on the commercial source of the vaccine. Accelerated schedules are possible if someone is traveling before the recommended immunization schedule can be completed; however, this is not approved by the U.S. Food and Drug Administration.

RG is 45 years old and has recently returned from a trip to China. While there he visited several small local markets, as well as a number of other typical tourist sites, including the Great Wall near Beijing. Two weeks after his return he developed a fever, which seemed only to defervesce intermittently with acetaminophen. During the past 2 days he has complained to his family of feeling more short of breath than usual and has had a crushing headache. Finally, tonight his overall condition worsens and he comes to the emergency department.

This is a worrisome presentation (particularly in view of recent evidence for infection by a number of transmissible emerging viruses, including severe acute respiratory syndrome [SARS], swine flu, avian flu, West Nile virus, and so on). He should be quarantined during workup! What should you do as part of the workup? What are the treatment options?

QUESTIONS FOR GROUP DISCUSSION

1. Although this patient certainly falls within a high risk for SARS, more common disorders are *still* more common. How would you ensure that this is not a typical viral infection and/or community-acquired pneumonia?

2. Given that his fever of the past 2 days only abates intermittently with acetaminophen how will you treat the fever?

3. This patient is feeling more short of breath than usual. What information would you hope to gain from a chest radiograph? What tests would you perform to determine how poorly the lungs are functioning? If sufficient supplemental oxygen is not possible by mask, how would you proceed?

4. Along with the fever and difficulty breathing, RG has a crushing headache. Explain why you would request computed tomography (CT) of his head and a lumbar puncture.

5. Having ruled out common infections, what emerging infectious agents should be high on the list of possibilities, particularly given his travel history? What tests would you request?

6. Essentially all the tests that you have requested come back without dramatic results (including the CT and lumbar puncture with cultures). The white blood cell count is minimally elevated (12,000/mm³, but still only 55% neutrophils and 40% lymphocytes (normal is ~60% neutrophils). What does this indicate regarding the type of pathogen with which RG is infected?

7. The chest radiograph shows hazy infiltrates throughout. This is consistent with the white blood cell differential (see question 6). Most importantly, your patient can only maintain an oxygen saturation greater than 92% on 60% oxygen given by re-breather mask. Therefore, it

is necessary to continue oxygen therapy and to monitor this patient's chest carefully. Explain how you would do this. Note that at this point you are still treating symptoms, not disease.

8. Serology comes back positive for West Nile virus and not for any of the other viruses of concern. What are the sequelae of West Nile viral infection? A vaccine is not available.

9. SARS is a coronavirus that has caused significant morbidity and mortality worldwide. Recent data suggest evidence for overexpression of the novel procoagulant fibroleukin in the lungs of SARS patients (a phenomenon seen also in the case of other single stranded RNA viruses, such as fulminant hepatitis C infection). What is fibroleukin? What is its normal role?

10. Discuss possible therapeutic avenues of approach regarding question 9.

RECOMMENDED APPROACH

Implication/Analysis of Family History

We are not provided with any family history; and given the urgency of the clinical presentation, the immediate goal is to treat the symptoms.

Implication/Analysis of Clinical History

RG is short of breath and has had intermittent fever for the past 2 days and a crushing headache. All of these symptoms are typical of viral infections. Despite his travel history, which must be kept in mind, we should consider first those infections that are common. Thus, you need to ensure this is not a typical infection (e.g., community-acquired pneumonia) and/or viral infection. However, he should be quarantined during workup. RG has a fever, which is only resolved intermittently; therefore, to get his temperature under control use simple measures (e.g., acetaminophen or nonsteroidal anti-inflammatory drugs) as well as sponging his body with warm water.

Common Infections

Common respiratory viral infections include influenza (types A and B), adenovirus, parainfluenza, rhinovirus, and respiratory syncytial virus (in infants). Nonculture tests are now available that provide results in minutes to hours instead of days using the conventional cell culture assays. More sophisticated assays (multiplex polymerase chain reaction [PCR]) for screening common viral infections of the nervous system have been developed in the United Kingdom, and, again, rapid results are possible. The most common cause of community (as opposed to health care facility)-acquired bacterial pneumonia is infection with *Streptococcus pneumoniae*, which can be determined using a rapid latex agglutination or immunochromographic assay.

Implications/Analysis of Laboratory Investigation

Routine blood work was ordered (e.g., complete blood cell count, electrolytes) as well as a chest radiograph. To determine the cause of the headaches, a CT scan was requested, as was a lumbar puncture to obtain cerebrospinal fluid (CSF) for culturing to determine if RG was infected with *Neisseria meningitidis*.

Blood Work, Chest Radiograph, CT

Results from the rapid diagnostic tests were all negative, indicating that the cause of RG's illness is not a common infection. Results of the blood work indicated that the white blood cell count was minimally elevated, with the differential showing 50% neutrophils and 45% lymphocytes (normal for neutrophils is 40% to 60%; for lymphocytes it is 20% to 40%). The fact that the differential count did not indicate an increase in neutrophils suggests that this is not likely to be a bacterial infection but rather a viremia (lymphocytosis). The chest radiograph showed hazy infiltrates throughout, again consistent with viral infection. CT of the head was normal, ruling out a brain tumor. Results from the cerebrospinal fluid

culture from the lumbar puncture to rule out meningitis (*N. meningitidis*) require several days.

Lung Function

To assess lung function, oxygen saturation with and without supplemental oxygen was requested. Sufficient oxygenation by mask delivery was evident and so intubation was not necessary. (In cases where intubation is required, appropriate precautions should be followed to protect the physician/technologist from respiratory secretions.) However, RG can only maintain an oxygen saturation greater than 92% on 60% oxygen given by re-breather mask. This is certainly in keeping with a significant respiratory compromise, and he needs to be monitored carefully with chest radiography and pulmonary function tests in an intensive care unit. An increase in lung infiltrate and respiratory distress would indicate a need for greater control of the airway (intubation).

Additional Laboratory Tests

Having ruled out common infections, it is time to test for transmissible emerging viruses including SARS, swine flu, avian flu, and West Nile virus. Serology (and PCR-DNA screening) should be sent to a specialized laboratory for SARS, as well as for other emerging viruses, including West Nile virus (see earlier).

DIAGNOSIS

Serology comes back (eventually) to indicate West Nile virus infection and not infection of any of the other viruses of concern.

THERAPY

Current therapies for West Nile virus infection have been disappointing (e.g., use of ribavirin and other novel antiviral agents).

Clinical trials to assess new therapies for patients infected with West Nile virus with serious neurologic complications are ongoing. Included in these experimental therapies are (1) IgG containing a high titer of anti–West Nile virus (Omr-IgG-am), (2) anti-sense compounds that target single-stranded RNA viruses such as West Nile, SARS, hepatitis C, dengue (AVI BioPharm NEUGENE), and (3) interferon alfa (Alferon) for West Nile meningoencephalitis.

ETIOLOGY: WEST NILE VIRUS

West Nile virus is a mosquito-borne virus that belongs to the family of flaviviruses, as do the yellow fever and dengue viruses. Individuals infected with West Nile virus may have no symptoms, whereas others may have fever and headache, become comatose, and have long-lasting neurologic damage, including muscle paralysis. Generally, most people make a complete recovery. A few will have longer-term neurologic dysfunction, probably reflecting cross-reactivity between immune response to virus and common neuronal antigens (see Cases 28 and 30).

Attempts to understand why there is such a discrepancy in response to West Nile virus infection have led to a search for susceptibility genes in murine models. A team of French scientists found a direct correlation between mortality and mutations in the gene encoding the enzyme "oligoadenylate synthetase." The activated form of this enzyme converts the latent endonuclease, RNase L, to its active form. West Nile virus has a single-stranded RNA genome, which is a substrate for RNase L. As yet, this mutation's association with West Nile virus has not been identified in humans.

SARS is a coronavirus that has caused significant morbidity/mortality worldwide (Fig. 48–1). A large effort is being made to develop a protective vaccine effective before and after exposure. In addition, better diagnostic and prognostic indicators are needed. Recent data suggest evidence for overexpression of the novel prothrombinase fibroleukin in the lungs of sick patients (a phenomenon seen also in the case of other single stranded RNA viruses (e.g., fulminant hepatitis C infection). Procoagulants and prothrombinases play an important role in triggering fibrin deposition and thrombosis in small vessels. Thus, measures to prevent fibroleukin overexpression are another important therapeutic avenue of approach.

Note that the incidence of disease in, and severity of infection in, immunocompromised individuals is extremely enhanced relative to healthy control populations (see Transplantation, Section V). Remember that, in fact, AIDS was recognized for what it was (an acquired immunodeficiency disease) because we had

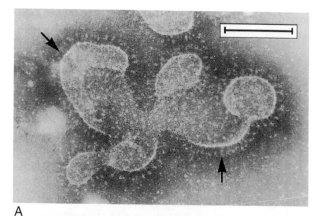

A

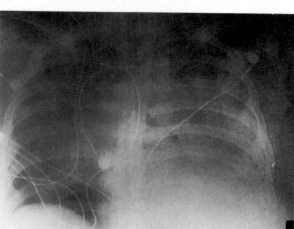

B

FIGURE 48–1 **A,** Negative-stain electron micrograph of a coronavirus such as SARS. **B,** Portable upright chest radiograph of a previously healthy female with viral pneumonia (in this case after adenovirus infection), showing consolidation of the left lower lobe and lingual segment, along with a left-sided pleural effusion. This would not be an atypical picture in SARS (in this case after coronavirus infection). (*A,* From Hart CA, Shears P: Color Atlas of Medical Microbiology, 2nd ed. St. Louis, Mosby, 2004; *B,* From Klinger JR, Sanchez MP, Curtin LA, et al: Multiple cases of life-threatening adenovirus pneumonia in a mental health care center. Am J Respir Crit Care Med 157:645–649, 1991.)

already gained experience with many of the presentations (Kaposi's sarcoma, *Pneumocystic carinii* (*jiroveci*) pneumonia) from looking after oncology patients and transplant survivors.

FURTHER READING

Ammann AJ: Leiner's disease and C5 deficiency. J Pediatr 81:1221, 1972.

Bernard GR, et al: Efficacy and safety of recombinant human activated protein C for severe sepsis. N Engl J Med 344:699, 2001.

Bouffard JP, et al: Neuropathy of the brain and spinal cord in human West Nile virus infection. Clin Neuropathol 23:59, 2004.

Cook DN, Pisetsky DS, Schwartz DA: Toll-like receptors in the pathogenesis of human disease. Nat Immunol 5:975, 2004.

Das UN: Is insulin an anti-inflammatory molecule? Nutrition 17:409, 2001.

Eskola J, et al: Efficacy of a pneumococcal conjugate vaccine against acute otitis media. N Engl J Med 344:403, 2001.

Gando S, et al: Activation of the extrinsic coagulation pathway in patients with severe sepsis and septic shock. Crit Care Med 26:2005, 1998.

Gioannini TL, et al: Isolation of an endotoxin-MD-2 complex that produced Toll-like receptor 4-dependent cell activation at picomolar concentrations. Proc Natl Acad Sci USA 101:4186, 2004.

Gould LH, FIkrig E: West Nile virus: A growing concern. J Clin Invest 113:1102, 2004.

Hogrefe WR, et al: Performance of immunoglobulin G (IgG) enzyme linked immunosorbent assays using a West Nile virus recombinant antigen (preM/E) for detection of West Nile virus- and other flavivirus specific antibodies. J Clin Microbiol 42:4641, 2004.

Kapoor AH, et al: Long persistence of West Nile virus (WNV) IgM antibodies in cerebral spinal fluid from patients with CNS disease. J Clin Virol 31:289, 2004.

Klee AL, et al: Long-term prognosis for clinical West Nile Virus infections. Emerg Infect Dis 10:1405, 2004.

Klugman KP, et al: A trial of a 9-valent pneumococcal conjugate vaccine in children with, and those without, HIV infection. N Engl J Med 349:1341, 2003.

Miyake K: Endotoxin recognition molecules: Toll like receptor-4-MD-2. Semin Immunol 16:11, 2004.

Nagi Y, et al: Essential role of MD-2 in LPS responsiveness and TLR4 distribution. Nat Immunol 3:667, 2002.

Ohnishi T, Muroi M, Tanamoto K: MD-2 is necessary for the Toll-like receptor 4 protein to undergo glycosylation essential for its translocation to the cell surface. Clin Diagn Lab Immunol 10:405, 2003.

Thomas L: Germs. N Engl J Med 287:553, 1972.

Watson JT, Gerber SI: West Nile virus: A brief review. Pediatr Infect Dis J 23:357, 2004.

Whitney CG, et al: Decline in invasive *pneumococcal* disease after the introduction of protein-polysaccharide conjugate vaccine. N Engl J Med 348:1737, 2003.

Whitney CG, Pickering LK: The potential of *pneumococcal* conjugate vaccines for children. Pediatr Infect Dis J 21:961, 2002.

Wise RP, et al: Postlicensure safety surveillance of 7-valent pneumococcal conjugate vaccine. JAMA 292:1702, 2004.

SECTION VII

Psychoneuroimmunology

Receptors That Share the Gamma (CD132) Chain

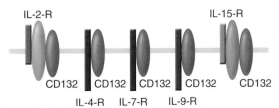

We have included this section in our book in recognition that society has acknowledged something which many scientists and clinicians seem loath to accept, that the immune system is but one of many physiologic systems, is integrated into a "whole," and is indeed influenced in a number of ways by "non-immunologic" cues. While we recognize that modern science seeks causal explanations for phenomena, we should be alert to the fact that while those explanations may not be forthcoming in our lifetime, the phenomena may yet be no less real.

Psychoneuroimmunology is a field that has had a tortuous path to credibility but that is slowly providing a sound scientific basis for observations that are often centuries or more old. In part the dichotomous relationship between observed biologic cellular (molecular) responses and behavior sprang from Descarte's insistence on the individuality of "mind" and "body." Conventional society tells us that this cannot be. How often do we acknowledge to ourselves that "stress," in any of its many manifestations (physical or otherwise), can render us susceptible to simple infections (the "flu")—see Case 51. A number of researchers over the past 20 or more years have even shown, in Pavlovian-type models, that certain immune responses can be brought under control of environmental "cues," rather like the salivation response Pavlov's dogs experienced in response to merely hearing their master's footsteps (which they anticipated would herald the arrival of food)—see Case 49.

What makes this area of sufficient importance for us to include these cases is that a scientific paradigm is now available that, correctly or not, can be used to help understand these phenomena. Only by further study will this area mature to its (we believe) rightful position in contemporary medicine. Whether we will eventually be able to manipulate immune responses in order to facilitate such beneficial responses as anti-tumor reactivity (over and above the effects of stress as an immunosuppressant—see Case 50), or diminished inflammation, remains to be seen.

INTERACTIONS BETWEEN THE CENTRAL NERVOUS SYSTEM AND THE IMMUNE SYSTEM

For many years conventional wisdom was that normal functioning of the immune system and the central nervous system (CNS) were independent of one another. Data showing that cells of the immune system express receptors for a number of CNS-active molecules, including catecholamines, histamine, endorphins, and so on, challenged this idea and led to speculation that this may not be the case under normal physiologic conditions. Early studies documented a correlation between catecholamine and steroid stress hormone levels in animals experiencing inescapable or escapable shock with or without a tumor implant.

Further extensions to these studies came from analyses of the functional significance of sympathetic innervation of lymphoid organs and from the application of the information so obtained to investigations of an animal model of multiple sclerosis (MS), experimental allergic encephalomyelitis (EAE), as well as clinical studies in MS patients themselves. In addition to affecting the peripheral immune system, sympathetic innervation has been documented to be of importance for the development of mucosal immunity.

CYTOKINES AND CHEMOKINES IN THE CENTRAL NERVOUS SYSTEM

Cytokines and chemokines are implicated in regulating immunity. Although it had been thought that chemokines function primarily to regulate cell trafficking, it is now clear that their function is considerably more complex than this. There is a large body of evidence implicating their importance in HIV infection, in cell activation, in autoimmune diseases, in neoplasia, and even in atherosclerosis.

A large body of data now indicates clearly that synthesis of these molecules is not restricted to cells of the immune system and, indeed, that some cytokines, chemokines, and their receptors have a significant impact on the CNS. These latter investigations focused on chemokines and cytokines involved in the pathogenesis of important neuroinflammatory diseases, ranging from MS and stroke to HIV encephalopathy.

Chemokines: Linking CNS and the Immune System

In addition to their role in pathologic states, chemokines and their receptors have an important role in cellular communication in both the normal adult and developing CNS. Stromal cell–derived factor-1/CXC12 (a chemokine), which is synthesized constitutively in the developing brain, seems to play an obligatory role in neuron migration during the formation of the granule cell layer of the cerebellum. In addition, many other chemokines are capable of directly regulating signal-transduction pathways involved in a variety of cellular functions within the CNS, ranging from synaptic transmission to growth.

Cytokines: Linking CNS and the Immune System

Cytokines have been found to be produced within the CNS (e.g., by glial cells and astrocytes, as well as by conventional lymphocytes within the CNS) and in the case of interleukin (IL)-1 and tumor necrosis factor (TNF) to modulate the development of nerve tissue cells. Because both IL-1 and TNF have been shown to cross the blood-brain barrier, these cytokines can affect the hypothalamus-pituitary-adrenal (HPA) axis, even after peripheral cytokine synthesis.

In addition to modulation of the development of nerve tissue cells, responses of these cells can also be regulated by cytokines. As one example of the latter, IL-4, IL-10, and transforming growth factor-β (TGFβ) have been documented to modify lipopolysaccharide (LPS) induction of inflammatory cytokines by glial cells.

Neuropeptides in the Immune System

Neuropeptides are short proteins that function either as neurotransmitters or as hormones. There is now abundant evidence that not only nerve tissue but also lymphoid tissue can express messenger ribonucleic acids (mRNAs) for a number of different neuropeptides. Included in these lymphoid tissues are those known to be crucial for the initiation of most immune responses, namely, macrophages and dendritic cells (antigen-presenting cells), sparking interest in the notion that neuropeptides might be implicated not merely in modulation of ongoing immune responses but also in their initiation.

Thymic Extracts

Analysis of expression of a number of neuropeptides, including prosomatostatin polypeptide in thymic extracts of mice showed a 10- to 20-fold enrichment in expression of peptides in low buoyant density cells, which also stained for the surface markers F4/80 (macrophage) or DEC205 (dendritic cells). Neuropeptides were differentially expressed by dendritic cells and macrophages in these normal mice.

Hepatobiliary System

In a separate anatomic study, the relationship between immunocytochemically identified nerve fibers and MHC class II–expressing antigen-presenting dendritic cells was investigated in the rat hepatobiliary system. Contacts between nerve fibers staining for the neuropeptide prosomatostatin, calcitonin gene–related peptide, calretinin, and vasoactive intestinal polypeptide (VIP) with dendritic cells were observed, which was consistent with a modulation of antigen presentation in this tissue by the autonomic nervous system.

Gut Tissue and Skin

In gut tissue, the neuropeptides prosomatostatin, VIP, and somatostatin are present in the nerve endings in myenteric plexus. Prosomatostatin is also present in nerve endings of cells within the skin and is thought to be present at abnormal concentrations in patients with atopic dermatitis, who have also been reported to show a marked imbalance in type 1 versus type 2 cytokine production, believed in turn to be responsible for some of the pathophysiology in this disease. In a separate study, VIP was shown to have an inhibitory effect on interferon gamma (IFNγ) (type 1 cytokine) and IL-4 (type 2 cytokine) production at physiologic concentrations.

Regulation of Cytokine Production by Prosomatostatin

In a contact hypersensitivity model, a prosomatostatin agonist and a prosomatostatin antagonist were injected intradermally to modify contact hypersensitivity to locally applied haptens. The prosomatostatin agonist enhanced contact hypersensitivity induced by conventional, but not optimal, sensitizing doses of hapten, whereas the prosomatostatin antagonist inhibited the induction of contact hypersensitivity by optimal sensitizing doses of hapten. These and other data were taken to infer once again that prosomatostatin agonist enhanced the *generation* of hapten-specific immunogenic signals from the dermis, although the role of local cytokine production in this model was not investigated. In a separate study prosomatostatin was found to have an enhancing effect on production of both IFNγ and IL-4 at physiologic concentrations (from 10^{-10} to 10^{-6} mol/L). IFNγ has been shown to influence the differentiation of Thp cells to Th1 cells, whereas IL-4 influences the shift to a Th2 phenotype.

Modulation of Inducible Nitric Oxide Synthase by Prosomatostatin

At least some of the immunomodulatory effects produced by macrophages are a reflection of immunomodulation occurring secondary to their altered release of low-molecular-weight molecules (reactive oxygen and nitrogen intermediates). To further address this issue, studies have focused on the effect of neuropeptide mediators on the activity of inducible nitric oxide synthase (iNOS) in macrophages. In LPS-activated macrophages, prosomatostatin stimulated nitric oxide production in a time- and concentration-dependent manner and this was blocked by a specific prosomatostatin receptor antagonist. Moreover, prosomatostatin stimulation increased the levels of both iNOS mRNA and iNOS protein, documenting that prosomatostatin can increase LPS-induced nitric oxide production in macrophages by augmenting the induction of iNOS expression.

Effect of Acute, Cold Stress on Prosomatostatin Modulation of iNOS

In an extension of these data the role of prosomatostatin on acute, cold stress–induced production of nitric oxide by peritoneal macrophages stimulated with LPS was examined. This group found that prosomatostatin enhanced nitric oxide from the acute, cold-stressed mice relative to the nonstressed mice These results further support a role for prosomatostatin in modulating production of nitric oxide by macrophages.

Effect of Prosomatostatin on Histamine Secretion in the Gut

Is there any independent evidence that prosomatostatin, or other neuropeptides, is implicated under physiologic conditions in gastrointestinal immunity? Mast cell hyperplasia (increase in number of mast cells) in the gut is a feature of inflammatory bowel disease, but the role of mast cells in this disease is still unclear. Because it is believed that mast cell/nerve interactions might impact on intestinal inflammation, one group has investigated whether prosomatostatin could cause histamine secretion from human gut mucosal mast cells. No induction of mast cell activation was seen in histologically normal mucosa from controls, whereas mucosal specimens taken from inflamed bowel tissue or from uninvolved tissue in a patient with Crohn's disease showed enhanced histamine secretion in the presence of prosomatostatin, either alone or in combination with anti-IgE. These data argue that mast cell/nerve interactions are indeed involved in histamine-releasing processes in the gut in inflammatory bowel disease.

Neurotrophins within the Immune System

Neurotrophins are a family of proteins that play a role in the growth and differentiation of neurons. Recently, the field of molecular communication between the CNS and the immune system has been expanded by documentation that neurotrophins, structurally related growth factors that include nerve growth factor (NGF), brain-derived neurotrophic factor (BDNF) and neurotrophins-3 and -4 (NT-3, NT-4), all of which have been reported to play roles in development, differentiation, and survival of neuronal subsets, can also be produced by, and can act upon, cells within the immune system. Under inflammatory conditions, for example, brain-derived neurotrophic factor synthesis has been detected in activated T cells and B cells, macrophages, and neurons.

Nerve Growth Factor Effects on Cells of the Immune System

NGF has been shown to promote growth and differentiation of mast cells and basophils. Analysis of the effect of NGF on responses of mature lymphocytes has provided evidence that it may modulate the threshold of responses to conventional immunologic stimuli, including those inducing synthesis of type 2 cytokines and IgE and thus predispose toward allergic-type responses. Finally, there are a number of reports concerning altered levels of NGF and other neurotrophins in a variety of autoimmune and/or inflammatory diseases, including systemic lupus erythematosus (SLE), MS, and bronchiolar lavage fluid of asthmatic patients after allergic challenge. Interestingly, a receptor for NGF, tyrosine kinase receptor A (trkA), has been found to be expressed predominantly in neonatal thymic tissue, consistent with reports that neurotrophin transcripts were highest during fetal life.

BEHAVIORAL CHANGES AND ALTERED IMMUNE RESPONSES

Perhaps even more provocative than the studies quoted earlier are those that have focused directly on the ability of behavioral changes themselves to modulate immunity. In an animal model system, the induction of experimental autoimmune encephalomyelitis (EAE) in rat strains preselected for their response to apomorphine as a selection criterion was explored.

High and low susceptibility rats were derived by selective breeding and designated APO-sus and APO-unsus, respectively. The APO-unsus rats were found to have a lower response to novel stress, as determined by lower locomotor activity and decreased activation of the HPA axis. In addition, these rats were susceptible to induction of EAE after immunization with myelin basic protein in Freund's adjuvant, whereas APO-sus rats were not. Because EAE is believed to be a type 1 cytokine–mediated phenomenon, it was of interest to find also that (in vitro) APO-sus rat cells were more likely to develop type 2 cytokine responses than cells from APO-unsus rats. A disparity in type 1 versus type 2 cytokine production has been observed in schizophrenia, although the relationship of such changes to disease remains unexplored.

Conditioned Responses

Classical conditioning paradigms have also been applied to study regulation of immune responses. These studies were spurred by findings in a taste aversion model in rats. Animals that had received immunization with a foreign antigen (sheep erythrocytes [SRBCs]) initially in the context of an unconditioned stimulus, cyclophosphamide (a nonspecific immunosuppressant), *and* a conditioned stimulus (saccharin) subsequently demonstrated decreased antibody responses to antigen (SRBCs) when injected in the context of saccharin without cyclophosphamide.

This suppressed response occurred independently of triggering of the HPA axis. Subsequent reports, however, showed that the decreased antibody response to SRBCs in the presence of saccharin (without cyclophosphamide) could be extinguished by repeated exposure to the conditioned stimulus (saccharin) in the absence of the unconditioned stimulus (cyclophosphamide).

These data have been reproduced in a variety of models, in which conditioned natural killer (NK) cell activation and even skin graft rejection responses were studied. There have, in addition, been a number of investigators who have applied this conditioning paradigm *to manipulate responses in animal models of clinical disease,* including SLE, malignancy, and infectious disease.

MECHANISMS RESPONSIBLE FOR BIOBEHAVIORAL CONTROL OF IMMUNITY?

The physiologic mechanism(s) behind conditioned immunity remains much of an enigma. To a large degree there remains a body of thought that explicitly or implicitly assumes that conditioned suppression of immunity reflects the operation of stress-induced responses (of the HPA axis). Glucocorticoid levels are elevated in, and often equated with, stress and have in addition been shown independently to decrease a number of immune responses. Thus, the idea that this should be (the sole) explanation for conditioning is perhaps an understandably attractive one. However, there are a number of pieces of evidence that can be cited to refute this notion.

Conditioning in the Absence of HPA Involvement

There are several reports of conditioned immunosuppression occurring in the absence of altered adrenocortical responses. As example, (1) studies examining the effect of circadian rhythmicity on the efficacy of conditioning showed that conditioned suppression was most easily elicited in animals at the trough (not peak) of their endogenous circulating corticosterone levels; (2) there are data showing that stimulation of animals to elicit increased adrenocortical stimulation leads to

enhanced (not suppressed) immune responses; (3) published experiments indicate that lithium chloride (LiCl), an agent that, like cyclophosphamide, evokes a profound taste aversion and elevated corticosterone levels, is ineffective as an unconditioned stimulus for conditioning antibody responses; (4) there are data showing that eliminating the differential environmental stimuli, likely stress inducing, components of taste aversion paradigms does not eliminate conditioned immunosuppression. However, none of these arguments necessarily negates the notion that conditioned immunosuppression reflects the operation of a *conditioned neuroendocrine change per se!*

Neuroimmune Mediators in Conditioning Models

If alterations in the HPA axis are not primarily responsible for the conditioned changes observed, what other factors might be implicated? Multiple processes are probably involved, and different factors may thus take on primary importance in different model systems/physiologic situations. Indeed, it is possible that different mechanisms are involved when conditioning is superimposed on a resting versus an activated immune system. This is particularly likely given that there is a plethora of potential neuroimmune mediators and because it is known already that the same immunomodulating agents bind to, and activate differentially, resting versus activated cells. Given the evidence that (1) the immune system is innervated, (2) leukocytes and neurons share numerous receptors for neuropeptides/neurotransmitters, and (3) lymphocytes and tissues of the nervous system produce and respond to many different common molecules, including cytokines, chemokines, neurotrophins, and conventional neuropeptides and/or neurotransmitters, it should not be surprising that there are, indeed, many potential mechanisms by which CNS/immune interactions occur in conditioned animals. There may be conditioned changes in neuroendocrine activation pathways that affect lymphocytes and their activation. There may alternatively be conditioned changes in the release of lymphocyte products, which in turn affect cells within the nervous system.

Dual Role of Cytokines

Recently, there has been a surge in interest in the potential dual role of cytokines in the CNS, acting both as CNS stimuli and modulators of inflammation.

As an example, transgenic mice overexpressing interferon alpha (IFNα) demonstrate many of the changes phenotypically characteristic of human neurodegenerative disorders, although they are (paradoxically) resistant to numerous neurotropic viruses. IL-6 has been found to promote production of arginine-vasopressin, which in turn leads to the syndrome of inappropriate secretion of antidiuretic hormone (SIADH), which is not uncommon in chronic inflammation. (In SIADH, the body retains water and so electrolyte levels may become low.)

Dual Role of Hormones

The dual action of brain-derived hormones has also been well documented. For instance, α-melanocyte–stimulating hormone inhibits an anti-inflammatory response, likely by regulation of NFκB/IκB). The wheel turns full circle once more with evidence that norepinephrine can induce differential cytokine gene expression from lymphocytes and that the sensitivity of lymphocytes to such signaling is critically dependent on their prior activation state.

Integration of our understanding of CNS/immune system interactions will likely become an increasingly more important issue for basic and clinical scientists.

LG is an 18-year-old girl in your practice with a history of seasonal allergies and, she says, multiple "bad responses" to many medications with rashes, wheezing, and general malaise. She has a known allergy to animal dander, including cats and dogs as well as rabbits (she had had one as a pet as a young child but was forced to give it up).

A patient in your practice, knowing your love for your German Shepherd dog who recently died, has purchased for you a gift of a porcelain statue of a full-sized shepherd that you have accorded a "pride of place" in the corner of your office. LG comes to visit for a routine physical and Papanicolaou test, but within a minute of being in the room develops severe signs of respiratory distress, relieved only by aggressive albuterol (Ventolin) inhalation in the adjacent examining room. She says it was "brought on" by the dog statue. Is this possible? Why?

QUESTIONS FOR GROUP DISCUSSION

1. What is classical conditioning? How is it induced experimentally?
2. At present, how can you eliminate the conditioned part of a response in humans?
3. In general terms, describe the experimental protocol and results of the guinea pig study regarding abrupt and not abrupt isolation stress on histamine release to a conditioned stimulus. How would you extrapolate that to human experiences?
4. Consider ischemic conditioning (see Case 43) and how you might extrapolate this to the results of question 3 and childhood experiences in general?
5. Describe the conditioning studies using epinephrine, a neutral sherbet, and NK cell activity. On the basis of this study, what activity of NK cells would you predict in acute stress responses?
6. Provide a rationale for the selection of IL-2 and IFNγ as dependent measures in the conditioned studies using cyclosporine. How could the results of this study be used to design studies to offset drug toxicity?
7. Explain why it is oversimplistic to suggest that inhibition of the hypothalamic-pituitary-adrenal (HPA) axis is the only explanation for conditioned immunosuppression.
8. Describe conditioning studies that indicate that β-adrenergic receptor activity is not required for the establishment of conditioned morphine-induced changes in immune status.
9. Describe conditioning studies that support the concept that endogenous opioid activity is involved in conditioned-stimulus–induced alterations of immune function.
10. What immune responses does blockade of glutamate release and/or uptake block?

RECOMMENDED APPROACH

Implications/Analysis of Family History

Although there is evidence for genetic associations for susceptibility to allergies, evidence for genetic susceptibility for conditioning in humans is lacking. However, studies with wild-type mice and laboratory mice lacking dopamine receptor D4 (D4R) have shown that mice lacking D4R showed heightened avoidance to classical fear conditioning. Future research may identify susceptibility genes in humans.

Implications/Analysis of Clinical History

Classical conditioning is deemed to have occurred when a particular stimulus (conditioned stimulus) evokes a similar response to that generated by an unconditioned stimulus, following pairing of these two stimuli. The number of pairings required to effect a conditioned response seems, in part, to depend on the strength of the emotional response at the time of the pairing.

In the absence of more information, we are unable to determine if LG's respiratory distress in the presence of the porcelain dog statue was due to a single emotional pairing (e.g., attacked by a dog when she was an infant and has no conscious memory of that experience) or whether this is the result of multiple pairings of another nature.

Implications/Analysis of Laboratory Studies

Whereas laboratory studies and/or allergen skin testing can identify the allergens to which this child is responding, these tests cannot possibly identify the objects that serve as conditioned stimuli.

Additional Laboratory Tests

Laboratory tests are not available to measure responses to conditional stimuli; however, psychological assessment should be considered.

DIAGNOSIS

The evidence to date (see later) is quite consistent with the clinical observation that this girl has a "conditioned" allergic response to animal dander, which can be elicited by visual cues alone.

THERAPY

The treatment at this stage would be of two kinds. You can continue to treat symptoms, and, as here, give this patient β-agonist therapy (and/or epinephrine) as appropriate during exacerbations. Alternatively, you could attempt to eliminate at least the conditioned part of this response, using behavioral therapy (extinction).

CONDITIONING OF VARIOUS IMMUNE PHENOMENA

Although there have been a number of studies concerning classical conditioning of a variety of immune phenomena in animals over the past several years, there are limited controlled experimental studies on conditioned immune responses in humans.

Conditioned Immune Phenomena: Guinea Pigs

Studies in the animal literature have attempted to model evidence for conditioned "allergic-type" responses. Learned histamine release has been one such model. In a classical conditioning procedure in which an immunologic challenge was paired with the presentation of an odor, guinea pigs subsequently showed a plasma histamine increase when presented with the odor alone.

Abrupt versus Nonabrupt Isolation Stress on Histamine Release

A guinea pig model investigated the effect of (abrupt and nonabrupt isolation, or relief from isolation) stress on classically conditioned histamine release, using ovalbumin as an unconditioned stimulus and dimethylsulfide (sulfur smelling) as a conditioned stimulus. Plasma histamine levels were monitored to assess responses.

The study consisted of two separate phases, with phase I serving as the conditioning phase and phase II as the test phase. Of the four groups in the study, two groups remained paired or single for both phases of the study. The remaining groups were either single for the first phase, then paired for the second, or vice versa.

Plasma histamine levels increased from baseline in response to the conditioned stimulus in all animals except for the animals that were paired in phase I and single in phase II. Although animals that were single in phase I and paired in phase II had histamine levels higher than the control group, the histamine level was still lower than that of guinea pigs, which were isolated or paired during *both* phases. Thus, a change of social relations, particularly isolation during the presentation of the conditioned stimulus, could produce a conditioned suppressive effect on immediate (asthmatic) responses.

CONDITIONED IMMUNE PHENOMENA: HUMAN STUDIES

Conditioned Increase in NK Cell Activity

Most of the published literature deals with studies exploring conditioning of NK cell activity in volunteer subjects. As an example, in one such study, subjects were exposed to a conditioning procedure in which a neutral sherbet was repeatedly paired with a subcutaneous injection of 0.2 mg epinephrine. After epinephrine administration an increase of NK cell activity could be observed (unconditioned response). On the conditioning test day the conditioned group showed increased NK cell activity after re-exposure of the sherbet combined with saline injection. No increase was found in control groups who previously received the sherbet in combination with saline (saline control) or with epinephrine in an unpaired manner (unpaired control). This study certainly supports the previously documented animal literature.

Conditioned Increase in Cytokine Secretion

In a further follow-up to the NK cell investigations (see earlier), healthy subjects in a double-blind, placebo-controlled study were conditioned in four sessions over 3 consecutive days, receiving the immunosuppressive drug cyclosporine as an unconditioned stimulus paired with a distinctively flavored drink each 12 hours. In the next week, re-exposure to the conditioned stimulus (drink), but now paired with placebo capsules (instead of cyclosporine), induced a suppression of immune functions, as analyzed by IL-2 and IFNγ mRNA expression, intracellular cytokine production, and *in vitro* release of IL-2 and IFNγ, as well as lymphocyte proliferation.

Whereas these data are consistent with the hypothesis that immunosuppression can be behaviorally conditioned in humans, it is important to note that at least one other group failed to replicate these data. Similarly, other workers reported a failure to condition allergic-type immune responses in human skin.

CONDITIONING OF IMMUNE RESPONSES: POSSIBLE MECHANISMS

Analysis of the biologic mechanism(s) implicated in classical conditioning of immune responses have taken several routes, depending on whether the cellular or biochemical aspects of the alterations in immunity are being studied.

Alterations in Cells, Receptors, and/or Environment in Conditioning

Several groups, using animal models, have reported changes in the cells/cellular receptors (and/or cellular environment) of conditioned animals that might contribute to changes in immune responses in this fashion. Included in such changes are alterations in the release of chemoattractants in conditioned mice, which might contribute to differences in cell migration. Indeed, data have confirmed that CNS control of cell migration is likely a fundamentally important mechanism for integration of the CNS/immune system axis, and there is evidence that a significant change in T cell population dynamics (resulting from altered cell migration) might underlie conditioned immunosuppression.

Alterations in Neuroendocrine Responses in Conditioning

Stressors (both physical and psychological) can influence antigen-specific as well as nonspecific reactions. Conditioning and stressful stimulation can alter the development and/or progression of a number of immunologically mediated pathophysiologic processes.

These behaviorally induced neural and endocrine responses alter various immune parameters, which interact with the concurrent immunologic events on which they are superimposed, and vice versa. Analyzing the causative interactions contributing to conditioned immunomodulation thus becomes very complicated, particularly since the neural or neuroendocrine pathways involved in the behavioral alteration of immune responses are largely known.

As discussed in more depth below, there is evidence that both conditioning and stressor-induced effects may result from the action of adrenocortical steroids, opioids, and catecholamines, among others, and all have been implicated in the mediation of *some* immunologic effects observed under *some* experimental conditions. An inability to generalize from one experimental study to another may reflect the fact that different conditioning and stressful environmental circumstances induce different constellations of neuroendocrine responses composing the milieu within which ongoing immune reactivity and the response to immunologic signals occur.

Alterations in the Hypothalamus-Pituitary-Adrenal Axis in Conditioning

Several studies using a serum corticosterone time course to examine possible involvement of glucocorticoids in conditioned immunosuppression detected no significant differences in serum corticosterone levels between nonconditioned controls and any conditioned group at any time point. These results support the hypothesis that conditioned immunosuppression is not linked to a rise in glucocorticoid levels. Further support for refuting the role of the HPA axis in conditioning comes from an animal model of conditioned immunosuppression, in which adrenalectomy failed to abort the conditioned suppression seen.

In another study, recombinant IL-1β, which is capable of stimulating the HPA axis to secrete corticosterone (an immunosuppressant), was paired with environmental cues in either a taste aversion or odor conditioning procedure. Animals receiving paired delivery of cues and IL-1 showed corticosterone production on re-exposure to cues, although no evidence was seen for altered CNS concentrations of IL-1 in conditioned animals, which might have reflected a peripheral effect (of IL-1 increases), subsequently eliciting a conditioned CNS response.

Sympathetic Nervous System and/or β-Adrenergic System in Conditioning

Evidence implicating the sympathetic nervous system in conditioning of immune responses also comes from animal studies. Rats receiving subtherapeutic cyclosporine rejected heart allografts at the same time as non–cyclosporine-treated rats. However, a behavioral conditioning regimen (using saccharin and cyclosporine) added to the subtherapeutic cyclosporine protocol produced a significant prolongation of graft survival. Additional data implicated altered production of interleukin-2 and IFNγ in these effects.

Peripheral β-Adrenergic Receptor Activity in Conditioning

Yet another animal study explored the involvement of peripheral β-adrenergic receptor activity in the establishment and expression of conditioned morphine-induced alterations of immune status. Animals received two conditioning sessions during which a subcutaneous injection of morphine sulfate was paired with exposure to a distinctive environment. On the test day, rats were re-exposed to the conditioned stimulus before sacrifice. As a variable, saline or nadolol was administered either before the training sessions or before the test session (nadolol [Nandol] is a β-adrenergic receptor inverse agonist).

Administration of nadolol before training did not affect the development of conditioned alterations of immune status. However, nadolol administration before testing completely attenuated the expression of a subset of the conditioned morphine-induced changes in immune status. Thus, although peripheral β-adrenergic receptor activity is not required for the establishment of conditioned morphine-induced alterations of immune status, it is involved in the expression of at least a subset of those responses. Other studies have suggested a role for central noradrenergic and dopaminergic systems in regulating the conditioned recall of NK cell responses.

Opioids/Opioid Receptors in Conditioning

Studies evaluating the effect of administration of the opiate receptor antagonists naltrexone and N-methylnaltrexone on the immunomodulatory effect of a conditioned stimulus that had been paired with electric footshock have been performed in animals. Naltrexone attenuated the conditioned stimulus–induced suppression of the *in vitro* proliferative response of splenic lymphocytes to several mitogens (concanavalin A, lipopolysaccharide, and a combination of ionomycin and phorbol myristate acetate) in a dose-dependent fashion. Naltrexone also attenuated the conditioned stimulus–induced reduction in NK cell activity. In contrast, the quaternary form of naltrexone, N-methylnaltrexone, failed to attenuate the conditioned stimulus–induced immunomodulatory effects. These data support the concept that endogenous opioid activity is involved in conditioned stimulus–induced alterations of immune function. Furthermore, the failure of N-methylnaltrexone to attenuate the conditioned stimulus–induced immunomodulatory effect suggests that the opioid receptors involved are located in the CNS.

GABA Signaling in Conditioning

The roles of glutamate and γ-aminobutyric acid (GABA) in recall of the conditioned NK cell response have also been examined. These results suggest that glutamate, but not GABA, was required for recall of the conditioned NK cell response. NMDA but not the kainate/AMPA receptors were suggested to be involved in the response. The levels of glutamate that were released, and/or taken up, also appeared to be critical, given the evidence that blockade of glutamate release and/or uptake abolished the conditioned NK cell response.

Altered Chemokine and/or Cytokines Production in Conditioning

While chemokines function primarily to regulate cell trafficking, it is now clear that their function is considerably more complex than this. They are of importance in HIV infection, in cell activation, in autoimmune diseases and neoplasia, and even in atherosclerosis. The potential role of altered chemokine synthesis in classical conditioning remains unknown.

MG, a 50-year-old mother of two, was recently diagnosed with breast cancer. Despite favorable histology and hormone receptor typing of the tumor, indicating a projected good response to taxol and other chemotherapy, and lack of any nodal involvement, she has had trouble coming to grips with the diagnosis. She has been referred to the psychiatric service for treatment of depression. In addition, recent blood work at the hospital, along with some functional studies, suggests a subtle impairment in immune functioning, which her general practitioner is concerned might impact on longer-term prognosis. What are your concerns? What is the evidence that MG's mental state might influence her disease? What might be done to address this issue?

QUESTIONS FOR GROUP DISCUSSION

1. There is a wealth of data indicating a link between clinical depression and immune function. What psychological factors have been identified as contributing to diminished survival in cancer patients?
2. Given the relationship identified in question 1, what adjunctive therapy would you recommend be used along with the primary treatment?
3. Assuming that you arrange for psychological counseling as adjunctive therapy for your patient, how would you monitor progression of treatment and its impact on disease progression? Is this the primary interceding variable between disease progression and mental state?
4. A recent trial has assessed evidence that adrenergic- and/or endorphin-mediated signals might be variables of importance in immunosuppression after cancer surgery. As such, what pharmacologic intervention would you recommend to improve immune functioning?
5. Which cells of the innate immune system play an important role in tumor killing? Consider your proposed intervention in question 4. What is the evidence that this drug intervention would enhance tumor killing?

RECOMMENDED APPROACH

Implications/Analysis of Family History

Although we are not provided with family history, there is evidence that susceptibility to cancer does have a genetic basis. Additionally, recent studies have identified a polymorphism in the 5-hydroxytryptamine transporter (5-HTT) gene that predisposes individuals to depression when faced with major life stresses.

The 5-HTT gene encodes the transporter protein required for serotonin reuptake into neurons.

Implications/Analysis of Clinical History

MG has been diagnosed with cancer, which is high on the list of stressors for anyone. The fact that her physician has referred her to a psychiatrist rather than psychologists for counseling is an indication that he considers this depression as profound and may require drug therapy.

Implications/Analysis of Laboratory Investigation

MG's blood work indicated that simple blood tests were normal, as were assays of innate immunity and electrophoresis of serum immunoglobulin. However, functional studies have revealed impaired NK cell cytotoxic activity, as well as diminished proliferative responses of B cells and T cells to mitogenic lectins.

These tests indicate that MG does not have a major immunologic defect but that the immune system is just not functioning optimally at this time. A number of studies have shown decreased NK cell activity in patients with a number of different cancers, so whether this decreased activity is secondary to the cancer or to depression is difficult to evaluate.

Depression has been linked to low serotonin levels, and thus antidepressants that prevent the reuptake of serotonin are prescribed for these patients. As such, one would expect that antidepressants that block the reuptake of serotonin (e.g., fluoxetine [Prozac]) would reverse immunosuppression, if a deficiency is the mechanism by which the immune system is depressed. However, studies in rodents have shown that acute administration of fluoxetine led to a decrease in mitogen-induced proliferation. This does not obviate a correlation between depression and decreases in lymphocyte proliferation but rather emphasizes that other genes may contribute to depression.

Additional Laboratory Tests

The question still remains—what is the primary interceding variable between disease progression and mental state? If one could identify this, then laboratory tests to evaluate changes after drug therapy could be initiated.

DIAGNOSIS

MG was diagnosed with depression.

THERAPY

MG's physician has referred her to a psychiatrist.

MENTAL HEALTH AND DISEASE

There is a growing realization that mental health can affect disease, both incidence (although data here are more tenuous) and prognosis. There is a wealth of data indicating a link between clinical depression and immune function. A variety of indices used to score depression (e.g., Beck Inventory) have been used to document this relationship. In general, individuals with poor self worth and feelings of hopelessness have been found to show diminished survival compared to controls, all other factors being equal, after diagnosis in a variety of different cancers, with breast cancer

being one of these. Accordingly, a major effort has been made to improve psychological factors as adjunctive therapy for cancer.

Monitoring Progression of Treatment

Less attention has been paid to how best to monitor progression of treatment. Should we be following immunologic parameters? Is this indeed the primary interceding variable between disease progression and mental state? Are there other variables we should be paying as much (or more) attention to? As one example, one might ask whether we should routinely take measurements of neurohormonal status in such patients.

Modulation of NK Cell Activity

A recent trial has assessed evidence that adrenergic and/or endorphin-mediated signals might be variables of importance in immunosuppression after cancer surgery and has suggested that we intervene (using β blockers/naltrexone) to improve immune functioning in this case, and thereby promote longer-term survival. Certainly, independent animal model data support evidence for a role for naltrexone in modulation of NK cell activity (a key player in tumor killing), whereas lymphocytes are known to possess adrenergic receptors that modulate their activity.

Conclusion

At this stage it is safest to conclude that this field is very much in its infancy and that a great deal more has to be learned before rational behavioral therapy (aimed at "improving" immune functioning in cancer patients) can be advocated.

KL is a 20-year-old first-year medical student who is visiting you for the fifth time in 4 months, with evidence of a viral-type respiratory infection. He has previously been a healthy individual, has all his vaccinations up to date, and has not traveled out of the country. He admits to finding his course study load "tiring and difficult" and has had to stay up at night on at least one occasion each week over the last month to prepare for tests. His roommate is well. His weight is stable. He is currently afebrile, with a dry cough. You order routine blood work and a chest radiograph, with all results returning as normal. What is the potential pathophysiology of this problem? What might you do about it?

C A S E

5 1

QUESTIONS FOR GROUP DISCUSSION

1. Many animal studies, designed with a goal of defining the effect of stress on immune responses, used adrenalectomy as a variable to analyze behaviorally induced changes in immunity. Provide a rationale for this approach.

2. Sleep deprivation in rodent models has led to both increased levels of corticosterone and significant changes in immune responses. How would you explain the fact that there is little evidence to suggest a correlation between immune dysfunction and altered serum corticosterone levels in these animals?

3. How would you rationalize the fact that cortisol levels are increased in both acute stress and chronic stress yet many reports indicate that acute stress enhances the immune system but that chronic stress is immunosuppressive.

4. In human studies, low levels of endotoxin lead to increased levels of cytokines (interleukin [IL]-1, IL-6, and tumor necrosis factor [TNF]). IL-1 and TNF are proinflammatory cytokines. Review the inflammatory process and discuss the role of these cytokines in the recruitment of cells to sites of infection or trauma.

5. In human studies (see question 4), low levels of endotoxin also lead to increased levels of cortisol. How would you explain the fact that cortisol, which has been shown to be an anti-inflammatory agent, does not abrogate the inflammatory effect of IL-1 and TNF?

6. Evidence has now accumulated for stress-associated changes in chemokine/cytokine levels, which may underlie some of these observed changes in cell migration. What cytokines are required for increased transmigration? Which chemokines are required to recruit monocytes and neutrophils into tissues?

7. A number of studies conducted on asymptomatic HIV-positive subjects before and after notification of HIV-1 antibody status measured immune system function in patients that were or were not involved in regular aerobic exercise or group, cognitive, or behavioral modification. Those who participated in interventions had lower or minimal decreases in immunologic parameters compared with controls. Describe a model that would explain this phenomenon.

RECOMMENDED APPROACH

Implications/Analysis of Family History

Although we are not provided with any family history, responses to sleep deprivation and stress may have a genetic component. Sleep deprivation is associated with increased levels of cortisol, a stress hormone, which correlate with alterations in immune function, as well as with depression. Recent studies with twins have shown a 62% heritability with respect to the levels of cortisol in stressed individuals.

Cortisol is secreted from the adrenal gland in response to adrenocorticotropic hormone (ACTH), which is released from the anterior pituitary in response to corticotropin-releasing factor (CRF) secreted by the hypothalamus.

Implications/Analysis of Clinical History

KL's clinical history indicates that he has had five viral-type respiratory infections in the past 4 months. Effective immune responses to viral infections require the activation of cell-mediated immunity, particularly NK cells, CD4+ T cells, and CD8+ T cells. The fact that KL has had so many viral infections suggests that these cells are not functioning at optimal levels.

Implications/Analysis of Laboratory Investigation

KL's blood work is normal as is his chest radiograph, suggesting that he does not have a major immunologic deficiency disorder. However, the fact that he is having so many viral infections does suggest that T cell and NK cell function is not optimal.

Additional Laboratory Tests

A relatively straight method to assess T cell function is an assay that measures T cell proliferation in response to mitogen stimulation. KL's T cell proliferative response in this assay was diminished relative to controls, as was the test to measure NK cell cytotoxicity.

DIAGNOSIS

KL was diagnosed with chronic stress.

THERAPY

Daily exercise or other approaches to relaxation (e.g., reading, listening to music, relaxation tapes) are recommended. In some cases, medication may be required.

EFFECT OF STRESS ON IMMUNE RESPONSES

Whereas the early field of investigations into behavior and immunity was replete with studies examining "stress," both psychological and/or physical, and its implication for immunosuppression, it rapidly became apparent that not all of the observations made in this area were easily subsumed under an umbrella of stress-induced effects. As noted in another case, in animal studies in particular, adrenalectomy, which would prevent release of cortisol, did not eliminate behaviorally induced changes in immunity and the changes did not follow the circadian rhythmicity of corticosteroid production. Furthermore, both acute and chronic stress lead to increases in cortisol, but acute stress is often reported as enhancing immune function whereas chronic stress is immunosuppressive.

This has great relevance to the large literature on behavior and susceptibility to infectious disease in the human population, which has been presumed to represent the ultimate "stress-related change." Once again, however, animal studies, as well as human studies, do not support such a simple model but rather imply more subtle changes in other neurohormonal/neurotransmitter-mediated immune changes.

Sleep Deprivation (Chronic Stress) and Serum Cortisol/Corticosterone

Note that different stressors, and their longevity, can, as mentioned many times, produce different changes in cortisol levels in humans. Acute stress can produce rapid changes in serum cortisol levels, whereas the effect of sleep deprivation (chronic stress) produces changes in a much slower fashion. In animal models, sleep loss is thought to be more stressful than in humans, and significant alterations in immune responses have been observed after sleep deprivation in mice. Nevertheless, there has been little evidence to suggest a correlation between immune dysfunction and altered serum corticosterone levels in such mice, despite profound alterations in cytokine levels. A similar dichotomy between cytokine changes and cortisol levels has also been reported in humans after exposure to low levels of endotoxin, which increase both cortisol and cytokines (IL-1, TNF, and IL-6).

Role of IL-1 and TNF in Cell Transmigration

There are some studies that can provide insight into the mechanism by which stress can affect immune function. Stress is known to produce profound changes in cellular redistribution/migration. Cell migration from circulation to the tissues occurs, in part, in response to the action of proinflammatory cytokines IL-1 and TNF on the vascular endothelium. IL-1 and TNF trigger biochemical signaling pathways that lead to the expression of adhesion molecules on the vascular endothelium. These adhesion molecules induce cell rolling and margination as a preliminary step to transmigration into the tissues. Recent evidence has now been accumulated for stress-associated changes in cytokine levels (and hence alteration in adhesion molecule expression), which may underlie some of these changes in cell migration.

Effect of Mental Stress and Sleep Deprivation on Cytokine Production

Mental stress has been reported to have an effect in altering cytokine production, including alterations in levels of IL-1, TNF, and IL-1 receptor antagonist (IL-1Ra). IL-1 and TNF are proinflammatory, whereas IL-1Ra competes with IL-1 for the IL-1R binding and so is inhibitory. Similar changes in these cytokines have been reported in medical students after academic stress. In association with the stress of infection there has been reported an association between stress levels and increased IL-6 production, beyond that accorded to infection *per se*.

Sleep deprivation itself, common among students, is a stressor and a modulator of cytokine/chemokine production, perhaps even independent of its stress-associated effects. There is a great deal of evidence indicating a role for the cytokines TNF and IL-1 in the regulation of normal sleep behavior with an association between sleep disruption, cortisol levels and IL-1 in an elderly human population.

Cytokines in Sleep Physiology

Numerous studies in humans have described interactions between cortisol, sleep deprivation, and cytokine changes, and it has been suggested that the activated hypothalamic-pituitary-adrenal (HPA) axis in humans stimulates arousal, whereas IL-1, IL-6, and TNF are possible mediators of excessive daytime sleepiness. Interferon gamma (IFNγ) may interact with TNF in producing altered sleep physiology, whereas more recent data have suggested a potential role for alterations in selected chemokines (CCL4/MIP-1β, but not CCL5/RANTES) in altered sleep in HIV-infected individuals.

Does Behavior Influence Infectious Disease Progression?

In the human field, research in AIDS has provided some additional insight into the possible influence of behavior on infectious disease. A number of studies conducted on asymptomatic HIV-positive subjects before and after notification of HIV-1 antibody status measured immune system function in patients who were or were not involved in aerobic exercise or group, cognitive, or behavioral modification. Those who participated in interventions had lower or minimal decreases in immunologic parameters compared with controls. One model under investigation theorizes that in the absence of aerobic conditioning or behavioral restructuring, a cascade of events (virologic and/or immunologic) occurs that decreases the individual's immunologic endocrine and neuropathic functioning. The patient's overall homeostasis (an interaction of physical and psychosocial factors) is proposed to be a key in preventing the initiation of a downward spiral that culminates in overt presentation of disease.

Effect of Examination Stress on Disease Susceptibility

Interesting and older studies investigated the role of stress on the susceptibility of human populations to infectious disease (influenza in particular). Cohorts of students about to take examinations were found to show enhanced susceptibility to disease, as well as an increased incidence of infection. In other studies, students were shown to have decreases in secretory IgA in saliva during acute examination stress. Again, the actual mechanisms(s) involved remain unknown.

FURTHER READING

Ader R, Cohen N: Behaviorally conditioned immunosuppression. Psychosom Med 37:333, 1975.

Bartels M, et al: Heritability of cortisol levels: Review and simultaneous analysis of twin studies. Psychoneuroimmunology 28:121, 2003.

Beishuizen A, Thijs LG: Endotoxin and the hypothalamo-pituitary-adrenal (HPA) axis. J Endotoxin Res 9:3, 2003.

Caspi A, et al: Influence of life stress on depression: Moderation by a polymorphism in the 5-HT gene. Science 310:291, 2003.

Clement Y, Catatayud F, Beizung C: Genetic basis of anxiety-like behaviour: A critical review. Brain Res Bull 57:57, 2002.

Davis CJ, Harding JW, Wright JW: REM sleep deprivation-induced deficits in the latency-to-peak induction and maintenance of long-term potentiation within the CA1 region of the hippocampus. Brain Res 973:293, 2003.

Dhabhar FS, McEwen BS: Enhancing versus suppressive effects of stress hormones on skin immune function. Proc Natl Acad Sci USA 96:1059, 1999.

Flint J: The genetic basis of neuroticism. Neurosci Biobehav Rev 28:307, 2004.

Hairston IS, et al: Sleep deprivation elevates plasma corticosterone levels in neonatal rats. Neurosci Lett 315:29, 2001.

Irie M, Nagata S, Endo Y: Effect of isolation on classical conditioned histamine release in guinea pigs. Neurosci Biobehav Rev 44:31, 2002.

Irie M, Nagata S, Endo Y: Tasting stress exacerbates classical conditioned histamine release in guinea pigs. Life Sci 72:689, 2002.

Karuagina A, et al: Hypothalamic-pituitary cytokine network. Endocrinology 145:104, 2004.

Katherine I, et al: Genetic screening for susceptibility to depression: Can we and should we? Aust NZ J Psychiatry 38:73, 2004.

Kuo JS, et al: The involvement of glutamate in recall of the conditioned NK cell responses. J Neuroimmunol 118:245, 2001.

Kusnecov AW, King MG, Husband AJ: Synergism of a compound unconditioned stimulus in taste aversion in conditioning. Physiol Behav 39:531, 1987.

Lesserman J: The effects of stressful life events, coping and cortisol on HIV infection. CNS Spectr 8:25, 2003.

Moraska A, et al: Elevated IL-1b contributes to antibody suppression produced by stress. J Appl Physiol 93:207, 2002.

Mouchantaf R, et al: Prosomatostatin is proteolytically processed at the amino terminal segment by subtilase SKI-1. Regul Pept 120:133, 2004.

Murray SE, et al: A genetic model of stress displays decreased lymphocytes and impaired antibody responses without altered susceptibility to *Streptococcus pneumoniae*. J Immunol 167:691, 2001.

Parker K, et al: Neuroendocrine aspects of hypercortisolism in major depression. Horm Behav 43:60, 2003.

Pelligrino TC, Bayer BM: Specific serotonin reuptake inhibitor-induced decreases in lymphocyte activity require endogenous serotonin release. Neuroimmunomodulation 8:179, 2000.

Redwine L, et al: Acute psychological stress: Effects on chemotaxis and cellular adhesion molecule expression. Psychosom Med 65:598, 2003.

Redwine L, et al: Differential immune cell chemotaxis responses to acute psychological stress in Alzheimer caregivers compared to non caregiver controls. Psychosom Med 66:770, 2004.

Shumake J, Gonzalez-Lima F: Brain systems underlying susceptibility to helplessness and depression. Neurosci Rev 2:198, 2003.

Sluyter F, Breivik T, Cools A: Manipulations in maternal environment reverse periodontitis in genetically predisposed rates. 9:931, 2002.

Steiner M, Lepage P, Dunn EJ: Serotonin and gender-specific psychiatric disorders. Int J Psychiatr Clin Pract 1:3, 1997.

Tomas L, et al: Absence of dopamine D4 receptors results in enhanced reactivity to unconditioned, but not conditioned fear. Eur J Neurol 15:158, 2002.

Zubenko GS, et al: Genome-wide linkage survey for genetic loci that influence the development of depressive disorders in families with recurrent, early onset, major depression. Am J Med Genet B Neuropsychiatr Genet 123B:1, 2003.

Reference Values

	Conventional Units (CU)	International Units (IU)	Percent			
			Neut	Lymph	Mono	Eos
Leukocytes						
(Total White Blood Cell)						
Pediatric						
1 year	$6.0\text{-}17.5 \times 10^3/mm^3$	$6.0\text{-}17.5 \times 10^9/L$	31	61	5	3
10 years	$4.5\text{-}13.5 \times 10^3/mm^3$	$5.0\text{-}14.5 \times 10^9/L$	54	38	4	2
Adult	$4.5\text{-}11.0 \times 10^3/mm^3$	$4.5\text{-}11.0 \times 10^9/L$	60	32	4	3
Conversion factor for IU: CU $\times 10^6$						
Note: $mm^3 = \mu L$						
Lymphocytes Total						
Pediatric						
1 year	$4.0\text{-}10.5 \times 10^3/mm^3$	$4.0\text{-}10.5 \times 10^9/L$				
10 years	$1.5\text{-}6.5 \times 10^3/mm^3$	$1.5\text{-}6.5 \times 10^9/L$				
Adult	$1.0\text{-}4.8 \times 10^3/mm^3$	$1.0\text{-}4.8 \times 10^9/L$				
Neutrophils Total						
Pediatric						
1 year	$1.5\text{-}8.5 \times 10^3/mm^3$	$1.5\text{-}8.5 \times 10^9/L$				
10 years	$1.8\text{-}8.0 \times 10^3/mm^3$	$1.8\text{-}8.0 \times 10^9/L$				
Adult	$1.8\text{-}7.7 \times 10^3/mm^3$	$1.8\text{-}7.7 \times 10^9/L$				
Monocytes Total						
Pediatric						
1 year	$0.05\text{-}1.1 \times 10^3/mm^3$	$0.05\text{-}1.1 \times 10^9/L$				
10 years	$0.00\text{-}0.8 \times 10^3/mm^3$	$0.00\text{-}0.8 \times 10^9/L$				
Adult	$0.00\text{-}0.8 \times 10^3/mm^3$	$0.00\text{-}0.8 \times 10^9/L$				
Platelets						
Pediatric						
Infant	$200\text{-}475 \times 10^3/mm^3$	$200\text{-}475 \times 10^9/L$				
Child	$150\text{-}450 \times 10^3/mm^3$	$150\text{-}450 \times 10^9/L$				
Adult	$150\text{-}400 \times 10^3/mm^3$	$150\text{-}400 \times 10^9/L$				

	Conventional Units (CU)	International Units (IU)
Hematocrit		
Vol red cells/Vol whole blood cells		
Pediatric		
6 mo-1yr	30-40%	
4-10 yr	31-43%	
Adult		
Male	42-52%	
Female	37-47%	
Hemoglobin'		
Pediatric		
1 mo	11.0-17.0 g/dL	6.82-10.54 mmol/L
6 mo	10.5-14.5 g/dL	6.51-8.99 mmol/L

	Conventional Units (CU)	International Units (IU)
Adult		
Male	14.0-18.0 g/dL	8.68-11.16 mmol/L
Female	12.0-16.0 g/dL	7.44-9.92 mmol/L

Conversion Factor for IU: CU × 0.62

Red Blood Cells (Range)

Pediatric (1 yr)		
Male	$3.5\text{-}4.9 \times 10^6/mm^3$	$3.5\text{-}4.9 \times 10^{12}/L$
Female	$3.4\text{-}5.0 \times 10^6/mm^3$	$3.5\text{-}5.0 \times 10^{12}/L$
Adult		
Male	$4.3\text{-}5.9 \times 10^6/mm^3$	$4.3\text{-}5.9 \times 10^{12}/L$
Female	$3.5\text{-}5.5 \times 10^6/mm^3$	$3.5\text{-}5.5 \times 10^{12}/L$

Conversion Factor for IU: CU × 10^6

Total Protein (Serum)

Pediatric		
Newborn	4.6-7.6 g/dL	46-76 g/L
Child	6.2-8.0 g/dL	62-80 g/L
Adult	6.0-8.5 g/dL	60-85 g/L

Conversion Factor for IU: CU × 10

Total Protein (Urine)   25-150 mg/24 hr

Serum Immunoglobulin

IgA

Pediatric		
Newborn	0-5 mg/dL	0.00-0.05 g/L
4-6 mo	10-46 mg/dL	0.10-0.46 g/L
6-8 yr	79-169 mg/dL	0.79-1.69 g/L
12-16 yr	85-211 mg/dL	0.85-2.11 g/L
Adult	139-261 mg/dL	1.39-2.61 g/L

Conversion Factor for IU: CU × 0.01

IgG

Pediatric		
Newborn	831-1231 mg/dL	8.31-12.31 g/L
4-6 mo	241-613 mg/dL	2.41-6.13 g/L
6-8 yr	667-1179 mg/dL	6.67-11.79 g/L
12-16 yr	822-1070 mg/dL	8.22-10.70 g/L
Adult	853-1463 mg/dL	8.53-14.63 g/L

IgM

Pediatric		
Newborn	6-16 mg/dL	0.06-0.16 g/L
4-6 mo	26-60 mg/dL	0.26-0.60 g/L
6-8 yr	40-90 mg/dL	0.40-0.90 g/L
12-16 yr	39-79 mg/dL	0.39-0.79 g/L
Adult	72-126 mg/dL	0.72-1.26 g/L

IgE   ± 2 SD   ±2 SD (kU/L) or (U/mL)

Pediatric		
Newborn	21.6 ng/mL	9
6 mo	72.0 ng/mL	30
6 yr	537.6 ng/mL	224
10 yr	787.2 ng/mL	328
Adult	305.8 ng/mL	127

One Mass Unit (U) = 2.4 ng IgE

Albumin (Serum)

Newborn	2.6-4.3 g/dL	26-43 g/L
Child	3.4-6.0 g/dL	34-60 g/L
Adult	3.1-4.3 g/dL	31-43 g/L

Conversion Factor for IU: CU × 10

	Conventional Units (CU)	International Units (IU)
Bilirubin		
(Direct, Conjugated, Soluble)		
Adult	0-0.4 mg/dL	6.85 µmol/L
Conversion Factor for IU: CU × 17.1		
Bilirubin (Total)		
Newborn	<12 mg/dL	<205.2 µmol/L
Adult	0.1-1.0 mg/dL	1.71-17.1 µmol/L
Conversion Factor for IU: CU × 17.1		
Calcium (Total)		
Children	8.0-11.0 mg/dL	2.00-2.75 mmol/L
Adult	8.5-10.5 mg/dL	2.13-2.63 mmol/L
Conversion Factor for IU: CU × 0.025		
Coagulation		
Activated partial thromboplastin time (aPTT)	20-34 sec	
Prothrombin time (PT)	10-13 sec	
International normalized ratio (INR)	2.0-3.0	
Creatinine		
Pediatric		
Child	0.3-0.7 mg/dL	26.52-61.88 µmol/L
Adolescent	0.5-1.0 mg/dL	44.20-88.4 µmol/L
Adult		
Female	0.5-1.2 mg/dL	44.20-106.08 µmol/L
Male	0.6-1.3 mg/dL	53.04-114.92 µmol/L
Conversion Factor for IU: CU × 88.4		
Glucose		
Pediatric	60-115 mg/dL	3.33-6.38 mmol/L
Adult	65-120 mg/dL	3.61-6.66 mmol/L
Conversion Factor for IU: CU × 0.05551		
Transaminases (Serum)		
Aspartate Aminotransferase (AST)		
(Newborn) Pediatric	20-60 U/L	0.34-1.02 µkat/L
Adult		
Male	10-40 U/L	0.17-0.68 µkat/L
Female	9-25 U/L	0.15-0.42 µkat/L
Alanine Aminotransferase (ALT)		
(Newborn) Pediatric	6-40 U/L	0.10-0.68 µkat/L
Adult		
Male	10-55 U/L	0.17-0.94 µkat/L
Female	7-30 U/L	0.12-0.51 µkat/L
IU = 1 µmol/min enzymatic activity for amount of enzyme		
IU = 16.667 × 10⁻⁹ katals (kat)		
Vitamin B_{12} deficiency	<100 pg/mL	<73.83 pmol/L

IU = 1 µmol/min enzymatic activity for amount of enzyme
IU = 16.667×10^{-9} katals (kat)

Conversion Factor for IU: CU × 0.7383
Data from:
Bakerman S, Bakerman P, Strausbuch P: Bakerman's ABC's of Interpretive Laboratory Data, 4th ed. Scottsdale, AZ, Interpretive Laboratory Data, 2002.
Bazaral M, Hamburger RN: Standardization and stability of immunoglobulin E (IgE). J Allergy Clin Immunol 49:189-191, 1972.
Beutler, E, et al (eds): Williams Hematology, 6th ed. New York, McGraw-Hill, 2001.
Kaplan LA, Pesce AJ: Clinical Chemistry. Toronto, Mosby, 1996.
Kratz A, Lewandrowski KB: Case records of the Massachusetts General Hospital. Weekly clinicopathological exercises. Normal reference laboratory values. N Engl J Med 339:1063-1072, 1998.

Multiple Choice Questions

Immunodeficiency Disorders

1. While on hospital rounds the attending physician indicates she was asked to assist in diagnosis of a child who has a range of medical problems, including decreased pigmentation of the skin and eyes, a history of recurrent and severe bacterial and viral infections, and a bleeding abnormality. She suggests that tests for giant granules, platelet dense bodies, and DNA analysis of the LYST gene might be informative. What defect was suspected?

    A. Chronic granulomatous disease

    B. Chronic mucocutaneous candidiasis

    C. Reticular dysgenesis

    D. Chédiak-Higashi syndrome

    E. Chronic myelogenous leukemia

2. HJ is a 4-year-old boy with recurrent sinus infections over the past few years. In preparation for a planned trip to the Far East he began a series of vaccinations with recombinant hepatitis B vaccine. Before the third vaccination, you test his titer of IgG antibody (from the previous immunizations) to assess the efficacy of the vaccination and find he has extraordinarily low titers (barely above the nonimmune level), with relatively high IgM titers. You would expect him also to

    A. Show generalized immunodeficiency

    B. Develop an immune response to pneumococcal polysaccharide vaccine

    C. Develop normal IgG responses to the Sabin poliovirus

    D. Generate IgG-dependent antibody-dependent cell-mediated cytotoxicity responses

    E. Generate a normal immune response to helminths

3. Chronic passive immunoglobulin administration is a reasonable therapy for all of the following immunodeficiency disorders EXCEPT:

    A. Bruton's type hypogammaglobulinemia

    B. Transient hypogammaglobulinemia of infancy

    C. IgG deficiency with high IgM

    D. Hypogammaglobulinemia

    E. Selective IgA deficiency

4. Peter is a 16-year-old boy whom you have seen in consultation for repeated episodes of spontaneous swelling of the lips over the past 3 to 5 years. Increased vascular permeability and edema play a role in this swelling, which is linked to a genetic defect in a complement regulatory protein. A deficiency in which one of the following would lead to these symptoms?

    A. C1 esterase inhibitor

    B. Anaphylatoxin inhibitor

    C. Factor D

    D. Properdin

    E. Factor H

5. A young infant in the Children's Hospital has been diagnosed with Omenn syndrome, a disorder in which recombinase genes RAG-1 and RAG-2 are mutated, or not expressed. These proteins would normally trigger

    A. Somatic mutation

    B. Isotype switching

    C. Alternative splicing

    D. Somatic recombination

    E. Memory cell formation

6. JD is an 8-year-old boy in your practice who has had a surprisingly high (eight) number of severe recurrent bacterial and fungal infections. Although each of these has responded to the appropriate medication, you are concerned to find the underlying cause of his problem. Routine analyses of serum immunoglobulins, B cell, and T cell counts (and function) showed no clear abnormality. Further testing revealed a dysfunction in phagocytosis such that ingested organisms were not totally destroyed. On the basis of this test, the physician explained to the family that RD had a genetic defect in an enzyme that was required to produce reactive oxygen intermediates. The most likely protein defect was in

    A. Cytochrome P450

    B. Lysosomal enzymes

    C. Inducible nitric oxide synthase

    D. CH50 test

    E. NADPH oxidase

7. A group of children with MHC class II deficiency form a cohort examined at two pediatric immunology units. Infections prompting diagnosis included those from both viruses and bacteria. Fungal infections, mainly candidiasis, were present in two thirds of the children and in half of these directly contributed to their death. Most of the children who were treated died, even with a bone marrow transplant. What disorder was most likely common to these patients?

   A. Severe combined immunodeficiency

   B. Systemic lupus erythematosus

   C. Bare lymphocyte syndrome

   D. Chronic mucocutaneous candidiasis

   E. Bruton's agammaglobulinemia

8. Three-year-old Johnny gets burned in a home accident and requires extensive skin grafting. The attending physician believes that Johnny will tolerate the graft with little (or no) immunosuppressive drugs because the child has an immunodeficiency disorder. Johnny most likely has

   A. DiGeorge syndrome

   B. Chronic mucocutaneous candidiasis

   C. X-linked agammaglobulinemia

   D. Chédiak-Higashi syndrome

   E. Chronic granulomatous disease

9. Peter is now 2 years old and has been well until being admitted to the hospital with two tender, swollen lumps in his groin. These are found to be staphylococcal-induced abscesses, and live bacteria are found to be present in phagocytic cells from the lesion. The numbers and appearance of circulating lymphocytes, leukocytes, and immunoglobulin levels are normal, as is the CH50 test. From what condition is Peter most likely to be suffering?

   A. Reticular dysgenesis

   B. Chronic granulomatous disease

   C. C5 deficiency

   D. C1 inhibitor deficiency

   E. Severe combined immunodeficiency

10. You are asked to provide a consult in the intensive care unit for a young girl with a documented episode of infection with *Neisseria meningitidis*. No family history is available (the girl was adopted), but review of her medical record from a forwarding hospital reveals an otherwise previously well child with three other episodes of *Neisseria* infection over 2 years. Which of the following is not a possible explanation of these findings?

   A. Low C3

   B. Low C6-C8

   C. Absent factor D

   D. Absent C1 inhibitor

   E. Low C5

11. A boy in your practice is born who is diagnosed with DiGeorge syndrome. DiGeorge syndrome is also called thymic aplasia (failure of the thymus to develop naturally), thymic hypoplasia (defective development of tissue), or third and fourth pharyngeal arch or pouch syndrome. Pathologically, the absence or incomplete development of the thymus characterizes DiGeorge syndrome. You would NOT expect this patient to have an increased incidence of infection with

    A. Viruses

    B. Fungi

    C. Parasites

    D. Intracellular bacteria

    E. Gram-negative bacteria (lipopolysaccharide)

12. A 20-year-old female diabetic, with hypothyroidism and irregular menses, complains of a chronic, recurrent rash for 6 months, with adherent white plaques in the mouth. There is no family history of immunodeficiency disorders, no history of connective tissue diseases, no travel, and no history of drug abuse. Purified protein derivative (PPD) testing is positive (she was exposed to *Mycobacterium tuberculosis* when working on an Indian reservation 4 years ago). Serum immunoglobulin, complement levels, and white blood cell counts were normal. She is possibly suffering from

    A. Selective IgM deficiency

    B. Chronic mucocutaneous candidiasis

    C. DiGeorge syndrome

    D. Chronic granulomatous disease

    E. Common variable immunodeficiency

13. John, a 14-month-old boy with severe gram-positive bacterial pneumonia, is referred to the Children's Hospital by the family physician. This is his third such infection in 4 months. He has two healthy sisters aged 3 and 5 years. The family lost a boy at 10 months of age to bacterial pneumonia 6 years ago. The family doctor has sent along some blood test results that show low serum immunoglobulin levels (all classes), few B cells, but normal numbers and functioning of T cells. Which one of the following is the most likely diagnosis?

A. X-linked hypogammaglobulinemia

B. Common variable hypogammaglobulinemia

C. Transient hypogammaglobulinemia of infancy

D. CD40 genetic defect

E. Severe combined immunodeficiency

14. A 25-year-old woman went to see her physician complaining of being tired and run down. Because of her lack of energy, she had given up her regular exercise program, a routine she had maintained for a number of years. Until a year ago she had been very active and considered herself in excellent physical condition. However, in the last year she had experienced several protracted colds and three vaginal yeast infections, which had not previously been a problem. During the physical examination the physician noted that several of her lymph nodes were enlarged, yet no present infection was evident. She admits to multiple sexual partners, and since she uses birth control pills she never uses condoms. The general practitioner ordered a series of tests to measure her immune system. Her tests revealed a lower than normal CD4+ T cell count. What type of infection would manifest in this manner?

A. HIV infection

B. Any virus

C. Bacterial

D. Fungal

E. Parasitic

15. In 1996 five young adults with a form of chronic granulomatous disease underwent gene therapy because they could not synthesize an essential subunit protein of the NADPH oxidase complex. In this clinical trial, white blood cells were removed from each patient and then the normal gene encoding the subunit protein of NADPH oxidase was inserted into these cells. The genetically altered cells were returned to the patients. When activated, the genetically altered phagocytes would produce molecules that they were unable to produce before the genetic alteration. One such molecule would be

A. Nitric oxide

B. Defensins

C. Hydrogen peroxide

D. Lactoferrin

E. Lysozyme

16. Sam weighed 7 pounds at birth and appeared the picture of health. He received vaccines normally given to North American children before he was 6 months of age and had no adverse reactions when immunized. At about 6 months of age, he became sick, lost weight, and developed severe diarrhea, accompanied by fever. In addition, he developed large white patches in his mouth (thrush) and had several episodes of ear infection (otitis media). Laboratory tests indicated normal serum immunoglobulins; normal numbers of B cells, natural killer cells, and CD8+ T cells; and marked abnormally low number of CD4+ T cells. What is a possible diagnosis?

A. Severe combined immunodeficiency

B. Acquired immunodeficiency syndrome

C. Chronic granulomatous disease

D. Leukocyte adhesion defect

E. X-linked agammaglobulinemia

17. A genetic disorder in which CD18, the β chain of integrins expressed on naive T cells, is not expressed on the cell surface would prevent which one of the following interactions between antigen-presenting cells and CD4+ T cells?

A. CD40/CD40L

B. CD80/CD28

C. MHC class II/CD4

D. ICAM-2/LFA-1

E. CD86/CD28

18. *Trypanosoma cruzi*, an obligate intracellular protozoan parasite, is the causative agent of Chagas' disease. This parasite invades a variety of cell types and replicates within the cytoplasm. Studies with knockout mice have shown that genetic defects in inducible nitric oxide synthase result in increased parasitic burden. You might anticipate a similar increase in parasite burden to be observed in mice with a mutation in one of the following receptors for

A. TGFβ

B. IFNγ

C. IL-10

D. IFNα

E. IL-6

19. The development of molecular genetics technology has revolutionized the study of many biologic processes. For example, genes can be inactivated at the level of the embryo to generate what is called "knockout" mice. Based on our present knowledge of B cell development, which one of the following steps in B cell maturation would not occur if the delta (δ) heavy chain constant gene was "knocked out"?

A. Somatic recombination of VDJ for the heavy chain

B. Somatic recombination of VJ for the light chain

C. Transcription of the pseudo light chain

D. Tolerance induction

E. Alternative splicing

20. SD, a 5-year-old child, has a history of pneumonia, sinusitis, and ear infection. The recurrent sinopulmonary infections responded well to antibiotics. Laboratory testing revealed that the serum levels of all antibody isotypes were normal except for IgA, which was undetectable. SD was diagnosed with "selective IgA deficiency." An appropriate therapeutic intervention for this patient would be regular prophylactic injections of

A. IgG

B. IgM

C. IgA

D. IVIG (all isotypes)

E. none of the above

21. Ms. D, a 40-year-old Native American, previously well, presents with a 4-month history of low-grade fever, cough, and weight loss. Blood work, including serum immunoglobulins and complement levels are normal. Urinalysis is normal. This would be a typical presentation of which form of immunodeficiency disorder/disease?

A. Severe combined immunodeficiency

B. Selective IgA deficiency

C. Complement disorders

D. Acquired deficiency (e.g., tuberculosis)

E. Leukocyte adhesion defect

22. The evolution of *Mycobacterium tuberculosis* as an intracellular pathogen has led to a complex relationship between it and its host, the human mononuclear phagocyte. The products of *M. tuberculosis*–specific T cells are essential for macrophage activation for intracellular mycobacterial killing. Which one of the following cytokines is most effective at activating macrophages to become super killers?

A. IL-2

B. IFNγ

C. IL-4

D. TGFβ

E. IL-10

23. A young mother living in Africa is HIV positive and has just given birth to a baby girl. As her physician you are to advise her whether to breast feed her infant. Because this is a region in Africa where many children die of gastrointestinal infections, you are in a dilemma as to what to advise. Furthermore, you know that breast feeding has been shown to be protective for the infant. Breast feeding protects the infant from infections because the mother's _____ are passively acquired by the nursing infant.

A. IgA antibodies (secretory IgA)

B. IgM antibodies

C. IgE antibodies

D. Natural killer cells

E. Hemagglutinins

24. A 5-year-old boy has been seen repeatedly by his physician for bacterial infections that have only been successfully resolved with treatment with antibiotics. These infections have consistently produced multiple and disseminated granulomas. The patient has high levels of serum antibody specific for various bacteria. The blood cell count is normal. A defect in which one of the following is consistent with these observations?

A. B cells

B. CD4+ T cells

C. NADPH oxidase

D. Complement

E. Inducible nitric oxide synthase

ANSWERS FOR IMMUNODEFICIENCY DISORDERS QUESTIONS

Questions	Answer choice	Questions	Answer choice
1.	D	13.	A
2.	B	14.	A
3.	E	15.	C
4.	A	16.	B
5.	D	17.	D
6.	E	18.	B
7.	C	19.	E
8.	A	20.	E
9.	B	21.	D
10.	D	22.	B
11.	E	23.	A
12.	B	24.	B

Hypersensitivity Reactions

1. A 19-year-old man is rushed to your emergency department from a local Chinese restaurant, after becoming acutely "ill" while eating shrimp. He is pale, cool, and clammy and has a low blood pressure. There is no medic-alert bracelet to be seen. You find he has wheezes throughout his lung fields, with poor air intake. His sister, who is with him, says this has never happened before, and no one in the family has ever been like this. The most likely reason for this reaction is

   A. Acute rejection of something he has eaten

   B. Delayed hypersensitivity reaction to something previously eaten

   C. Acute hypersensitivity reaction (anaphylaxis)

   D. Serum sickness

   E. Anxiety

2. Eosinophilia (increase in number of eosinophils) is a characteristic feature of a number of pathologic conditions, including parasitic infections. To understand the role of various cytokines in this process, "knockout" mice have been generated and then challenged with *Trichinella spiralis*, a parasite. You would predict that knocking out the gene for which one of the following cytokines would result in the greatest increase in parasitic burden and poor patient prognosis?

   A. IL-1

   B. IL-2

   C. IL-3

   D. IL-4

   E. IL-5

3. All the following are type III hypersensitivity reactions EXCEPT

   A. Hemolytic disease of the newborn

   B. Farmer's lung

   C. Rheumatoid arthritis

   D. Serum sickness

   E. Systemic lupus erythematosus

4. While playing tennis on a warm day a young man felt a wasp on his arm and brushed it off, but still received a mild sting, which he ignored. Ten minutes later he felt dizzy and began to itch under his arms and on his scalp. When he broke out in hives and felt tightness in his chest, he headed for the hospital. On the way he felt cold and clammy and collapsed on the seat of the taxi. In the emergency department his pulse was barely detectable. Which one of the following treatments is most appropriate at this time?

   A. Cromolyn sodium

   B. Epinephrine

   C. Penicillin

   D. Antihistamines

   E. Anticoagulant

5. Susan, ABO blood type "O," has chronic anemia and has received washed red blood cell transfusions for "chronic" anemia of "undetermined etiology." While she receives this last transfusion, she develops fever, abdominal pain, and hypotension. You stop the transfusion, and treat appropriately. The call from the laboratory confirms an error in matching. This immune reaction is a typical hypersensitivity reaction designated

   A. Type I
   B. Type II
   C. Type III
   D. Type IV

6. You are doing a follow-up evaluation on a young man for blood in the urine after a seemingly innocent upper respiratory viral infection. When an acute deterioration in some of his renal function tests occurs, you ask for a renal biopsy. This shows signs of immune complex deposition along the basement membrane as a result of excessive numbers of circulating antigen/antibody complexes. This patient is likely experiencing a

   A. Type IV hypersensitivity reaction
   B. Type III hypersensitivity reaction
   C. Type II hypersensitivity reaction
   D. Type I hypersensitivity reaction

7. A 28-year-old woman is seen in your office with complaints of fatigue, shortness of breath on exertion, and general loss of appetite over the last 8 to 10 months following a flu-like illness. Routine blood work shows a significant anemia (hemoglobin less than 50% of normal) and a positive Coombs' test. A likely diagnosis is

   A. Type I hypersensitivity
   B. Type II hypersensitivity
   C. Type III hypersensitivity
   D. Type IV hypersensitivity

8. A patient with a history of "wheezing" sees you because of chronically itchy skin, with some intermittent reddened and raised areas of the skin. Blood work shows a low-grade eosinophilia. You would not be surprised to find all of the following in this person EXCEPT:

   A. Multiple positive reactions to allergen testing
   B. Elevated serum IgE
   C. Elevated production of IL-4
   D. Elevated production of IL-5
   E. Elevated IFNγ

9. A patient who sustained a severe snakebite was brought to the emergency department. He was given equine antivenom gamma globulin and responded well to treatment. Within 5 days, the patient developed a slight fever and hives. This patient is likely beginning to experience a reaction consistent with which one of the following:

   A. Type I hypersensitivity
   B. Type II hypersensitivity
   C. Type III hypersensitivity
   D. Type IV hypersensitivity

10. Ms. Allen has experienced generalized fatigue, pallor, and intermittent chest pains of 4 months' duration. She has been taking a new medication over this time and she is now found to be profoundly anemic. These findings are most consistent with

   A. New-onset rheumatoid arthritis
   B. Antibodies binding to the drug (hapten) on red blood cells
   C. Pneumonia
   D. Anxiety disorder
   E. Antibodies binding to glycophorin on red blood cells

ANSWERS FOR HYPERSENSITIVITY REACTIONS QUESTIONS

Questions	Answer choice	Questions	Answer choice
1.	C	6.	B
2.	E	7.	B
3.	A	8.	E
4.	B	9.	C
5.	B	10.	B

Autoimmunity

1. You are in the process of developing novel antibodies for use in autoimmune disorders. After extensive studies in patients with multiple sclerosis (MS), you conclude that a major (unknown) antigen incites expansion of a family of Vβ8 T cells. You believe that infusion of anti-Vβ8 antibodies would benefit the patient because the treatment would eliminate

   A. Only the CD4+ T cell and CD8+ T cell clones specific for the MS antigens

   B. Only Vβ8 CD4+ T cells irrespective of specificity

   C. Only Vβ8 CD8+ T cells irrespective of specificity

   D. Several clones of Vβ8 CD8+ T cells and CD4+ T cells irrespective of the specificity

   E. Only Vβ8 CD4+ T cell clones specific for the MS antigens

2. Three hundred thirty-nine patients with active rheumatoid arthritis were given a placebo or CTLA4Ig at 10-mg/kg body weight. Treatment with CTLA4Ig was well tolerated and patients showed statistically significant improvement in all scales of outcome measures. (All 339 patients received methotrexate as well.) With which molecule(s) would this soluble fusion protein bind on antigen-presenting cells?

   A. CD80

   B. CD86

   C. B7-1

   D. B7-2

   E. All of the above

3. Rheumatoid arthritis is a systemic inflammatory disease that causes joint damage and disability. Current therapies target the products of activated macrophages (tumor necrosis factor [TNF] and interleukin-1 [IL-1]). Both IL-1 and TNF play an important role in the recruitment of neutrophils and monocytes to the site of inflammation. One of the most widely accepted therapies is a genetically engineered protein that "mops up" TNF. Which disease recurs in some individuals using this form of therapy?

   A. Inflammatory bowel disease

   B. Gram-negative pneumonia

   C. Tuberculosis

   D. Rheumatoid arthritis

   E. Influenza infections

4. Brenda is a 25-year-old married African American. Over the last 5 months she has noticed increasing swelling in her legs and she has had intermittent severe headaches, unrelated to menses. Also, she has noticed that her urine is dark and "frothy," which when tested indicated the presence of protein (creatinine) and red blood cells. Despite her and her husband's wishes, she has been unable to conceive for 5 years and has had three spontaneous first-trimester abortions. Laboratory testing indicated several autoantibodies, including anti-DNA, anti-platelet, anti-leukocyte, and anti-phospholipid. Which one of the following complement proteins/tests would not be decreased during the active stage of disease?

   A. C3

   B. C4

   C. CH50 test

   D. Factor B

   E. C2

5. You are evaluating a 43-year-old patient who has requested a reversal of his vasectomy. He has high levels of anti-sperm antibodies. The reason underlying the production of these autoantibodies is most likely to be:

   A. Cross-reacting antibodies following a viral infection

   B. Release of sequestered antigen as a result of the vasectomy

   C. Polyclonal activation following ingestion of kidney beans

   D. Polyclonal activation due to superantigen

   E. Inappropriate class II MHC expression on antigen-presenting cells

6. A young man comes into your office with complaints of intermittent hemoptysis for 2 months, associated with some blood in his urine. He is a nonsmoker and was previously in excellent health. He also describes a weight gain (10 lb) over the past 3 weeks, with "puffy eyes" in the morning. Sample blood work reveals a profoundly elevated serum creatinine concentration. Lung biopsy shows serum immunoglobulin on basement membranes. These symptoms are suggestive of

   A. Acute myocardial infarction

   B. Goodpasture's' syndrome

   C. Graves' disease

   D. DiGeorge syndrome

7. You are treating a patient with multiple sclerosis. A number of novel treatments are under consideration for autoimmune disorders and included in these are oral "feeding" of the putative disease-inciting agent, in this case myelin-associated antigen. The scientific rationale for this therapy includes all of the following EXCEPT

A. Oral immunization can induce tolerance

B. Oral immunization may reverse a presumed Th1/Th2 imbalance in autoimmunity

C. Multiple sclerosis is known to be caused by dietary deficiencies

D. Oral immunization can increase levels of immuno-suppressive cytokines

8. Judy, who is only 24, has had recurrent hot flashes over the past 6 months. Her appetite and energy level have increased, although she has not gained weight. She notices her heart beating faster quite frequently. Her blood glucose concentration is normal, but she notices her eyes seem to be "bulging." Which of the following is likely to help in making a diagnosis?

A. Check urine for sugar

B. Measure serum cortisol

C. Measure levels of T3 and T4

D. Shilling test

E. CH50 test

9. Mrs. Jenkins, a 32-year-old African American, consulted with her physician with complaints of malaise, lethargy, and body aches. During the interview with the physician it became clear that her body aches and lethargy had been coming on for some time. The body aches seem to involve both joints and muscles and could not be localized to any specific part of the body. Mrs. Jenkins was also concerned about her weight loss and a red raised patchy rash on her face. Office urinalysis reveals significant proteins in the urine. Which of the following diseases would you suspect?

A. Systemic lupus erythematosus

B. Myasthenia gravis

C. Chronic fatigue syndrome

D. Acquired immunodeficiency syndrome

E. Graves' disease

10. XP is a 60-year-old woman who has had erosive deforming rheumatoid arthritis for 20 years. Rheumatoid arthritis is an inflammatory condition. XP has failed all conventional treatments (including anti-inflammatory medications, gold, and methotrexate). You are considering her for inclusion in a clinical trial. Which one of the following antibody therapies would you not consider?

A. Anti-TNF

B. Anti-IL-1

C. Anti-IFNγ

D. Anti-IL-12

E. Anti-IL-10

ANSWERS FOR AUTOIMMUNITY QUESTIONS

Questions	Answer choice	Questions	Answer choice
1.	D	6.	B
2.	E	7.	C
3.	C	8.	C
4.	D	9.	A
5.	B	10.	E

Tumor Immunology

1. Cytokine secretion by CD4+ T cells and CD8+ T cells isolated from 12 patients with prostate cancer and 7 healthy subjects was measured. An increase in IL-10 expression and a decrease in IL-2 expression was observed in patients with prostate cancer but not in healthy subjects. Based on these results a polarization toward which one of the following cells would you suspect?

   A. Th1
   B. Th2
   C. Tc1
   D. Th0
   E. NK

2. Your patient, a 60-year-old previously healthy man, presents with fatigue (×4 months), weight loss, and abdominal fullness over the same period. The physician's presumptive diagnosis is chronic myelogenous leukemia. If the physician is correct, laboratory/cytogenic tests would reveal

   A. No abnormalities
   B. Translocation between chromosomes 9 and 22
   C. Decreased white blood cell count
   D. Decreased platelet count
   E. Expression of ZAP-70 in B cells

3. Your patient with choriocarcinoma is found to have increased βhCG levels. Treatment with methotrexate leads to a decrease in these levels. At about 4 weeks of treatment the levels begin to rise. This is most consistent with

   A. Tumor recurrence
   B. Smoking cessation
   C. Random laboratory error
   D. Normal pregnancy

4. A patient with B cell lymphoma is receiving therapy aimed at targeting the (unique) surface immunoglobulin expressed on his tumor cells. Used in this way, the immunoglobulin is an example of

   A. An oncofetal antigen
   B. A virally induced tumor antigen
   C. Tumor-specific antigen
   D. Tumor-associated antigen

5. You are a family physician for a patient with melanoma who has failed all conventional therapy. She asks that you inform her of available "novel" options currently being explored. Included in these are all of the following EXCEPT

   A. Transfecting tumor cells with the IL-2 gene and re-infusion
   B. Transfecting tumor cells with the TNFα gene and re-infusion
   C. Culturing tumor cells alone and re-infusion along with immunosuppressive drugs
   D. Culturing tumor infiltrating lymphocytes (TIL) and re-infusion to the patient

6. CEA is found to be elevated in cancer of the gastrointestinal tract, as well as in breast tissue, stomach, and some lung cancers and in patients with emphysema. Its expression is also increased in a number of nonspecific diseases of the gastrointestinal tract. John's religious beliefs prevent him from drinking alcoholic beverages. He is an ex-smoker. After resection of a primary bowel cancer, you decide to follow CEA levels because

   A. CEA is useful for monitoring tumor recurrence in this scenario
   B. CEA levels will predict if he has begun smoking again
   C. Increased CEA levels will predict new-onset hepatic cirrhosis
   D. A rise then a fall in CEA levels after surgery predicts metastasis

7. Bob has had a malignancy for a number of years now and is not doing well. He wishes to have experimental therapy at a large teaching hospital. His physician explains to him that he is going to remove his macrophages and transfect them with a gene that will cause increased expression of class I MHC. This should result in an increased percentage of tumor killing by

   A. NK cells
   B. CTL cells
   C. Both NK and CTL cells
   D. Neither NK nor CTL cells
   E. Macrophages

8. One immunotherapy for renal carcinoma requires the culturing of cells obtained from tumor resection. When these cells are generated in the presence of the appropriate cytokine, LAK cells are generated. This cytokine is

   A. IL-1
   B. IL-2
   C. IL-3
   D. IL-4
   E. IL-5

9. Lung cancer cells often metastasize (spread) from the lung to the brain. These cells enter the blood circulation and enter tissues at the new site. Which one of the following would NOT be a consideration in selecting therapies to block the entry of cancer cells into the tissues?

   A. Antibodies that block adhesion molecules

   B. A fusion protein (Enbrel) that binds TNF

   C. Anti-IL-1 Fab_2 fragments

   D. Liposomes carrying the gene for kallikrein

   E. Antibodies to selected chemokines

10. A 44-year-old male friend is newly diagnosed with CLL (B-cell chronic lymphocytic leukemia). He hears that there may be a new treatment available using anti-idiotype vaccination. This treatment is based on the infusion of antibodies that recognize

    A. T cell β chain

    B. T cell α chain

    C. Sequence within Fc region

    D. Sequence within Fab region

    E. $Fc\alpha$ receptors

ANSWERS FOR TUMOR IMMUNOLOGY QUESTIONS

Questions	Answer choice	Questions	Answer choice
1.	B	6.	A
2.	B	7.	B
3.	A	8.	B
4.	C	9.	D
5.	C	10.	D

Transplantation

1. Pat had a heart transplant 5 years ago. At her last follow-up appointment (2 weeks ago) she was stable, with a normal cardiogram, and had had no change in her medications for 2 years. She has had no signs of rejection (as determined by protocol biopsy) in 4 years. She is maintained on low doses of prednisone and cyclosporine. She was admitted to the hospital last night with symptoms suggestive of a stroke. You believe this is most likely an effect of

   A. Second-hand smoke

   B. Her recent (3 years ago) decision to switch to a vegetarian diet

   C. A side effect of the long-term prednisone treatment

   D. An acute rejection episode

   E. Chronic rejection

2. A patient on your transplant service is enrolled in a study designed to investigate levels of cytokines produced during various stages of transplantation/acceptance/rejection. A patient showing elevated levels of IL-2 in the grafted organ would most likely be undergoing

   A. "A healing in" process associated with a graft acceptance

   B. Acute graft rejection

   C. Cytotoxic reaction to immunosuppressive drugs

   D. Systemic infection

   E. Hyperacute rejection

3. A child receives a bone marrow transplant from an HLA-identical sibling. After successful engraftment, 3 weeks later the child has diarrhea and a rash on the palms and soles of the feet, spreading to the trunk, with jaundice. Administration of an anti–T cell serum plus cyclosporine produces improvement. What is the most likely cause?

   A. Inadequate numbers of donor cells were transfused

   B. Reaction of donor lymphocytes with antigens on the recipient's cells

   C. Long-term effects of original drug ingestion

   D. Viral infection (CMV)

   E. Failure of graft to "take"

4. A patient of yours returns to the intensive care unit from the operating room after her third renal transplant in the past 10 years. The two previous grafts failed as a result of chronic rejection. Thirty minutes later she complains of severe abdominal cramps, has a fever, and becomes

hypotensive (low blood pressure). She is returned immediately to the operating room. She is not bleeding, but her graft shows extensive thrombosis. She did not receive transfusion during the surgery. What is the most likely explanation?

A. Acute rejection

B. Graft versus host reaction

C. Hyperacute rejection

D. Chronic rejection because she is now conditioned to this type of rejection

E. Type I hypersensitivity reaction

5. A patient on your transplant service, a recipient of a kidney graft last year who has been on immunosuppressive therapy, has complained of vague abdominal pain for several months. She has had multiple investigations to ensure her graft is functioning well with no evidence of rejection. A recent CT scan of the abdomen suggests a mass in the liver. Biopsy evidence would most likely indicate which type of cancer?

A. Lymphoma

B. Retinoblastoma

C. Wilms' tumor

D. Neurofibromatosis

E. Colon cancer

6. MB recently received an HLA-matched bone marrow transplant for treatment of acute leukemia. While initial blood work after transplantation suggested a good reconstitution of the T cell component of his immune system, over the following days he develops a general lethargy, some jaundice, and a significant desquamating rash. You suspect that you are dealing with a so-called acute graft versus host disease (GvHD) reaction. Which one of the following cytokines is unlikely to be associated with acute GvHD?

A. IFNγ

B. TNFα

C. IL-2

D. IL-4

E. IL-1

7. A baboon heart has just been transplanted into one of your patients. She develops a fever, myalgias, and diffuse chest pain within 2 hours of surgery. Which of the following is the most likely explanation for her problem? These are signs of

A. Hyperacute autograft rejection response

B. Acute allograft rejection response

C. Chronic isograft rejection

D. Hyperacute rejection of a xenograft

E. Chronic allograft rejection

8. A 3-month-old boy with X-linked severe combined immunodeficiency (XSCID) has been transplanted with bone marrow from his 2-year-old sister. She shares 2/4 HLA-A and B-loci and is mismatched at 2/4 HLA-DP and DR loci. Three weeks later he becomes unwell, with diarrhea, sloughing of his skin, an erythematous rash over his body, and tender, swollen feet. His lymphocyte count has been steadily rising since 1 week after transplant. What do you suspect?

A. Acute rejection of the graft

B. Host versus graft disease

C. Graft versus host disease

D. Failure of transplant to take; the symptoms are due to the death of transplanted marrow cells

E. Epstein-Barr virus (human herpesvirus 4) infection

9. John is 4 weeks post renal transplant, undergoing an episode of acute rejection. Appropriate treatment might include all of the following EXCEPT

A. Cyclosporine

B. Tacrolimus

C. Anti–IL-10 antibody

D. Anti-CD3 antibody

E. Anti–IL-2 receptor antibody

10. Xenotransplantation is an emerging medical technology that offers promise for the treatment of human diseases. Transplantation of pig hearts into humans, however, requires that genes encoding human complement proteins are introduced into the pig (transgenic pigs). These proteins would protect the transplanted pig heart from damage resulting from complement activation immediately after grafting. The human genes selected would most likely be

A. Anaphylatoxin inhibitor and properdin

B. Factor B and factor D

C. Properdin and CD4bp

D. CD59 and decay accelerating factor

E. Factor I and factor D

ANSWERS FOR TRANSPLANTATION QUESTIONS

Questions	Answer choice	Questions	Answer choice
1.	C	6.	D
2.	B	7.	D
3.	B	8.	C
4.	C	9.	C
5.	A	10.	D

Immunization

1. A young mother receives a tetanus/diphtheria toxoid booster immunization in the fourth month of her pregnancy. The child is breast fed from birth. At 2 days of age the child has IgG antibody titers against both of these toxoids. There is no IgM or IgA anti-tetanus or anti-diphtheria toxoid titer. This is an example of which ONE of the following:

   A. Active immunization of the child because of its exposure to the toxoids when the mother received the booster

   B. A combination of active and passive immunization of the child

   C. Passive immunization attributable to maternal antibody crossing the placenta

   D. The result is incorrect because the child has not had time to develop antibodies of any type at this age.

   E. The result is incorrect because most antibody in the serum at that age comes from colostrum, which is high in IgA.

2. Bruce has received surgical nephrectomy for a renal cell carcinoma. He is about to undergo an experimental treatment protocol in which some of his dendritic cells are removed and allowed to endocytose the isolated tumor cells. When these cells are re-injected into the patient, the dendritic cells will present tumor antigens to T cells. This is an example of

   A. Shamanism

   B. Passive immunotherapy

   C. Active immunotherapy

   D. Passive vaccination

   E. Conventional chemotherapy

3. A vaccine is being developed for trials in HIV infection. In recent studies it is found that a novel molecule isolated from the viral coat protein stimulates CD4+ Th2 production in monkeys and in human volunteers. However, when immunized animals are challenged they remain fully susceptible to infection, and the "leader" of the clinical trials group concludes this molecule will not be valuable. One explanation for why the animals are not protected is that immunization with a viral coat protein does not stimulate

   A. CD8+ T cell immunity

   B. B cell immunity

   C. NK cell reactivity

   D. Antigen-presenting cells

   E. Thp cells specific for viral coat protein

4. Adam is the son of a missionary working in Africa, where infections with *Mycobacterium tuberculosis* are rampant. As protection, immunization with *Mycobacterium bovis* was recommended for the family. Adam was not immunized because previous testing had determined that he had a deficiency of a particular cytokine receptor. Which cytokine receptor was most likely deficient?

   A. IL-4R

   B. TGFβ-R

   C. IFNγ-R

   D. IFNα/β-R

   E. IL-10-R

5. CK is a virologist who has been recruited to Zaire to work for 6 weeks as a volunteer because a severe hemorrhagic disease has broken out there. The suspected organism is the Ebola virus. Although CK has received all appropriate immunization, there is no vaccine available for protection against Ebola. Therefore, in addition to bringing protective gear, CK receives an injection of antibodies pooled from individuals who have recovered from the disease. The pooled antibodies, which should protect CK during his entire stay in Zaire, are of which isotype?

A. IgA

B. IgG

C. IgE

D. IgD

E. IgE

6. The administration of vaccines is not without hazard. Which one of the following vaccines is least likely to affect adversely an immunocompromised host?

A. Recombinant hepatitis B protein

B. Bacille Calmette-Guérin (BCG)

C. Sabin polio

D. Salk polio

E. Measles

7. Joan is a 17-year-old girl who comes to your emergency department in the terminal stages of delivery. You determine this to be an uneventful pregnancy (she is now 39 weeks of gestation). She has had essentially no antenatal care. She delivered a healthy baby boy, and the delivery itself is uncomplicated. You order the nurse to give Joan an injection of RhoGam. The rationale for this is that you are concerned that the

A. Mother is Rh– and the baby is Rh+

B. Father is Rh+ and the baby is Rh–

C. Mother is Rh+ and the baby is Rh–

D. Father is Rh– and the baby is Rh+

E. Father and the baby are both Rh–, while the mother is Rh+

8. A cancer patient needs immunoprophylaxis against possible hepatitis B virus exposure. You decide on antibody prophylaxis followed by active hepatitis B virus immunization. All the following are correct EXCEPT:

A. This represents an example of passive immunization.

B. Any transferred IgM (high-molecular-weight aggregate) must be given intramuscularly to avoid complement activation.

C. Hepatitis B immune globulin is ineffective after acute exposure.

D. Hepatitis B vaccine immunization should be given at a different site from administration of hepatitis B immune globulin.

9. A heroin addict, in her last month of pregnancy, is diagnosed with a right lower lobe pneumonia. Response leads to the formation of IgG antibodies. The fetus would be immunologically protected when born owing to

A. Active artificial immunity

B. Active natural immunity

C. Passive natural immunity

D. Passive artificial immunity

E. No protection of the fetus would occur.

10. Jane, a 15-month-old infant, was brought to her family practice clinic for her routine well-child examination. During the course of the office visit, Jane received her first measles immunization. For successful immunization leading to formation of specific memory cells, all the following cell types would need to be activated EXCEPT

A. T cells

B. B cells

C. Dendritic cells

D. Eosinophils

E. Natural killer cells

ANSWERS FOR IMMUNIZATION QUESTIONS

Questions	Answer choice	Questions	Answer choice
1.	C	6.	A
2.	C	7.	A
3.	A	8.	C
4.	C	9.	C
5.	B	10.	D

Note: Page numbers followed by f refer to figures; page numbers followed by t refer to tables.